# THE DIETER'S CALORIE COUNTER

*Also by Corinne T. Netzer*

THE BRAND-NAME CARBOHYDRATE GRAM COUNTER
THE CHOLESTEROL CONTENT OF FOOD
THE COMPLETE BOOK OF FOOD COUNTS
THE CORINNE T. NETZER 1992 CALORIE COUNTER
THE FAT CONTENT OF FOOD
THE CORINNE T. NETZER ENCYCLOPEDIA OF FOOD VALUES
THE CORINNE T. NETZER DIETER'S DIARY

# THE DIETER'S CALORIE COUNTER

CORINNE T. NETZER

3rd Edition,
Revised & Updated

A DELL TRADE PAPERBACK

A DELL TRADE PAPERBACK

Published by
Dell Publishing
a division of
Bantam Doubleday Dell Publishing Group, Inc.
666 Fifth Avenue
New York, New York 10103



ISBN: 0-440-50321-3

Printed in the United States of America

Published simultaneously in Canada

June 1992

10 9 8 7 6 5 4 3 2 1

BVG

# INTRODUCTION

The third edition of *The Dieter's Calorie Counter* is a compilation of basic foods, brand-name foods, and fast foods—all integrated and alphabetized.

Because this book is alphabetized, you should have no difficulty finding whatever food you want to look up. However, there are instances where you may have to look in more than one place. If you are looking for a specific food and cannot find it immediately, look for it under a category, such as cakes, pies, pasta sauce, rolls, etc. Wherever sensible, I have cross-referenced listings, but the pressure of space has made it impossible to do so for every item.

All the foods included in *The Dieter's Calorie Counter* are listed in useful household portions. And similar foods are generally listed in uniform measures. However, this was not possible—or even reasonable—in certain cases. All breads, for example, could have been listed in a standard one-ounce measure, but that would mean you would have to weigh a slice of bread in order to determine its calorie content. Hence, breads and various other foods are listed by the unit (piece of slice or portion, etc.) as packaged by the manufacturer. This means that, although you can determine the calories in individual slices of bread, you should *not* compare different brands and varieties of breads (or other foods listed by the piece) because they may vary a great deal in size.

Since the purpose of the book is to help you lose weight, remember also to compare only foods that are listed in similar measures. Do not compare foods listed in *dis*similar measures. This rule particularly applies to the confusion between measures by capacity and measures by weight. Eight ounces is a measure of how much something weighs; one cup is a measure of how much space it occupies. A cup of lightweight food, such as popcorn for example, weighs about one ounce; but eight ounces of popcorn would fill many cups.

Naturally, you can convert a similar unit of measure into a smaller or larger amount. The following table may be useful in making such conversions.

**Equivalents by Capacity**

(all measures level)

| | | |
|---|---|---|
| 1 quart | = | 4 cups |
| 1 cup | = | 8 fluid ounces |
| | = | ½ pint |
| | = | 16 tablespoons |
| 2 tablespoons | = | 1 fluid ounce |
| 1 tablespoon | = | 3 teaspoons |

**Equivalents by Weight**

| | | |
|---|---|---|
| 1 pound | = | 16 ounces |
| 3.57 ounces | = | 100 grams |
| 1 ounce | = | 28.35 grams |

The material contained in *The Dieter's Calorie Counter* is based on information from the United States government, from producers and processors of brand-name foods, and from fast-food restaurant chains. The data contained herein are the latest available as this book goes to press. Bear in mind, however, that the food industry often changes recipes and sizes and may discontinue a product or add new ones. In the future I will revise and update this book to keep you completely informed.

Good luck and good dieting.

CORINNE T. NETZER

# ABBREVIATIONS & SYMBOLS IN THIS BOOK

| | |
|---|---|
| cont. | container |
| diam. | diameter |
| fl. | fluid |
| ″ | inch |
| < | less than |
| lb. | pound |
| oz. | ounce |
| pkg. | package |
| pkt. | packet |
| qt. | quart |
| tbsp. | tablespoon |
| tsp. | teaspoon |
| w/ | with |

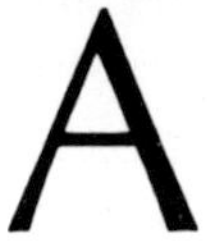

| FOOD AND MEASURE | CALORIES |
|---|---|
| **Abalone:** | |
| raw, meat only, 4 oz. | 119 |
| flour-coated, fried, 4 oz. | 214 |
| **Acapulco dip:** | |
| (*Ortega*), 1 oz. | 8 |
| **Acerola:** | |
| 1 medium, .2 oz. | 2 |
| trimmed, ½ cup | 16 |
| **Acerola juice,** fresh: | |
| 6 fl. oz. | 36 |
| **Acorn squash,** see "Squash" | |
| **Ale,** see "Beer, ale, and malt liquor" | |
| **Alfalfa seeds:** | |
| (*Arrowhead Mills*), 1 cup | 40 |
| **Alfalfa seeds, sprouted,** raw: | |
| ½ cup | 5 |
| **Alfredo sauce:** | |
| canned (*Progresso* Authentic Pasta Sauces), ½ cup | 340 |
| mix (*French's Pasta Toss*), 2 tsp. | 25 |
| mix (*Lawry's* Pasta Alfredo), 1 pkg. | 226 |
| refrigerated (*Contadina Fresh*), 6 oz. | 540 |
| **Allspice,** ground: | |
| 1 tsp. | 5 |
| **Almond:** | |
| dried, 1 oz. or 24 kernels | 167 |
| dried, slivered, 1 cup packed | 795 |
| dried, blanched (*Planters*), 1 oz. | 170 |

| FOOD AND MEASURE | CALORIES |
|---|---|

*Almond, continued*

dry-roasted, kernels, 1 cup .... 810
dry-roasted (*Planters*), 1 oz. .... 170
oil-roasted, 1 oz. or 22 kernels .... 176
toasted, 1 oz. .... 167

**Almond butter:**

raw (*Hain* Natural), 2 tbsp. .... 190
blanched, toasted (*Hain*), 2 tbsp. .... 220
honey and cinnamon, 1 tbsp. .... 96
smooth (*Westbrae Natural*), 2 tbsp. .... 190

**Almond meal:**

partially defatted, 1 oz. .... 116

**Almond paste:**

1 oz. .... 127

**Almond powder:**

full-fat, 1 oz. .... 168
partially defatted, 1 oz. .... 112

**Amaranth:**

raw, trimmed, ½ cup .... 4
boiled, drained, ½ cup .... 14

**Amaranth seed:**

(*Arrowhead Mills*), 2 oz. .... 200

**Amber jack,** meat only:

raw, 4 oz. .... 96

**Anchovy:**

fresh, European, raw, meat only, 4 oz. .... 148
canned, in oil, drained, 1.6 oz., yield from 2-oz. can .... 95
canned, in oil, drained, 5 medium .... 42

**Anise seed:**

1 tsp. .... 7

**Apple:**

fresh, raw, 1 medium, 2¾" diam., 3 per lb. .... 81
fresh, raw, unpeeled, sliced, ½ cup .... 32

| FOOD AND MEASURE | CALORIES |
|---|---|
| fresh, raw, peeled, sliced, ½ cup | 31 |
| fresh, boiled, peeled, sliced, ½ cup | 46 |
| canned: | |
| in water (*White House*), 4 oz. | 40 |
| in water, chipped (*White House*), 4 oz. | 50 |
| sliced, dessert (*Lucky Leaf/Musselman's*), 4 oz. | 70 |
| sliced, sweetened (*White House*), 4 oz. | 54 |
| rings, spiced (*White House*), 3.5 oz. | 180 |
| baked, whole (*Lucky Leaf/Musselman's*), 1 apple | 110 |
| baked style (*White House*), 3.5 oz. | 118 |
| dehydrated, sulfured, uncooked, ½ cup | 104 |
| dried, sulfured, uncooked, 10 rings, 2.3 oz. | 155 |
| dried, sulfured, cooked, unsweetened, ½ cup | 72 |
| dried, sliced, uncooked (*Del Monte*), 2 oz. | 140 |
| dried, chunks (*Sun-Maid/Sunsweet*), 2 oz. | 150 |
| frozen, sliced, ½ cup | 41 |
| frozen, heated, sliced, ½ cup | 48 |

**Apple, escalloped,** frozen:

| | |
|---|---|
| (*Stouffer's*), 4 oz. | 130 |

**Apple, glazed,** frozen:

| | |
|---|---|
| in raspberry sauce (*The Budget Gourmet* Side Dish), 5 oz. | 110 |

**Apple butter:**

| | |
|---|---|
| (*Bama*), 2 tbsp. | 25 |
| (*Tap'n Apple*), 1 oz. | 45 |
| (*White House*), 1 oz. | 50 |
| all varieties (*Smucker's*), 1 tsp. | 12 |

**Apple cider,** 6 fl. oz.:

| | |
|---|---|
| (*Indian Summer*) | 80 |
| cinnamon (*Indian Summer*) | 90 |
| sparkling (*Lucky Leaf*) | 80 |
| canned or frozen, diluted (*Tree Top*) | 90 |

**Apple cobbler:**

| | |
|---|---|
| deep dish (*Awrey's*), 1 piece | 320 |
| frozen (*Pet-Ritz*), ⅙ pkg. | 290 |
| frozen (*Stilwell*), 4 oz. | 200 |

| FOOD AND MEASURE | CALORIES |
|---|---|
| **Apple crisp,** frozen: | |
| (*Pepperidge Farm* Berkshire), 4¾ oz. | 250 |
| (*Weight Watchers*), 3.5 oz. | 190 |
| **Apple danish,** 1 piece: | |
| (*Awrey's* Round), 4.5 oz. | 390 |
| (*Awrey's* Square), 3 oz. | 220 |
| fried (*Hostess* Breakfast Bake Shop) | 400 |
| frozen (*Pepperidge Farm*), 2.25 oz. | 220 |
| frozen (*Sara Lee* Individual), 1.3 oz. | 120 |
| frozen (*Sara Lee Free & Light*), ⅛ pkg. | 130 |
| **Apple drink:** | |
| (*Hi-C* Candy Apple Cooler), 6 fl. oz. | 94 |
| **Apple dumpling,** frozen: | |
| (*Pepperidge Farm*), 3 oz. | 260 |
| **Apple fritter,** frozen: | |
| (*Mrs. Paul's*), 2 pieces | 240 |
| **Apple fruit roll:** | |
| (*Flavor Tree*), 1 piece | 75 |
| **Apple fruit square,** frozen: | |
| (*Pepperidge Farm*), 1 piece | 220 |
| **Apple juice,** 6 fl. oz., except as noted: | |
| (*Indian Summer*) | 90 |
| (*Kraft* Pure 100%) | 80 |
| (*Minute Maid* Juices to Go), 9.6 fl. oz. | 145 |
| (*Minute Maid On The Go*), 10 fl. oz. | 152 |
| (*Mott's*) | 88 |
| (*Mott's* Natural Style) | 76 |
| (*Ocean Spray*) | 90 |
| (*Red Cheek* Natural/100% Pure) | 97 |
| (*S&W* 100% Pure Unsweetened) | 85 |
| (*TreeSweet*) | 90 |
| (*Tropicana* 100% Pure), 8 fl. oz. | 116 |
| (*Veryfine* 100%), 8 fl. oz. | 107 |
| (*White House*) | 87 |
| blend (*Libby's Juicy Juice*) | 90 |

| FOOD AND MEASURE | CALORIES |
|---|---|
| sparkling (*Welch's*) | 100 |
| canned, chilled, or frozen, diluted (*Tree Top*) | 90 |
| chilled or frozen, diluted (*Minute Maid*) | 91 |
| **Apple juice cocktail:** | |
| (Welch's Orchard), 10 fl. oz. | 170 |
| **Apple pastry pocket:** | |
| (*Tastykake*), 3 oz. | 323 |
| **Apple punch:** | |
| (*Red Cheek*), 6 fl. oz. | 113 |
| **Apple and spice bake,** frozen: | |
| (*Pepperidge Farm* Dessert Lights), 4¼ oz. | 170 |
| **Apple sticks,** frozen: | |
| breaded, fried (*Farm Rich*), 4 oz. | 260 |
| **Apple turnover:** | |
| frozen (*Pepperidge Farm*), 1 piece | 300 |
| refrigerated (*Pillsbury*), 1 piece | 170 |
| **Apple-cherry juice:** | |
| (*Musselman's* Breakfast Cocktail), 6 fl. oz. | 100 |
| (*Red Cheek*), 6 fl. oz. | 113 |
| **Apple-cherry-berry drink:** | |
| (*Veryfine*), 8 fl. oz. | 130 |
| **Apple-citrus juice:** | |
| canned or frozen, diluted (*Tree Top*), 6 fl. oz. | 90 |
| **Apple-cranberry cider:** | |
| (*Indian Summer*), 6 fl. oz. | 100 |
| **Apple-cranberry drink:** | |
| (*Mott's*), 9.5-oz. can | 167 |
| **Apple-cranberry juice:** | |
| (*Apple & Eve*), 6 fl. oz. | 80 |
| (*Lucky Leaf*), 6 fl. oz. | 130 |
| (*Mott's*), 6 fl. oz. | 83 |
| canned or frozen, diluted (*Tree Top*) | 100 |

| FOOD AND MEASURE | CALORIES |
|---|---|

**Apple-cranberry juice cocktail:**

(*Veryfine*), 8 fl. oz. .......... 130

**Apple-grape juice:**

(*Libby's Juicy Juice*), 6 fl. oz. .......... 90
(*Mott's*), 6 fl. oz. .......... 86
(*Red Cheek*), 6 fl. oz. .......... 109
canned or frozen, diluted (*Tree Top*), 6 fl. oz. .......... 100

**Apple-grape juice cocktail:**

(*Musselman's* Breakfast), 6 fl. oz. .......... 110
(*Welch's Orchard* Cocktails-In-A-Box), 8.45 fl. oz. .......... 150
canned or frozen, diluted (*Welch's Orchard*), 6 fl. oz. .......... 110

**Apple-grape-cherry juice cocktail:**

(*Welch's Orchard*), 6 fl. oz. .......... 110
(*Welch's Orchard* Cocktails-In-A-Box), 8.45 fl. oz. .......... 150
frozen, diluted (*Welch's Orchard*), 6 fl. oz. .......... 90

**Apple-grape-raspberry juice cocktail:**

(*Welch's Orchard*), 6 fl. oz. .......... 100
(*Welch's Orchard* Cocktails-In-A-Box), 8.45 fl. oz. .......... 140
frozen, diluted (*Welch's Orchard*), 6 fl. oz. .......... 90

**Apple-orange-pineapple juice cocktail:**

(*Welch's Orchard*), 10 fl. oz. .......... 180
(*Welch's Orchard* Cocktails-In-A-Box), 8.45 fl. oz. .......... 140
bottled or frozen, diluted (*Welch's Orchard*), 6 fl. oz. .......... 100

**Apple-pear juice:**

canned or frozen, diluted (*Tree Top*), 6 fl. oz. .......... 90

**Apple-raspberry drink:**

(*Mott's*), 9.5-fl.-oz. can .......... 150

**Apple-raspberry juice:**

(*Mott's*), 6 fl. oz. .......... 83
(*Red Cheek*), 6 fl. oz. .......... 113
canned or frozen, diluted (*Tree Top*), 6 fl. oz. .......... 80

**Apple-raspberry juice cocktail:**

(*Veryfine*), 8 fl. oz. .......... 110

| FOOD AND MEASURE | CALORIES |
|---|---|
| **Apple-white grape juice cocktail:** | |
| frozen, diluted (*Welch's* No Sugar Added), 6 fl. oz. | 40 |
| **Applesauce:** | |
| (*Del Monte*), ½ cup | 90 |
| (*Del Monte Lite*), ½ cup | 50 |
| (*Hunt's Snack Pack*), 4.25 oz. | 80 |
| (*Mott's*), 6 oz. | 150 |
| (*Mott's* Chunky), 6 oz. | 86 |
| (*Mott's* Natural), 6 oz. | 80 |
| (*S&W*), ½ cup | 90 |
| (*S&W* Unsweetened/*S&W/Nutradiet*), ½ cup | 55 |
| (*Stokely*), ½ cup | 90 |
| (*Stokely* Unsweetened), ½ cup | 45 |
| (*Tree Top* Original), ½ cup | 80 |
| (*White House* Regular or Chunky), 4 oz. | 80 |
| (*White House* Unsweetened or in Apple Juice), 4 oz. | 50 |
| cinnamon (*Mott's*), 6 oz. | 152 |
| **Apricot:** | |
| fresh, untrimmed, 1 lb. | 202 |
| fresh, 3 medium, 12 per lb. | 51 |
| fresh, halves, ½ cup | 37 |
| canned, ½ cup: | |
| whole, peeled or halves, unpeeled (*Del Monte*) | 100 |
| halves, unpeeled (*Del Monte Lite*) | 60 |
| in water, halves, unpeeled (*S&W/Nutradiet*) | 35 |
| in water, whole, peeled (*S&W/Nutradiet*) | 28 |
| in juice, unpeeled (*Libby Lite*) | 60 |
| in heavy syrup, halves, unpeeled (*S&W*) | 110 |
| in heavy syrup, whole, peeled (*S&W*) | 100 |
| dehydrated, sulfured, uncooked, ½ cup | 192 |
| dehydrated, sulfured, cooked, ½ cup | 156 |
| dried (*Del Monte*), 2 oz. | 140 |
| dried (*Sun-Maid/Sunsweet*), 2 oz. | 140 |
| dried, sulfured, uncooked, 10 halves, 1.2 oz. | 83 |
| dried, sulfured, cooked, unsweetened, halves, ½ cup | 106 |
| frozen, sweetened, ½ cup | 119 |
| **Apricot fruit roll:** | |
| (*Flavor Tree*), 1 piece | 76 |

| FOOD AND MEASURE | CALORIES |
|---|---|
| **Apricot nectar:** | |
| (*Del Monte*), 6 fl. oz. | 100 |
| (*Libby's*), 6 fl. oz. | 110 |
| (*S&W*), 6 fl. oz. | 100 |
| **Apricot-pineapple nectar:** | |
| (*S&W/Nutradiet*), 4 fl. oz. | 35 |
| ***Arby's:*** | |
| sandwiches, 1 serving: | |
| beef 'n cheddar, 7 oz. | 455 |
| chicken breast, 6.5 oz. | 493 |
| ham 'n cheese, 5.5 oz. | 292 |
| roast beef, regular, 5.2 oz. | 353 |
| roast beef, super, 8.3 oz. | 501 |
| roast chicken club, 8.3 oz. | 610 |
| turkey deluxe, 7 oz. | 375 |
| french fries, 2.5 oz. | 246 |
| potato cakes, 3 oz. | 204 |
| shake, Jamocha, 11.5 oz. | 368 |
| **Arrowhead:** | |
| raw, 1 medium corm, 2⅝" diam. | 12 |
| boiled, drained, 1 medium corm | 9 |
| **Arrowroot,** powdered: | |
| (*Tone's*), 1 tsp. | 10 |
| **Artichoke,** globe or French: | |
| fresh, boiled, drained, 1 medium, 11.3 oz. raw | 60 |
| fresh, boiled, drained, hearts, ½ cup | 42 |
| canned, hearts, marinated (*S&W*), 3.5 oz. | 225 |
| frozen, hearts (*Birds Eye* Deluxe), 3 oz. | 30 |
| frozen, hearts (*Seabrook*), 3 oz. | 25 |
| **Arugula:** | |
| fresh (*Frieda* of California), 1 oz. | 7 |
| **Asparagus:** | |
| fresh, raw, untrimmed, 1 lb. | 54 |
| fresh, boiled, drained, 4 spears, ½" diam. at base | 15 |
| fresh, boiled, drained, cuts and spears, ½ cup | 22 |

| FOOD AND MEASURE | CALORIES |
|---|---|
| canned, ½ cup: | |
| (*Stokely* Regular/No Salt or Sugar Added) | 20 |
| green (*Green Giant*) | 20 |
| spears, all green or green tipped (*Del Monte*) | 20 |
| spears, all green (*S&W* Fancy) | 18 |
| spears, colossal, all green (*S&W* Fancy) | 20 |
| points, all green (*S&W/Nutradiet*) | 17 |
| white (*Green Giant*) | 16 |
| frozen, spears (*Southern*), 3.5 oz. | 27 |
| frozen, spears or cuts (*Birds Eye*), 3.3 oz. | 25 |
| frozen, spears or cuts (*Frosty Acres*), 3.3 oz. | 25 |
| frozen, cuts (*Green Giant Harvest Fresh*), ½ cup | 25 |

**Asparagus pilaf,** frozen:

| | |
|---|---|
| (*Green Giant* Microwave Garden Gourmet), 1 pkg. | 190 |

**Au jus gravy:**

| | |
|---|---|
| canned (*Franco-American*), 2 oz. | 10 |
| canned (*Heinz*), 2 oz. or ¼ cup | 18 |
| mix, prepared (*French's*), ¼ cup | 10 |
| mix, prepared (*Lawry's*), 1 cup | 84 |
| mix, prepared (*McCormick/Schilling*), ¼ cup | 20 |

**Avocado:**

| | |
|---|---|
| California, whole, 8 oz. or 1 medium | 306 |
| California, pureed, ½ cup | 204 |
| Florida, whole, 1 lb. or 1 medium | 339 |
| Florida, pureed, ½ cup | 129 |

**Avocado dip:**

| | |
|---|---|
| (*Kraft*), 2 tbsp. | 50 |

# B

| FOOD AND MEASURE | CALORIES |
|---|---|
| **Bacon,** cooked: | |
| 4.5 oz., yield from 1 lb. raw | 732 |
| (*Black Label*), 2 slices | 60 |
| (*Kahn's American Beauty*), 2 slices | 100 |
| (*Oscar Mayer*/*Oscar Mayer* Lower Salt), 1 slice | 33 |
| (*Oscar Mayer* Center Cut), 1 slice | 25 |
| (*Oscar Mayer* Thick Sliced), 1 slice | 58 |
| (*Range Brand*), 2 slices | 110 |
| (*Red Label*), 3 slices | 110 |
| **Bacon, Canadian-style:** | |
| unheated (*Jones Dairy Farm*), 1 slice | 25 |
| grilled, 2 slices, yield from 2 unheated 1-oz. slices | 86 |
| (*Hormel* Sliced), 1 oz. | 45 |
| (*Light & Lean*), 2 slices | 35 |
| (*Oscar Mayer*), .8-oz. slice | 28 |
| **Bacon, substitute,** heated: | |
| beef (*Sizzlean*), 2 strips | 70 |
| pork (*Sizzlean*), 2 strips | 90 |
| pork, brown sugar cured (*Sizzlean*), 2 strips | 110 |
| turkey (*Louis Rich*), 1 slice | 32 |
| **"Bacon," vegetarian,** frozen: | |
| (*Morningstar Farms* Breakfast Strips), 3 strips | 80 |
| (*Worthington Stripples*), 4 strips | 120 |
| **Bacon bits:** | |
| (*Hormel*), 1 tbsp. | 30 |
| (*Libby's Bacon Crumbles*), 1 tbsp. | 25 |
| (*Oscar Mayer*), ¼ oz. | 20 |
| imitation (*Bac*Os*), 2 tsp. | 25 |
| **Bacon and horseradish dip:** | |
| (*Kraft*), 2 tbsp. | 60 |
| (*Kraft* Premium), 2 tbsp. | 50 |

| FOOD AND MEASURE | CALORIES |
|---|---|

**Bacon and onion dip:**

(*Kraft* Premium), 2 tbsp. . . . . . . . . . . . . . . . . . . 60

**Bagel,** frozen, 1 piece:

all varieties (*Lender's* Bagelettes) . . . . . . . . . . . . 70
all varieties, except plain and onion (*Lender's* Big'n Crusty),
3⅛ oz. . . . . . . . . . . . . . . . . . . . . . . . 250
plain (*Lender's* Big'n Crusty, 3⅛ oz. . . . . . . . . . . 240
plain (*Sara Lee*), 3.1 oz. . . . . . . . . . . . . . . . 230
plain, egg, or rye (*Lender's*), 2 oz. . . . . . . . . . . 150
blueberry (*Lender's*), 2.5 oz. . . . . . . . . . . . . . 190
cinnamon and raisin (*Sara Lee*), 3.1 oz. . . . . . . . . 240
cinnamon raisin or egg (*Sara Lee*), 2.5 oz. . . . . . . . 200
egg (*Sara Lee*), 3.1 oz. . . . . . . . . . . . . . . . . 250
garlic, onion, or pumpernickel (*Lender's*), 2 oz. . . . . 160
oat bran (*Lender's*), 2.5 oz. . . . . . . . . . . . . . . 170
oat Bran (*Sara Lee*), 2.5 oz. . . . . . . . . . . . . . . 180
onion (*Lender's* Big'n Crusty), 3⅛ oz. . . . . . . . . . 230
onion or poppy seed (*Sara Lee*), 3.1 oz. . . . . . . . . 230
onion, plain, or poppy seed (*Sara Lee*), 2.5 oz. . . . . . 190
poppy seed or sesame seed (*Lender's*), 2 oz. . . . . . . 160
raisin'n honey (*Lender's*), 2.5 oz. . . . . . . . . . . . 200
sesame seed (*Sara Lee*), 3.1 oz. . . . . . . . . . . . . 240
soft (*Lender's*), 2.5 oz. . . . . . . . . . . . . . . . . 210
wheat'n raisin (*Lender's*), 2.5 oz. . . . . . . . . . . . 190

**Baking powder:**

(*Davis*), 1 tsp. . . . . . . . . . . . . . . . . . . . . . 8

**Balsam-pear:**

leafy tips, raw, ½ cup . . . . . . . . . . . . . . . . . . 7
leafy tips, boiled, drained, ½ cup . . . . . . . . . . . . 10
pods, raw, ½″ pieces, ½ cup . . . . . . . . . . . . . . . 8
pods, boiled, drained, ½″ pieces, ½ cup . . . . . . . . . 12

**Bamboo shoots:**

fresh, raw, ½″ slices, ½ cup . . . . . . . . . . . . . . . 21
fresh, boiled, drained, ½″ slices, ½ cup . . . . . . . . . 8
canned (*La Choy*), 1.5 oz. . . . . . . . . . . . . . . . . 8

| FOOD AND MEASURE | CALORIES |
|---|---|
| **Banana** (see also "Plantain"): | |
| fresh, unpeeled, 1 lb. | 271 |
| fresh, 1 medium, 8¾" long, 6.2 oz. | 105 |
| dehydrated, 1 oz. | 98 |
| red, fresh, 1 medium, 7¼" long | 118 |
| red, fresh, sliced, ½ cup | 68 |
| **Banana nectar:** | |
| (*Libby's*), 6 fl. oz. | 110 |
| **Barbecue loaf:** | |
| (*Oscar Mayer*), 1-oz. slice | 46 |
| **Barbecue sauce:** | |
| (*Estee*), 1 tbsp. | 18 |
| (*Hunt* Original), 1 tbsp. | 20 |
| (*Kraft/Kraft* Hot), 2 tbsp. | 45 |
| (*Kraft Thick'n Spicy* Original), 2 tbsp. | 50 |
| all varieties (*Enrico's*), 1 tbsp. | 18 |
| all varieties (*French's Cattleman's*), 1 tbsp. | 25 |
| all varieties (*Heinz* Thick and Rich), 1 tbsp. | 20 |
| all varieties (*Ott's*), 1 tbsp. | 14 |
| all varieties, except original hickory smoke, or mesquite smoke (*Kraft Thick'n Spicy*), 2 tbsp. | 60 |
| Cajun style (*Golden Dipt*), 1 fl. oz. | 90 |
| garlic (*Kraft*), 2 tbsp. | 40 |
| hickory smoke (*Kraft*), 2 tbsp. | 45 |
| hickory or mesquite smoke (*Kraft Thick'n Spicy*), 2 tbsp. | 50 |
| hickory smoke, w/onion bits (*Kraft*), 2 tbsp. | 50 |
| hickory smoke, regular or hot (*Kraft*), 2 tbsp. | 40 |
| honey (*Hain*), 1 tbsp. | 14 |
| Italian seasoning, Kansas City, or onion (*Kraft*), 2 tbsp. | 50 |
| mesquite smoke (*Kraft*), 2 tbsp. | 45 |
| Oriental (*La Choy*), 1 tbsp. | 16 |
| **Barbecue seasoning:** | |
| (*McCormick/Schilling* Spice Blends), ¼ tsp. | <1 |
| **Barley,** pearled: | |
| raw (*Arrowhead Mills*), 2 oz. | 200 |
| raw (*Quaker Scotch* Brand Quick), ⅓ cup | 172 |

| FOOD AND MEASURE | CALORIES |
|---|---|
| raw, medium (*Quaker Scotch* Brand), ¼ cup | 172 |
| cooked, 1 cup | 193 |
| **Barracuda:** | |
| raw, meat only, 4 oz. | 107 |
| **Basil, dried:** | |
| 1 tsp. | 4 |
| **Bass,** fresh, meat only: | |
| freshwater, raw, 4 oz. | 128 |
| sea, baked, broiled, or microwaved, 4 oz. | 141 |
| sea or striped, raw, 4 oz. | 108 |
| **Batter mix** (see also specific listings): | |
| (*Golden Dipt*), 1 oz. | 100 |
| **Bay leaf,** dried: | |
| crumbled, 1 tsp. | 2 |
| **Bean curd,** see "Tofu" | |
| **Bean dip:** | |
| hot or onion (*Hain*), 4 tbsp. | 70 |
| Mexican (*Hain*), 4 tbsp. | 60 |
| **Bean mix,** prepared: | |
| Cajun, and sauce (*Lipton*), ½ cup | 160 |
| chicken, and sauce (*Lipton*), ½ cup | 150 |
| **Bean salad,** canned: | |
| four bean (*Joan of Arc/Read*), ½ cup | 100 |
| green bean, German-style (*Joan of Arc/Read*), ½ cup | 90 |
| three bean (*Green Giant*), ½ cup | 70 |
| three bean (*Joan of Arc/Read*), ½ cup | 90 |
| **Bean sprouts:** | |
| kidney, raw, ½ cup | 27 |
| kidney, boiled, drained, 4 oz. | 37 |
| mung, raw, ½ cup | 16 |
| mung, boiled, drained, ½ cup | 13 |

| FOOD AND MEASURE | CALORIES |
|---|---|
| *Bean sprouts, continued* | |
| navy, raw, ½ cup | 35 |
| navy, boiled, drained, 4 oz. | 88 |
| pinto, raw, 1 oz. | 18 |
| pinto, boiled, drained, 4 oz. | 25 |
| canned (*La Choy*), 2 oz. | 6 |
| canned, mung (*La Choy*), 2 oz. | 8 |

**Beans, adzuki:**

| | |
|---|---|
| boiled, ½ cup | 147 |
| canned, sweetened, ½ cup | 351 |

**Beans, baked** (see also specific bean listings):

| | |
|---|---|
| (*Allens*), ½ cup | 170 |
| (*Campbell's* Home Style), 8 oz. | 220 |
| (*Grandma Brown's*), 1 cup | 301 |
| (*Grandma Brown's Saucepan*), 1 cup | 307 |
| (*S&W* Brick Oven), ½ cup | 160 |
| (*Van Camp's*), 1 cup | 260 |
| (*Van Camp's Deluxe*), 1 cup | 320 |
| plain or vegetarian: | |
| (*Allens*), ½ cup | 110 |
| (*B&M*/*B&M* 50% Less Sodium), 8 oz. | 230 |
| (*Campbell's*), 7¾ oz. | 170 |
| (*Van Camp's* Vegetarian Style), 1 cup | 210 |
| w/miso (*Health Valley* Vegetarian), 4 oz. | 90 |
| barbecue (*B&M*), 8 oz. | 260 |
| barbecue (*Campbell's*), 7⅞ oz. | 210 |
| Boston (*Health Valley* Regular/No Salt Added), 4 oz. | 213 |
| brown sugar (*Van Camp's*), 1 cup | 290 |
| chili, hot (*Campbell's*), 7¾ oz. | 180 |
| w/franks (*Van Camp's Beanee Weenee*), 1 cup | 326 |
| honey, hot 'n spicy, or maple (*B&M*), 8 oz. | 240 |
| molasses-brown sugar sauce (*Campbell's* Old Fashioned), 8 oz. | 230 |
| pea (*B&M*), 8 oz. | 270 |
| w/pork: | |
| (*Allens* Extra Fancy), ½ cup | 125 |
| (*Allens* Extra Standard), ½ cup | 90 |
| (*Allens* Fancy), ½ cup | 110 |
| (*Campbell's*), 8 oz. | 200 |

| FOOD AND MEASURE | CALORIES |
|---|---|
| (*Joan of Arc*), ½ cup | 90 |
| (*Hormel Micro-Cup*), 7½ oz. | 254 |
| (*Hunt's*), 4 oz. | 140 |
| (*S&W*), ½ cup | 130 |
| (*Van Camp's*), 1 cup | 220 |
| tomato (*B&M*), 8 oz. | 230 |
| vegetarian, see "plain or vegetarian," above | |
| western style (*Van Camp's*), 1 cup | 207 |

**Beans, black:**

| | |
|---|---|
| boiled, ½ cup | 113 |
| canned (*Progresso*), ½ cup | 90 |

**Beans, broad:**

| | |
|---|---|
| fresh, boiled, drained, 4 oz. | 64 |
| dry, boiled, ½ cup | 93 |

**Beans, butter,** see "Beans, lima"

**Beans, chili,** canned:

| | |
|---|---|
| (*Hunt's*), 4 oz. | 100 |
| (*S&W*), ½ cup | 130 |
| caliente style (*Green Giant/Joan of Arc*), ½ cup | 100 |
| in chili gravy (*Dennison's*), 7.5 oz. | 180 |
| hot (*Allens*), ½ cup | 90 |
| Mexican style (*Allens*), ½ cup | 135 |
| Mexican style (*Van Camp's*), 1 cup | 210 |
| in sauce (*Hormel*), 5 oz. | 130 |
| spiced (*Gebhardt*), 4 oz. | 113 |

**Beans, cranberry:**

| | |
|---|---|
| dry, boiled, ½ cup | 120 |

**Beans, fava,** canned:

| | |
|---|---|
| (*Progresso*), ½ cup | 90 |

**Beans, great northern:**

| | |
|---|---|
| dry, boiled, ½ cup | 104 |
| canned (*Allens*), ½ cup | 105 |
| canned (*Joan of Arc*), ½ cup | 80 |
| canned, w/pork (*Allens*), ½ cup | 100 |
| canned, w/pork (*Luck's*), 7.25 oz. | 220 |

| FOOD AND MEASURE | CALORIES |
|---|---|

**Beans, green:**

fresh, raw, untrimmed, 1 lb. .............................. 123
fresh, raw, ½ cup .............................. 17
fresh, boiled, drained, ½ cup .............................. 22
canned, ½ cup:
(*Stokely* Regular/No Salt or Sugar Added) .............................. 20
whole (*S&W* Vertical Pack/Stringless) .............................. 20
whole, cut, or French style (*Del Monte*) .............................. 20
cut (*Featherweight*) .............................. 25
cut (*S&W/Nutradiet/S&W* Premium Golden/Blue Lake) .............................. 20
cut, French style, or kitchen sliced (*Green Giant*) .............................. 16
cut, Italian (*Del Monte*) .............................. 25
almondine (*Green Giant*) .............................. 45
dilled (*S&W*) .............................. 60
seasoned, French style (*Del Monte*) .............................. 20
frozen:
(*Green Giant*), ½ cup .............................. 14
whole (*Birds Eye* Deluxe), 3 oz. .............................. 25
whole (*Birds Eye* Farm Fresh), 4 oz. .............................. 30
whole (*Southern*), 3.5 oz. .............................. 33
cut (*Birds Eye* Portion Pack), 3 oz. .............................. 25
cut (*Green Giant Harvest Fresh*), ½ cup .............................. 16
cut (*Stokely Singles*), 3 oz. .............................. 30
cut or French style (*Birds Eye*), 3 oz. .............................. 25
French style (*Southern*), 3.5 oz. .............................. 34
Italian (*Birds Eye*), 3 oz. .............................. 30
petite (*Birds Eye* Deluxe), 2.6 oz. .............................. 20
in butter sauce (*Green Giant* One Serving), 5.5 oz. .............................. 60
in butter sauce, cut (*Green Giant*), ½ cup .............................. 30
packaged, w/potatoes and mushrooms, in sauce
(*Green Giant Pantry Express*), ½ cup .............................. 50

**Beans, green, combinations,** frozen:

Bavarian, w/spaetzle (*Birds Eye* International), 3.3 oz. .............................. 100
French, w/toasted almonds (*Birds Eye* Combinations), 3 oz. .............................. 50
and mushroom, creamy (*Green Giant* Garden Gourmet), 1 pkg. .............................. 220
mushroom casserole (*Stouffer's*), 4.75 oz. .............................. 160

**Beans, hyacinth:**

fresh, boiled, drained, ½ cup .............................. 22
dry, boiled, ½ cup .............................. 114

| FOOD AND MEASURE | CALORIES |
|---|---|
| **Beans, kidney:** | |
| dry, red, boiled, ½ cup | 112 |
| canned, ½ cup, except as noted: | |
| (*S&W/Nutradiet*) | 90 |
| red (*Hunt's*), 4 oz. | 120 |
| red (*Progresso*) | 100 |
| red, dark (*S&W* Lite 50% Less Salt/Premium) | 120 |
| red, dark or light (*Allens*) | 105 |
| red, dark or light (*Joan of Arc/Green Giant*) | 90 |
| red, dark or light (*Stokely*) | 110 |
| red, dark, light, or New Orleans (*Van Camp's*), 1 cup | 180 |
| baked, red (*B&M*), 8 oz. | 250 |
| white (*Progresso* Cannellini) | 80 |
| **Beans, lima:** | |
| fresh, raw, trimmed, ½ cup | 88 |
| fresh, boiled, drained, ½ cup | 104 |
| canned, ½ cup, except as noted: | |
| (*Featherweight*) | 80 |
| (*Joan of Arc*) | 80 |
| (*S&W*) | 100 |
| (*Stokely* Regular/No Salt or Sugar Added) | 80 |
| butterbeans (*Van Camp's*), 1 cup | 160 |
| butterbeans, large (*Allens*) | 110 |
| green (*Del Monte*) | 70 |
| green, all varieties (*Allens*) | 90 |
| green, small (*S&W* Fancy) | 80 |
| green, small, w/pork, (*Luck's*), 7.5 oz. | 220 |
| w/ham (*Dennison's*), 7.5 oz. | 250 |
| w/pork (*Luck's*), 7.5 oz. | 230 |
| frozen: | |
| (*Green Giant*), ½ cup | 100 |
| (*Green Giant Harvest Fresh*), ½ cup | 80 |
| baby (*Birds Eye*), 3.3 oz. | 130 |
| baby, butter (*Seabrook*), 3.3 oz. | 140 |
| baby or speckled (*Southern*), 3.5 oz. | 135 |
| Fordhook (*Birds Eye*), 3.3 oz. | 100 |
| Fordhook (*Southern*), 3.5 oz. | 105 |
| speckled (*Seabrook*), 3.3 oz. | 120 |
| tiny (*Seabrook*), 3.3 oz. | 110 |

| FOOD AND MEASURE | CALORIES |
|---|---|
| *Beans, lima, frozen, continued* | |
| in butter sauce (*Green Giant*), ½ cup | 100 |
| in butter sauce, baby (*Stokely Singles*), 4. oz. | 140 |
| **Beans, lima, mature:** | |
| dry, baby, boiled, ½ cup | 115 |
| dry, large, boiled, ½ cup | 108 |
| canned, w/liquid | 95 |
| **Beans, Mexican,** canned: | |
| (*Old El Paso* Mexe-Beans), ½ cup | 163 |
| **Beans, mung:** | |
| boiled, ½ cup | 107 |
| **Beans, navy:** | |
| boiled, ½ cup | 129 |
| canned (*Allens*), ½ cup | 160 |
| **Beans, pink:** | |
| boiled, ½ cup | 125 |
| **Beans, pinto:** | |
| dry, boiled, ½ cup | 117 |
| canned: | |
| (*Allens*), ½ cup | 105 |
| (*Gebhardt*), 4 oz. | 197 |
| (*Green Giant/Joan of Arc*), ½ cup | 90 |
| (*Old El Paso*), ½ cup | 100 |
| (*Progresso*), ½ cup | 110 |
| baked style, w/pork (*Lucks*, 15 oz.), 7.5 oz. | 220 |
| picante style (*Green Giant/Joan of Arc*), ½ cup | 100 |
| frozen (*Seabrook*), 3.2 oz. | 160 |
| **Beans, red,** canned: | |
| (*Allens*), ½ cup | 115 |
| (*Green Giant/Joan of Arc*), ½ cup | 90 |
| (*Van Camp's*), 1 cup | 190 |
| small (*Hunt's*), 4 oz. | 90 |
| small, baked (*B&M*), 8 oz. | 223 |

| FOOD AND MEASURE | CALORIES |
|---|---|

**Beans, refried:**

| | |
|---|---|
| (*Little Pancho*), ½ cup | 80 |
| canned: | |
| (*Bearitos* Organic), 1 oz. | 30 |
| (*Gebhardt*), 4 oz. | 130 |
| (*Old El Paso*), ¼ cup | 55 |
| (*Rosarita*), 4 oz. | 100 |
| w/cheese (*Old El Paso*), ¼ cup | 36 |
| w/green chilies (*Old El Paso*), ¼ cup | 49 |
| jalapeño (*Gebhardt*), 4 oz. | 110 |
| regular or spicy (*Del Monte*), ½ cup | 130 |
| w/sausage (*Old El Paso*), ¼ cup | 180 |
| spicy (*Bearitos* Organic), 1 oz. | 31 |
| spicy (*Old El Paso*), ¼ cup | 35 |
| spicy or vegetarian (*Rosarita*), 4 oz. | 120 |
| vegetarian (*Old El Paso*), ¼ cup | 70 |

**Beans, Roman,** canned:

| | |
|---|---|
| (*Progresso*), ½ cup | 110 |

**Beans, shellie,** canned:

| | |
|---|---|
| (*Stokely*), ½ cup | 35 |

**Beans, string or snap,** see "Beans, green"

**Beans, wax,** see "Beans, green"

**Beans, white:**

| | |
|---|---|
| boiled, ½ cup | 125 |
| boiled, small, ½ cup | 127 |
| canned, w/liquid, ½ cup | 153 |

**Beans, yellow eye,** canned:

| | |
|---|---|
| baked (*B&M*), 8 oz. | 326 |

**Beans and frankfurter dinner,** frozen:

| | |
|---|---|
| (*Banquet*), 10 oz. | 520 |
| (*Morton*), 10 oz. | 350 |
| (*Swanson*), 10½ oz. | 440 |

**Béarnaise sauce:**

| | |
|---|---|
| (*Great Impressions*), 2 tbsp. | 192 |

| FOOD AND MEASURE | CALORIES |
|---|---|
| **Beechnuts,** shelled: | |
| dried, 1 oz. | 164 |
| **Beef**[1], choice grade, meat only, 4 oz.: | |
| brisket, flat half, braised, separable lean and fat | 413 |
| brisket, flat half, braised, lean only | 252 |
| brisket, point half, braised, separable lean and fat | 458 |
| brisket, point half, braised, lean only | 296 |
| chuck, arm pot roast, braised, separable lean and fat | 395 |
| chuck, arm pot roast, lean only | 255 |
| chuck, blade roast, braised, lean and fat | 412 |
| chuck, blade roast, braised, lean only | 298 |
| flank steak, trimmed to 0″ fat, broiled, lean only | 235 |
| ground: | |
| extra lean, raw | 265 |
| extra lean, broiled, medium | 290 |
| lean, raw | 300 |
| lean, broiled, medium | 308 |
| regular, raw | 352 |
| regular, broiled, medium | 328 |
| porterhouse (short loin), broiled, separable lean and fat | 346 |
| porterhouse (short loin), broiled, lean only | 247 |
| rib, large end, roasted, separable lean and fat | 434 |
| rib, large end, roasted, lean only | 284 |
| rib, small end, roasted, separable lean and fat | 416 |
| rib, small end, roasted, lean only | 263 |
| rib, shortrib, braised, separable lean and fat | 534 |
| rib, shortrib, braised, lean only | 335 |
| rib eye, small end, broiled, separable lean and fat | 348 |
| rib eye, small end, broiled, lean only | 255 |
| round, bottom, braised, separable lean and fat | 322 |
| round, bottom, braised, lean only | 249 |
| round, eye of, roasted, separable lean and fat | 273 |
| round, eye of, roasted, lean only | 198 |
| round, tip, roasted, separable lean and fat | 280 |
| round, tip, roasted, lean only | 213 |
| round, top, braised, separable lean and fat | 295 |
| round, top, braised, lean only | 242 |
| round, top, broiled, separable lean and fat | 254 |

[1]Retail cuts; trimmed to ¼″ fat, except as noted.

| FOOD AND MEASURE | CALORIES |
|---|---|
| round, top, broiled, lean only | 214 |
| round, top, roasted, separable lean and fat | 245 |
| shank crosscuts, simmered, separable lean and fat | 298 |
| shank crosscuts, simmered, lean only | 228 |
| sirloin, top, broiled, separable lean and fat | 305 |
| sirloin, top, broiled, lean only | 229 |
| T-bone steak (short loin), broiled, separable lean and fat | 338 |
| T-bone steak (short loin), broiled, lean only | 243 |
| tenderloin, broiled, separable lean and fat | 345 |
| tenderloin, broiled, lean only | 252 |
| tenderloin, roasted, separable lean and fat | 384 |
| tenderloin, roasted, lean only | 262 |
| top loin (short loin), broiled, separable lean and fat | 338 |
| top loin (short loin), broiled, lean only | 243 |

**Beef, corned:**

| | |
|---|---|
| (*Eckrich* Slender Sliced), 1 oz. | 40 |
| (*Healthy Deli*), 1 oz. | 35 |
| (*Healthy Deli* St. Paddy's), 1 oz. | 24 |
| (*Hillshire Farm*), 1 oz. | 31 |
| (*Oscar Mayer*), .6-oz. slice | 17 |
| brisket, cured, cooked, 4 oz. | 285 |
| loaf, jellied, 1-oz. slice | 46 |
| canned (*Libby's,* 12 oz.), 2.4 oz. | 160 |

**Beef, corned, hash,** canned:

| | |
|---|---|
| (*Dinty Moore*), 2 oz. | 130 |
| (*Libby's,* 15 oz.), 7.5 oz. | 400 |
| (*Mary Kitchen,* 15 oz.), 7.5 oz. | 360 |

**Beef, corned, spread,** canned:

| | |
|---|---|
| (*Hormel*), ½ oz. | 35 |

**Beef, dried:**

| | |
|---|---|
| cured, 1 oz. | 47 |

**Beef, roast,** see "Beef" and "Beef luncheon meat"

**Beef, roast, hash:**

| | |
|---|---|
| canned (*Mary Kitchen*), 7½ oz. | 350 |
| frozen (*Stouffer's*), 10 oz. | 380 |

| FOOD AND MEASURE | CALORIES |
|---|---|

**Beef, roast, spread,** canned:

(*Hormel*), ½ oz. .... 31
(*Underwood*), 2⅛ oz. .... 140
(*Underwood* Light), 2⅛ oz. .... 90
mesquite smoked (*Underwood*), 2⅛ oz. .... 126

**Beef, variety meats,** see specific listings

**"Beef," vegetarian:**

canned:
slices (*Worthington* Savory Slices), 2 slices .... 100
steak (*Worthington Prime Stakes*), 3.25-oz. piece .... 160
steak (*Worthington Vegetable Steaks*), 2½ pieces .... 110
stew (*Worthington* Country Stew), 9.5 oz. .... 220
frozen:
(*Worthington Stakelets*), 2.5-oz. piece .... 150
corned, roll (*Worthington*), 2.5 oz. .... 150
corned, slices (*Worthington*), 4 slices or 2 oz. .... 120
pie (*Worthington*), 8-oz. pie .... 360
roll (*Worthington*), 4 slices or 2.5 oz. .... 130
roll, smoked (*Worthington*), 3 slices or 2 oz. .... 120

**Beef dinner,** frozen:

(*Banquet Extra Helping*), 16 oz. .... 870
(*Swanson*), 11.25 oz. .... 310
in barbecue sauce (*Swanson*), 11 oz. .... 460
chopped (*Banquet*), 11 oz. .... 420
chopped steak (*Swanson Hungry Man*), 16.75 oz. .... 640
enchilada, see "Enchilada dinner"
meat loaf, see "Meat loaf dinner"
Mexicana (*The Budget Gourmet*), 12.8 oz. .... 560
patty, charbroiled (*Freezer Queen*), 10 oz. .... 300
patty, cheese, sandwich (*Kid Cuisine*), 6.25 oz. .... 400
pepper steak (*Armour Classics Lite*), 11.25 oz. .... 220
pepper steak (*Healthy Choice*), 11 oz. .... 290
pepper steak (*Le Menu*), 11.5 oz. .... 370
pot roast, Yankee (*Armour Classics*), 10 oz. .... 310
pot roast, Yankee (*The Budget Gourmet*), 11 oz. .... 380
pot roast, Yankee (*Healthy Choice*), 11 oz. .... 260
pot roast, Yankee (*Le Menu*), 10 oz. .... 330

| FOOD AND MEASURE | CALORIES |
|---|---|
| Salisbury steak: | |
| (*Armour Classics*), 11.25 oz. | 350 |
| (*Armour Classics Lite*), 11.5 oz. | 300 |
| (*Banquet*), 11 oz. | 500 |
| (*Banquet Extra Helping*), 18 oz. | 910 |
| (*Freezer Queen*), 10 oz. | 380 |
| (*Healthy Choice*), 11.5 oz. | 300 |
| (*Le Menu* LightStyle), 10 oz. | 280 |
| (*Morton*), 10 oz. | 300 |
| (*Swanson*), 10.75 oz. | 400 |
| (*Swanson Hungry Man*), 16.5 oz. | 680 |
| w/gravy and mushrooms (*Stouffer's Dinner Supreme*), 11⅝ oz. | 400 |
| w/mushroom gravy (*Banquet Extra Helping*), 18 oz. | 890 |
| parmigiana (*Armour Classics*), 11.5 oz. | 410 |
| sirloin (*The Budget Gourmet*), 11.5 oz. | 410 |
| short ribs, boneless (*Armour Classics*), 9.75 oz. | 380 |
| sirloin: | |
| chopped (*Le Menu*), 12.25 oz. | 430 |
| chopped (*Swanson*), 10.75 oz. | 340 |
| roast (*Armour Classics*), 10.45 oz. | 190 |
| tips (*Armour Classics*), 10.25 oz. | 230 |
| tips (*Healthy Choice*), 11.75 oz. | 290 |
| tips (*Le Menu*), 11.5 oz. | 400 |
| tips, in Burgundy sauce (*The Budget Gourmet*), 11 oz. | 310 |
| sliced (*Morton*), 10 oz. | 220 |
| sliced (*Swanson Hungry Man*), 15.25 oz. | 450 |
| sliced, gravy and (*Freezer Queen*), 10 oz. | 210 |
| steak Diane (*Armour Classics Lite*), 10 oz. | 290 |
| Stroganoff (*Armour Classics Lite*), 11.25 oz. | 250 |
| Stroganoff (*Le Menu*), 10 oz. | 430 |
| Swiss steak (*The Budget Gourmet*), 11.2 oz. | 450 |
| Swiss steak (*Swanson*), 10 oz. | 350 |
| tamale, see "Tamale dinner" | |

**Beef entree,** canned (see also "Beef entree, packaged"):

| | |
|---|---|
| chow mein (*La Choy* Bi-Pack), ¾ cup | 70 |
| pepper Oriental (*La Choy* Bi-Pack), ¾ cup | 80 |
| stew: | |
| (*Dinty Moore*, 24 oz.), 8 oz. | 220 |
| (*Estee*), 7.5 oz. | 210 |
| (*Featherweight*), 7.5 oz. | 160 |

| FOOD AND MEASURE | CALORIES |
|---|---|
| *Beef entree, canned, stew, continued* | |
| (*Hormel/Dinty Moore Micro-Cup*), 7.5 oz. | 190 |
| (*Libby's*, 15 oz.), 7.5 oz. | 160 |
| (*Wolf* Brand), 1 scant cup | 180 |

**Beef entree,** frozen:

| | |
|---|---|
| (*Banquet* Platters), 10 oz. | 460 |
| and broccoli, w/rice (*La Choy Fresh & Lite*), 11 oz. | 260 |
| casserole (*Pillsbury Microwave Classic*), 1 pkg. | 430 |
| Champignon (*Tyson Gourmet Selection*), 10.5 oz. | 370 |
| chop suey, w/rice (*Stouffer's*), 12 oz. | 300 |
| creamed, chipped (*Banquet Cookin' Bags*), 4 oz. | 100 |
| creamed, chipped (*Freezer Queen Cook-In-Pouch*), 5 oz. | 80 |
| creamed, chipped (*Stouffer's*), 5.5 oz. | 230 |
| Dijon, w/pasta and vegetables (*Right Course*), 9.5 oz. | 290 |
| enchilada, see "Enchilada entree" | |
| fiesta, w/corn pasta (*Right Course*), 8⅞ oz. | 270 |
| London broil, in mushroom sauce (*Weight Watchers*), 7.37 oz. | 140 |
| meat loaf, see "Meat loaf entree" | |
| Oriental (*The Budget Gourmet* Slim Selects), 10 oz. | 290 |
| Oriental, w/vegetables and rice (*Lean Cuisine*), 8⅝ oz. | 250 |
| patty, charbroiled, mushroom gravy and: | |
| (*Banquet Cookin' Bags*), 5 oz. | 210 |
| (*Banquet Family Entrees*), 8 oz. | 290 |
| (*Freezer Queen Cook-In-Pouch*), 5 oz. | 90 |
| (*Freezer Queen Family Suppers*), 7 oz. | 180 |
| patty, onion gravy and (*Banquet Family Entrees*), 8 oz. | 300 |
| patty, onion gravy and (*Freezer Queen Family Suppers*), 7 oz. | 200 |
| pepper Oriental (*Chun King*), 13 oz. | 310 |
| pepper steak: | |
| (*Dining Lite*), 9 oz. | 260 |
| (*Healthy Choice*), 9.5 oz. | 250 |
| (*Tyson Gourmet Selection*), 11.25 oz. | 330 |
| green, w/rice (*Stouffer's*), 10.5 oz. | 330 |
| w/rice (*The Budget Gourmet*), 10 oz. | 300 |
| w/rice and vegetables (*La Choy Fresh & Lite*), 10 oz. | 280 |
| and peppers, w/rice (*Freezer Queen* Single Serve), 9 oz. | 260 |
| pie: | |
| (*Banquet*), 7 oz. | 510 |
| (*Banquet* Supreme Microwave), 7 oz. | 440 |
| (*Morton*), 7 oz. | 430 |

| FOOD AND MEASURE | CALORIES |
|---|---|
| (*Stouffer's*), 10 oz. | 500 |
| (*Swanson* Pot Pie), 7 oz. | 370 |
| (*Swanson Hungry Man* Pot Pie), 16 oz. | 610 |
| pot roast, homestyle (*Right Course*), 9.25 oz. | 220 |
| ragout, w/rice pilaf (*Right Course*), 10 oz. | 300 |
| Salisbury steak: | |
| (*Dining Lite*), 9 oz. | 200 |
| (*Swanson* Homestyle Recipe), 10 oz. | 320 |
| charbroiled, w/vegetable medley (*Freezer Queen* Single Serve), 9 oz. | 330 |
| gravy and (*Banquet Cookin' Bags*), 5 oz. | 190 |
| gravy and (*Banquet Family Entrees*), 8 oz. | 300 |
| gravy and (*Freezer Queen Cook-In-Pouch*), 5 oz. | 160 |
| gravy and (*Freezer Queen Family Suppers*), 7 oz. | 200 |
| in gravy (*Stouffer's*), 9⅞ oz. | 250 |
| w/Italian sauce and vegetables (*Lean Cuisine*), 9.5 oz. | 280 |
| Romana (*Weight Watchers*), 8.75 oz. | 190 |
| sirloin (*The Budget Gourmet* Slim Selects), 9 oz. | 280 |
| supreme (*Tyson Gourmet Selection*), 10 oz. | 430 |
| short ribs (*Tyson Gourmet Selection*), 11 oz. | 470 |
| short ribs, in gravy (*Stouffer's*), 9 oz. | 350 |
| sirloin, in herb sauce (*The Budget Gourmet* Slim Selects), 10 oz. | 290 |
| sirloin, roast (*The Budget Gourmet*), 9.5 oz. | 330 |
| sirloin tips: | |
| in Burgundy sauce (*Swanson* Homestyle Recipe), 7 oz. | 160 |
| w/country vegetables (*The Budget Gourmet*), 10 oz. | 310 |
| and mushrooms, in wine sauce (*Weight Watchers*), 7.5 oz. | 220 |
| sliced, barbecue sauce and (*Banquet Cookin' Bags*), 4 oz. | 100 |
| sliced, gravy and: | |
| (*Banquet Cookin' Bags*), 4 oz. | 100 |
| (*Banquet Family Entrees*), 8 oz. | 160 |
| (*Freezer Queen Cook-In-Pouch*), 4 oz. | 60 |
| (*Freezer Queen Deluxe Family Suppers*), 7 oz. | 130 |
| steak, breaded (*Hormel*), 4 oz. | 370 |
| steak, Ranchero (*Lean Cuisine*), 9.25 oz. | 270 |
| stew (*Banquet Family Entrees*), 7 oz. | 140 |
| stew (*Freezer Queen Family Suppers*), 7 oz. | 150 |
| Stroganoff: | |
| (*The Budget Gourmet* Slim Selects), 8.75 oz. | 280 |
| (*Weight Watchers*), 8.5 oz. | 290 |

| FOOD AND MEASURE | CALORIES |
|---|---|
| *Beef entree, frozen, Stroganoff, continued* | |
| w/parsley noodles (*Stouffer's*), 9.75 oz. | 390 |
| sauce, and noodles (*Banquet Family Entrees*), 7 oz. | 190 |
| Szechuan (*Chun King*), 13 oz. | 340 |
| Szechwan, w/noodles and vegetables (*Lean Cuisine*), 9.25 oz. | 260 |
| teriyaki: | |
| (*Chun King*), 13 oz. | 380 |
| (*Dining Lite*), 9 oz. | 270 |
| w/rice and vegetables (*La Choy Fresh & Lite*), 10 oz. | 240 |
| in sauce, w/rice and vegetables (*Stouffer's*), 9.75 oz. | 290 |
| tortellini, see "Tortellini dishes, frozen" | |

**Beef entree,** packaged, 1 serving:

| | |
|---|---|
| pepper steak, Oriental (*Hormel Top Shelf*) | 290 |
| ribs, boneless (*Hormel Top Shelf*) | 440 |
| roast, tender (*Hormel Top Shelf*) | 240 |
| Salisbury steak, w/potatoes (*Hormel Top Shelf*) | 254 |
| Stroganoff (*Hormel Top Shelf*) | 320 |
| sukiyaki (*Hormel Top Shelf*) | 330 |

**Beef gravy,** canned:

| | |
|---|---|
| (*Franco-American*), 2 oz. | 25 |
| w/chunky beef (*Hormel Great Beginnings*), 5 oz. | 136 |

**Beef jerky** (see also "Sausage sticks"):

| | |
|---|---|
| (*Frito-Lay's*), .21 oz. | 25 |
| (*Frito-Lay's* Tender), .7 oz. | 120 |
| (*Hormel* Lumberjack), 1 oz. | 101 |
| (*Pemmican Arrowhead*), 1 piece, approx. .7 oz. | 70 |
| (*Pemmican Steakers*), 1 pouch, approx. 1.1 oz. | 80 |
| (*Pemmican Steakers*), 1 strip, approx. 1.37 oz. | 40 |
| (*Pemmican Tender Brave/Chief/Trail/Tribe* Packs), 1 oz. | 80 |
| (*Pemmican Tender Tomahawk*), 1 piece, approx. .25 oz. | 20 |
| (*Slim Jim*), 1 piece, approx. .14 oz. | 20 |
| (*Slim Jim Big Jerk*), 1 piece, approx. .25 oz. | 25 |
| (*Slim Jim Giant Jerk*), 1 piece, approx. .63 oz. | 60 |
| natural, jalapeño, peppered, or *Tabasco* (*Pemmican*), 1.1 oz. | 90 |
| natural style (*Pemmican*), 1 oz. | 80 |
| regular or *Tabasco* (*Slim Jim Super Jerk*), 1 piece | 30 |
| teriyaki, natural style (*Pemmican*), 1 oz. | 80 |

| FOOD AND MEASURE | CALORIES |
|---|---|

**Beef luncheon meat,** 1 oz., except as noted:

| | |
|---|---|
| (*Eckrich* Slender Sliced) | 35 |
| corned, see "Beef, corned" | |
| loaf, jellied (*Hormel* Perma-Fresh), 2 slices | 90 |
| roast: | |
| (*Healthy Deli*) | 30 |
| (*Oscar Mayer* Thin Sliced), .4-oz. slice | 14 |
| Italian (*Healthy Deli*) | 31 |
| oven-roasted, cured (*Hillshire Farm* Deli Select) | 31 |
| top round, oven-roasted (*Boar's Head*) | 40 |
| top round, oven-roasted (*Boar's Head* Deluxe) | 45 |
| sandwich steak (*Steak-Umm*), 2 oz. | 180 |
| smoked (*Hillshire Farm* Deli Select) | 31 |
| smoked (*Oscar Mayer*), .5-oz. slice | 14 |
| smoked, cured (*Hormel*) | 50 |
| smoked, cured, dried (*Hormel*) | 45 |

**Beef marinade seasoning mix:**

| | |
|---|---|
| (*Lawry's*), 1 pkg. | 49 |

**Beef pie,** see "Beef entree, frozen"

**Beef pocket sandwich,** frozen:

| | |
|---|---|
| and broccoli (*Lean Pockets*), 1 pkg. | 250 |
| 'n cheddar (*Hot Pockets*), 5 oz. | 370 |

**Beef seasoning mix:**

| | |
|---|---|
| ground, w/onions (*French's*), ¼ pkg. dry | 25 |

**Beef stew,** see "Beef entree, canned" and "Beef entree, frozen"

**Beef stew seasoning mix:**

| | |
|---|---|
| (*French's*), ⅙ pkg. | 25 |
| (*Lawry's*), 1 pkg. | 131 |
| (*McCormick/Schilling*), ¼ pkg. | 33 |

**Beef Stroganoff seasoning mix:**

| | |
|---|---|
| (*McCormick/Schilling*), ¼ pkg. | 32 |

**Beef suet,** see "Suet"

| FOOD AND MEASURE | CALORIES |
|---|---|
| **Beer, ale, and malt liquor,** 12 fl. oz.: | |
| (*Anheuser Marzen*) | 168 |
| (*Beck's*) | 148 |
| (*Bud Light*) | 110 |
| (*Budweiser*) | 144 |
| (*Busch*) | 144 |
| (*Carlsberg*) | 149 |
| (*Carlsberg* Light) | 110 |
| (*Coqui* Malt Liquor) | 208 |
| (*Dribeck's*) | 94 |
| (*King Cobra* Malt Liquor) | 182 |
| (*Knickerbocker*) | 140 |
| (*LA*) | 114 |
| (*Lite*) | 96 |
| (*Lite* Genuine Draft) | 98 |
| (*Löwenbräu* Dark Special/*Löwenbräu* Special) | 158 |
| (*McSorley's* Ale) | 166 |
| (*Meister Brau*) | 141 |
| (*Meister Brau* Light) | 98 |
| (*Michelob*) | 156 |
| (*Michelob* Classic Dark) | 158 |
| (*Michelob* Dry) | 133 |
| (*Michelob* Light) | 134 |
| (*Miller* Genuine Draft/*Miller High Life*) | 147 |
| (*Miller Magnum*) | 162 |
| (*Milwaukee's Best*) | 133 |
| (*Milwaukee's Best* Light) | 98 |
| (*Natural* Light) | 110 |
| (*Prior* Double Dark) | 171 |
| (*Rheingold*) | 148 |
| (*Rheingold* Light) | 96 |
| (*Rolling Rock* Light) | 104 |
| (*Rolling Rock* Premium) | 145 |
| (*Schmidt* Light) | 96 |
| (*Schmidt's*) | 148 |
| (*Schmidt's* Classic) | 144 |
| (*Tiger Head* Ale) | 166 |
| **Beer batter mix:** | |
| (*Golden Dipt*), 1 oz. | 100 |

| FOOD AND MEASURE | CALORIES |
|---|---|
| **Beerwurst** (see also "Salami, beer"): | |
| beef, 1 oz. | 92 |
| pork, 1 oz. | 67 |
| **Beet:** | |
| fresh, raw, whole, 2 medium, 2" diam. | 71 |
| fresh, boiled, drained, 2 medium | 31 |
| fresh, boiled, drained, sliced, ½ cup | 26 |
| canned, ½ cup: | |
| whole, sliced, or cut (*Stokely/Stokely* No Salt/Sugar) | 40 |
| whole, sliced, diced, or julienne (*S&W/S&W* Premium) | 40 |
| whole, tiny, or sliced (*Del Monte* Regular/No Salt) | 35 |
| sliced (*Featherweight*) | 45 |
| sliced (*S&W/Nutradiet*) | 35 |
| diced (*Stokely*) | 35 |
| Harvard (*Stokely*) | 70 |
| pickled (*Stokely*) | 100 |
| pickled (*Stokely,* Jars) | 90 |
| pickled, whole, extra small (*S&W*) | 70 |
| pickled, crinkle sliced (*Del Monte*) | 80 |
| pickled, w/red wine vinegar (*S&W* Regular/Party) | 70 |
| **Beet greens:** | |
| raw, 1" pieces, ½ cup | 4 |
| boiled, drained, 1" pieces, ½ cup | 20 |
| **Berliner:** | |
| beef and port, 1 oz. | 65 |
| **Berry drink:** | |
| (*Hawaiian Punch* Very Berry), 6 fl. oz. | 90 |
| wild (*Hi-C*), 6 fl. oz. | 92 |
| mix, prepared, blend (*Crystal Light* Sugar Free), 8 fl. oz. | 4 |
| **Berry juice** (see also specific listings): | |
| (*Libby's Juicy Juice*), 6 fl. oz. | 90 |
| **Berry juice drink:** | |
| wild (*Tropicana* Sparkler), 8 fl. oz. | 110 |
| **Biscuit,** 1 piece, except as noted: | |
| (*Wonder*) | 80 |
| (*Awrey's* 2" Round or Square), 1 oz. | 80 |

| FOOD AND MEASURE | CALORIES |
|---|---|
| *Biscuit, continued* | |
| (*Awrey's* 3″ Square), 2 oz. | 160 |
| (*Awrey's* Sliced or Unsliced), 2 oz. | 160 |
| country (*Awrey's* 3″), 2 oz. | 160 |
| frozen (*Bridgford*), 2 oz. | 180 |
| refrigerated: | |
| (*Ballard Ovenready*) | 50 |
| (*Big Country/1869 Brand Butter Tastin'*) | 100 |
| (*Pillsbury* Big Premium Heat 'n Eat), 2 pieces | 280 |
| (*Pillsbury* Country) | 50 |
| (*Roman Meal*), 2 pieces | 180 |
| baking powder or buttermilk (*1869 Brand*) | 100 |
| butter or buttermilk (*Pillsbury*) | 50 |
| buttermilk (*Ballard Ovenready*) | 50 |
| buttermilk (*Hungry Jack* Extra Rich) | 50 |
| buttermilk (*Pillsbury* Heat 'n Eat), 2 pieces | 170 |
| buttermilk (*Pillsbury* Tender Layer) | 50 |
| buttermilk, flaky or fluffy (*Hungry Jack*) | 90 |
| buttermilk or Southern style (*Big Country*) | 100 |
| flaky (*Hungry Jack*) | 80 |
| flaky (*Hungry Jack Butter Tastin'*) | 90 |
| flaky, honey (*Hungry Jack*) | 90 |
| fluffy (*Pillsbury* Good 'n Buttery) | 90 |
| oat bran, honey nut (*Roman Meal*) | 131 |
| white (*Roman Meal* Premium) | 127 |
| mix: | |
| (*Arrowhead Mills*), 2 oz. | 100 |
| (*Bisquick*), ½ cup | 240 |
| (*Martha White BixMix*), 1 piece, prepared | 100 |
| buttermilk (*Health Valley* Biscuit & Pancake), 1 oz. | 100 |

## **Black bean dinner,** canned:

| | |
|---|---|
| western, w/vegetables (*Health Valley Fast Menu*), 7.5 oz. | 120 |

## **Blackberry:**

| | |
|---|---|
| fresh, ½ cup | 37 |
| canned, in water (*Allens*), ½ cup | 25 |
| canned, in heavy syrup, ½ cup | 118 |
| frozen, unsweetened, ½ cup | 49 |

| FOOD AND MEASURE | CALORIES |
|---|---|

**Blackberry cobbler,** frozen:

| | |
|---|---|
| (*Pet-Ritz*), 1/6 pkg. | 250 |
| (*Stilwell*), 4 oz. | 280 |

**Blackened redfish seasoning,** see "Fish seasoning and coating mix"

**Black-eyed peas** (see also "Cowpeas"):

| | |
|---|---|
| canned, fresh, plain, or w/snaps (*Allens*), 1/2 cup | 100 |
| canned, mature (*Joan of Arc/Green Giant*), 1/2 cup | 90 |
| canned, mature, plain or w/pork (*Allens*), 1/2 cup | 105 |
| canned, mature, w/pork (*Luck's*), 7.5 oz. | 200 |
| frozen (*Seabrook*), 3.3 oz. | 130 |
| frozen (*Southern*), 3.5 oz. | 136 |

**Blood sausage:**

| | |
|---|---|
| 1 oz. | 107 |

**Bloody Mary mix:**

| | |
|---|---|
| bottled (*Holland House* Smooth N' Spicy), 1 fl. oz. | 3 |

**Blue cheese dip:**

| | |
|---|---|
| (*Kraft* Premium), 2 tbsp. | 50 |

**Blueberry:**

| | |
|---|---|
| fresh, 1/2 cup | 41 |
| canned, in heavy syrup (*S&W*), 1/2 cup | 111 |
| frozen, unsweetened, 1/2 cup | 39 |
| frozen, sweetened, 1/2 cup | 94 |

**Blueberry cobbler:**

| | |
|---|---|
| deep dish (*Awrey's*), 1/8 pie | 310 |
| frozen (*Pet-Ritz*), 1/6 pkg. | 370 |

**Blueberry pie,** see "Pie, frozen" and "Pie, snack"

**Blueberry turnover,** frozen:

| | |
|---|---|
| (*Pepperidge Farm*), 1 piece | 310 |

**Bluefish,** meat only, raw:

| | |
|---|---|
| 4 oz. | 140 |

| FOOD AND MEASURE | CALORIES |
|---|---|

**Boar, wild,** meat only:

roasted, 4 oz. .... 181

**Bockwurst:**

raw, 1 link, 7 links per lb. .... 200

**Bok choy,** see "Cabbage, Chinese"

**Bologna:**

(*Boar's Head* Lower Salt), 1 oz. .... 80
(*Eckrich/Eckrich Smorgas Pac/Eckrich* Sandwich), 1-oz. slice .... 100
(*Eckrich* German Brand), 1-oz. slice .... 80
(*Eckrich Lite*), 1 oz. .... 70
(*Eckrich* Thick Sliced, 12 oz.), 1.7-oz. slice .... 160
(*Eckrich* Thick Sliced, 1 lb.), 1.8-oz. slice .... 170
(*Hillshire Farm* Large), 1 oz. .... 90
(*Hillshire Farm* Ring), 1 oz. .... 89
(*Hormel* Coarse Ground, 1 lb.), 2 oz. .... 160
(*Hormel* Fine Ground, 1 lb.), 2 oz. .... 170
(*Hormel* Perma-Fresh), 2 slices .... 180
(*Kahn's* Deluxe Club/Giant Deluxe), 1 slice .... 90
(*Kahn's* Deluxe Club Family Pack), 1 slice .... 70
(*Kahn's* Giant Thick Deluxe), 1 slice .... 110
(*Kahn's* Thick Deluxe), 1 slice .... 140
(*Kahn's* Thin Sliced Deluxe), 1 slice .... 60
(*Light & Lean*), 2 slices .... 140
(*Light & Lean* Thin Sliced), 2 slices .... 70
(*Oscar Mayer*), 1-oz. slice .... 90
(*Oscar Mayer*), 1.6-oz. slice .... 144
(*Oscar Mayer* Light), 1-oz. slice .... 64
(*Pilgrim's Pride*), 1-oz. slice .... 59
beef:
 (*Boar's Head*), 1 oz. .... 74
 (*Eckrich*), 1-oz. slice .... 90
 (*Eckrich* Thick Sliced), 1.5-oz. slice .... 130
 (*Hebrew National* Original Deli Style), 1 oz. .... 90
 (*Hormel* Coarse Ground, 1 lb.), 2 oz. .... 160
 (*Hormel* Perma-Fresh), 2 slices .... 170
 (*Kahn's/Kahn's Giant/Kahn's* Pounder), 1 slice .... 90
 (*Kahn's* Family Pack), 1 slice .... 70
 (*Oscar Mayer*), 1-oz. slice .... 89

| FOOD AND MEASURE | CALORIES |
|---|---|
| (*Oscar Mayer*), 1.6-oz. slice | 143 |
| (*Oscar Mayer* Light), 1-oz. slice | 64 |
| garlic flavored (*Oscar Mayer*), 1 oz. | 90 |
| Lebanon (*Oscar Mayer*), .8-oz. slice | 46 |
| beef and cheddar (*Kahn's*), 1 slice | 90 |
| beef and pork (*Healthy Deli*), 1 oz. | 41 |
| w/cheese (*Eckrich*), 1-oz. slice | 90 |
| w/cheese (*Oscar Mayer*), .8-oz. slice | 74 |
| garlic (*Eckrich*), 1-oz. slice | 90 |
| garlic (*Kahn's*), 1 slice | 90 |
| ham, see "Ham bologna" | |
| pork and beef (*Boar's Head*), 1 oz. | 80 |
| turkey, see "Turkey bologna" | |

**"Bologna," vegetarian,** frozen:

| | |
|---|---|
| (*Worthington Bolono*), 2 slices or 1.3 oz. | 60 |

**Bolognese sauce:**

| | |
|---|---|
| canned (*Progresso* Authentic Pasta Sauces), ½ cup | 150 |
| refrigerated (*Contadina Fresh*), 7.5 oz. | 230 |

**Bonito,** meat only:

| | |
|---|---|
| Caribbean, raw, 4 oz. | 156 |
| Japanese, raw, 4 oz. | 147 |

**Borage:**

| | |
|---|---|
| raw, 1" pieces, ½ cup | 9 |
| boiled, drained, 4 oz. | 28 |

**Bouillon** (see also "Soup canned," and "Soup mix"):

| | |
|---|---|
| beef, cube or instant (*Steero*), 1 cube or tsp. | 6 |
| beef, cube or instant (*Wyler's*), 1 cube or tsp. | 6 |
| beef, instant (*Lite-Line* Low Sodium), 1 tsp. | 12 |
| beef or chicken (*Featherweight*), 1 tsp. | 18 |
| beef or chicken (*Weight Watchers* Broth Mix), 1 pkt. | 8 |
| brown (*G. Washington's* Seasoning & Broth), 1 pkt. | 6 |
| chicken, cube or instant (*Steero*), 1 cube or tsp. | 8 |
| chicken, cube or instant (*Wyler's*), 1 cube or tsp. | 8 |
| chicken, instant (*Lite-Line* Low Sodium), 1 tsp. | 12 |
| golden (*G. Washington's* Seasoning & Broth), 1 pkt. | 6 |
| onion (*G. Washington's* Seasoning & Broth), 1 pkt. | 12 |
| onion flavor, instant (*Wyler's*), 1 tsp. | 10 |

| FOOD AND MEASURE | CALORIES |
|---|---|
| *Bouillon, continued* | |
| vegetable (*G. Washington's* Seasoning & Broth), 1 pkt. | 12 |
| vegetable flavor, instant (*Wyler's*), 1 tsp. | 6 |
| **Bourbon,** see "Liquor" | |
| **Boysenberry:** | |
| fresh, see "Blackberry" | |
| canned, in heavy syrup, ½ cup | 113 |
| frozen, unsweetened, ½ cup | 33 |
| **Boysenberry juice:** | |
| (*Smucker's* Naturally 100%), 8 fl. oz. | 120 |
| **Brains:** | |
| beef, simmered, 4 oz. | 181 |
| lamb, braised, 4 oz. | 164 |
| pork, braised, 4 oz. | 156 |
| veal, braised, 4 oz. | 154 |
| **Bran,** see "Cereal" and specific grain listings | |
| **Brandy,** see "Liquor" | |
| **Bratwurst:** | |
| (*Eckrich*) 1 link | 310 |
| (*Hillshire Farm* Fully Cooked), 2 oz. | 170 |
| (*Kahn's*), 1 link | 190 |
| fresh or smoked (*Hillshire Farm*), 2 oz. | 190 |
| smoked (*Eckrich Lite* Bratwurst Links), 1 link | 190 |
| spicy (*Hillshire Farm*), 2 oz. | 180 |
| **Braunschweiger:** | |
| (*Hormel*), 1 oz. | 80 |
| (*Oscar Mayer/Oscar Mayer* German Brand), 1 oz. | 96 |
| (*Oscar Mayer* Tube), 1 oz. | 97 |
| (*Oscar Mayer* Slices), .9-oz. slice | 89 |
| **Brazil nuts, shelled:** | |
| 1 oz., 6 large or 8 medium | 186 |
| **Bread,** 1 slice, except as noted: | |
| apple walnut (*Arnold*) | 64 |
| (*Arnold Bran'nola* Original) | 85 |

| FOOD AND MEASURE | CALORIES |
|---|---|
| barbecue (*Colombo* Brand BBQ Loaf), 2 oz. | 139 |
| bran, whole (*Brownberry* Natural) | 58 |
| bran and oat (*Oatmeal Goodness* Light) | 40 |
| brown and serve (*du Jour Austrian/French*) | 70 |
| (*Brownberry Bran'nola*) | 85 |
| (*Brownberry* Health Nut) | 71 |
| cinnamon oatmeal (*Oatmeal Goodness*) | 90 |
| cinnamon raisin (*Arnold*) | 67 |
| cinnamon raisin (*Weight Watchers*) | 60 |
| cinnamon swirl (*Pepperidge Farm*) | 90 |
| date nut roll (*Dromedary*), ½" slice | 80 |
| French: | |
| (*DiCarlo* Parisian) | 70 |
| extra sour (*Colombo* Brand), 2 oz. | 150 |
| extra sour, sliced (*Colombo* Brand), 2 oz. | 153 |
| sweet (*Colombo* Brand French Stick), 2 oz. | 154 |
| twin (*Pepperidge Farm* Hearth), 1 oz. | 80 |
| garlic (*Colombo* Brand), 2 oz. | 185 |
| grain: | |
| mixed (*Roman Meal* Round Top) | 67 |
| mixed (*Roman Meal* Thin Sliced Sandwich) | 55 |
| multi (*Roman Meal* Sun Grain) | 68 |
| multi (*Weight Watchers*) | 40 |
| nutty (*Arnold Bran'nola*) | 85 |
| nutty (*Brownberry Bran'nola* Nutty Grains) | 85 |
| seven (*Pepperidge Farm* Hearty Slice), 2 slices | 180 |
| (*Hollywood* Dark or Light) | 70 |
| honey bran (*Pepperidge Farm,* 1½ lb.) | 90 |
| Italian: | |
| (*Arnold* Francisco International), 1-oz. slice | 72 |
| (*Brownberry* Light) | 44 |
| (*Wonder* Family) | 70 |
| brown and serve (*Pepperidge Farm* Hearth), 1 oz. | 80 |
| light (*Arnold* Bakery) | 45 |
| thick sliced (*Arnold* Francisco International) | 66 |
| (*Monk's* Hi-Fibre) | 70 |
| oat (*Arnold/Brownberry Bran'nola* Country) | 90 |
| oat, crunchy (*Pepperidge Farm,* 1½ lb.), 2 slices | 190 |
| oat bran: | |
| (*Awrey's*) | 50 |
| (*Roman Meal* Split-Top) | 68 |

| FOOD AND MEASURE | CALORIES |
|---|---|
| *Bread, oat bran, continued* | |
| (*Weight Watchers*) | 40 |
| honey (*Roman Meal*) | 71 |
| honey nut (*Roman Meal*) | 72 |
| oatmeal: | |
| (*Pepperidge Farm*) | 70 |
| (*Pepperidge Farm*, 1½ lb.) | 90 |
| (*Pepperidge Farm* Light Style) | 45 |
| (*Pepperidge Farm* Very Thin) | 40 |
| and bran (*Oatmeal Goodness*) | 90 |
| light (*Arnold* Bakery) | 44 |
| sunflower seed (*Oatmeal Goodness*) | 90 |
| orange raisin (*Brownberry*) | 67 |
| pita, oat bran (*Sahara*), ½ piece | 66 |
| pita, wheat, whole (*Sahara*), 1 piece | 150 |
| pita, white (*Sahara*), ½ piece or 1 mini piece | 79 |
| pumpernickel (*Arnold*) | 70 |
| pumpernickel (*Pepperidge Farm* Family) | 80 |
| pumpernickel (*Pepperidge Farm* Party), 4 slices | 60 |
| raisin: | |
| bran (*Brownberry*) | 61 |
| cinnamon (*Brownberry*) | 66 |
| w/cinnamon (*Monk's*) | 70 |
| w/cinnamon, swirl (*Pepperidge Farm*) | 90 |
| walnut (*Brownberry*) | 68 |
| rice bran (*Roman Meal*) | 70 |
| rice bran, golden (*Monk's*) | 70 |
| rice bran, honey nut (*Roman Meal*) | 71 |
| rye: | |
| (*Braun's Old Allegheny*) | 70 |
| (*Pepperidge Farm* Family) | 80 |
| (*Weight Watchers*) | 40 |
| (*Wonder*) | 70 |
| all varieties (*Beefsteak*) | 70 |
| caraway (*Brownberry* Natural) | 73 |
| Dijon (*Pepperidge Farm*) | 50 |
| dill (*Arnold*) | 71 |
| Jewish, seeded (*Levy's*) | 76 |
| Jewish, seedless (*Levy's*) | 75 |
| party (*Pepperidge Farm*), 4 slices | 60 |

| FOOD AND MEASURE | CALORIES |
|---|---|
| seedless (*Brownberry* Natural Thin Sliced) | 45 |
| seedless (*Pepperidge Farm* Family) | 80 |
| sesame wheat (*Pepperidge Farm,* 1½ lb.), 2 slices | 190 |
| sourdough (*DiCarlo*) | 70 |
| sourdough French (*Boudin*), 2 slices or 2 oz. | 130 |
| sunflower and bran (*Monk's*) | 70 |
| Vienna (*Pepperidge Farm* Hearth Thick Sliced) | 70 |
| Vienna (*Pepperidge Farm* Light Style) | 45 |
| wheat: | |
| (*Arnold* Brick Oven) | 57 |
| (*Brownberry* Hearth), 1 oz. | 70 |
| (*Brownberry* Natural) | 80 |
| (*Country Grain*) | 70 |
| (*Fresh & Natural*) | 70 |
| (*Home Pride* Butter Top/7 Grain/Stoneground) | 70 |
| (*Pepperidge Farm,* 1½ lb.) | 90 |
| (*Pepperidge Farm* Family, 2 lb.) | 70 |
| (*Pepperidge Farm* Light Style) | 45 |
| (*Pepperidge Farm* Very Thin) | 35 |
| (*Weight Watchers*) | 40 |
| all varieties (*Beefsteak*) | 70 |
| apple honey (*Brownberry*) | 69 |
| cracked (*Pepperidge Farm*) | 70 |
| cracked (*Wonder*) | 70 |
| dark (*Arnold Bran'nola*) | 83 |
| hearty (*Arnold/Brownberry Bran'nola*) | 88 |
| honey wheatberry (*Arnold*) | 77 |
| light golden (*Arnold* Bakery) | 44 |
| oatmeal (*Oatmeal Goodness*) | 90 |
| oatmeal (*Oatmeal Goodness* Light) | 40 |
| soft (*Brownberry*) | 74 |
| sprouted (*Pepperidge Farm*) | 70 |
| whole (*Arnold* Stoneground 100%) | 48 |
| whole (*Daily*), 2 oz. | 140 |
| whole (*Monk's* 100% Stone Ground) | 70 |
| whole (*Pepperidge Farm* Thin Sliced) | 60 |
| whole (*Wonder* Family/100%/Regular/Soft) | 70 |
| whole (*Wonder* High Fiber/Light) | 40 |
| white: | |
| (*Arnold* Brick Oven) | 61 |
| (*Arnold* Country White) | 98 |

| FOOD AND MEASURE | CALORIES |
|---|---|
| *Bread, white, continued* | |
| (*Arnold* Light Premium) | 42 |
| (*Beefsteak* Robust) | 70 |
| (*Brownberry* Light Premium) | 42 |
| (*Brownberry* Natural) | 59 |
| (*Home Pride* Butter Top) | 70 |
| (*Monk's*) | 60 |
| (*Pepperidge Farm* Country, 1½ lb.), 2 slices | 190 |
| (*Pepperidge Farm* Large Family Thin Sliced) | 70 |
| (*Pepperidge Farm* Sandwich), 2 slices | 130 |
| (*Pepperidge Farm* Thin Sliced, 1 lb.) | 80 |
| (*Pepperidge Farm* Thin Sliced, 8 oz.) | 70 |
| (*Pepperidge Farm* Toasting) | 90 |
| (*Pepperidge Farm* Very Thin) | 40 |
| (*Weight Watchers*) | 40 |
| (*Wonder*) | 70 |
| (*Wonder* High Fiber/Light) | 40 |
| (*Wonder* Thin Sliced) | 50 |
| w/buttermilk (*Wonder*) | 70 |
| extra fiber (*Arnold* Brick Oven) | 55 |
| **Bread, canned,** brown: | |
| (*S&W* New England), 2 slices | 76 |
| (*B&M/Friends*), 1.6 oz. | 92 |
| w/raisins (*B&M/Friends*), 1.6 oz. | 94 |
| **Bread, sweet, mix[1]:** | |
| banana (*Pillsbury*), 1/12 loaf | 170 |
| blueberry nut (*Pillsbury*), 1/12 loaf | 150 |
| cherry nut (*Pillsbury*), 1/12 loaf | 180 |
| cornbread: | |
| (*Aunt Jemima* Easy), 1 serving | 196 |
| (*Dromedary*), 3 tbsp. dry | 100 |
| (*Dromedary*), 2″ × 2″ square | 130 |
| (*Martha White* Cotton Pickin'), ¼ pan | 170 |
| (*Pillsbury/Ballard*), ⅛ recipe | 140 |
| white (*Robin Hood/Gold Medal* Pouch Mix), ⅙ mix | 150 |
| yellow (*Martha White* Light Crust), 2 oz. dry | 140 |
| yellow (*Robin Hood/Gold Medal* Pouch Mix), ⅙ mix | 150 |

[1]Prepared according to basic package directions, except as noted.

| FOOD AND MEASURE | CALORIES |
|---|---|
| cranberry or date (*Pillsbury*), 1⁄12 loaf | 160 |
| date nut (*Dromedary*), 1⁄12 loaf | 183 |
| gingerbread (*Betty Crocker* Classic), 1⁄9 mix | 220 |
| gingerbread (*Pillsbury*), 3″ square | 190 |
| nut (*Pillsbury*), 1⁄12 loaf | 170 |
| **Bread dough:** | |
| frozen, honey walnut or white (*Bridgford*), 1 oz. | 76 |
| frozen, white (*Rich's*), 2 slices | 120 |
| refrigerated (*Roman Meal*), 1-oz. slice | 85 |
| refrigerated, cornbread twists (*Pillsbury*), 1 twist | 70 |
| refrigerated, French, crusty (*Pillsbury*), 1″ slice | 60 |
| refrigerated, wheat or white (*Pipin' Hot*), 1″ slice | 70 |
| **Breadcrumbs:** | |
| plain (*Devonsheer*), 1 oz. | 108 |
| plain or Italian (*Progresso*), 2 tbsp. | 60 |
| Italian style (*Devonsheer*), 1 oz. | 104 |
| Italian style, whole wheat (*Jaclyn's*), ½ oz. | 28 |
| **Breadfruit:** | |
| peeled and seeded, ½ cup | 114 |
| **Breadfruit seeds,** shelled: | |
| raw, 1 oz. | 54 |
| boiled, 1 oz. | 48 |
| roasted, 1 oz. | 59 |
| **Breadsticks,** 1 piece, except as noted: | |
| plain (*Stella D'Oro*) | 41 |
| onion (*Stella D'Oro*) | 40 |
| pizza (*Fattorie & Pandea*), 3 pieces | 59 |
| pizza (*Stella D'Oro*) | 43 |
| sesame (*Fattorie & Pandea*), 3 pieces | 65 |
| sesame (*Stella D'Oro*) | 51 |
| wheat (*Stella D'Oro*) | 42 |
| wheat, whole (*Fattorie & Pandea*), 3 pieces | 57 |
| refrigerated, soft (*Pillsbury*) | 100 |
| refrigerated, regular or soft (*Roman Meal*) | 117 |
| **Breakfast, frozen,** see specific listings | |
| **Breakfast strips,** see "Bacon, substitute" | |

| FOOD AND MEASURE | CALORIES |
|---|---|

## Broccoli:

| | |
|---|---|
| fresh, raw, 1 spear, 8.7 oz. | 42 |
| fresh, raw, chopped, ½ cup | 12 |
| fresh, boiled, drained, 1 spear, 6.3 oz. | 51 |
| fresh, boiled, drained, chopped, ½ cup | 22 |
| frozen: | |
| all cuts (*Birds Eye*), 3.3 oz. | 25 |
| spears (*Green Giant Harvest Fresh*), ½ cup | 20 |
| spears, baby (*Birds Eye* Deluxe), 3.3 oz. | 30 |
| spears, whole (*Birds Eye* Farm Fresh), 4 oz. | 30 |
| florets (*Birds Eye* Deluxe), 3.3 oz. | 25 |
| cuts (*Birds Eye* Portion Pack), 3 oz. | 20 |
| cuts (*Green Giant* Polybag), ½ cup | 12 |
| cuts (*Green Giant Harvest Fresh*), ½ cup | 16 |
| cuts (*Stokely Singles*), 3 oz. | 25 |
| chopped (*Southern*), 3.5 oz. | 28 |
| in butter sauce (*Green Giant* One Serving), 4.5 oz. | 45 |
| in butter sauce, spears (*Birds Eye* Combinations), 3.3 oz. | 45 |
| in butter sauce, spears (*Green Giant*), ½ cup | 40 |
| in cheese sauce (*Birds Eye* Combinations), 5 oz. | 130 |
| in cheese sauce (*Freezer Queen Side Dishes*), 4.5 oz. | 48 |
| in cheese sauce (*Green Giant*), ½ cup | 60 |
| in cheese sauce, cuts (*Green Giant* One Serving), 5 oz. | 70 |
| in cheese sauce, cuts (*Stokely Singles*), 4 oz. | 80 |

## Broccoli and cheese in pastry:

| | |
|---|---|
| frozen (*Pepperidge Farm*), 1 piece | 230 |

## Broccoli combinations, frozen:

| | |
|---|---|
| and carrots: | |
| baby, and water chestnuts (*Birds Eye* Farm Fresh), 4 oz. | 45 |
| baby whole, and chestnuts (*Stokely Singles*), 3 oz. | 30 |
| and cauliflower: | |
| (*Stokely Singles*), 3 oz. | 20 |
| medley (*Green Giant Valley Combinations*), ½ cup | 30 |
| cauliflower and carrots: | |
| (*Birds Eye* Farm Fresh), 4 oz. | 35 |
| baby (*Stokely Singles*), 3 oz. | 25 |
| no sauce (*Green Giant* One Serving), 4 oz. | 25 |
| in butter sauce (*Birds Eye* Combinations), 3.3 oz. | 45 |

| FOOD AND MEASURE | CALORIES |
|---|---|
| in butter sauce (*Green Giant*), ½ cup | 30 |
| w/cheese sauce (*Birds Eye* Combinations), 4.5 oz. | 110 |
| in cheese sauce (*Birds Eye For One*), 5 oz. | 110 |
| in cheese sauce (*Green Giant* One Serving), 5 oz. | 70 |
| in cheese-flavored sauce (*Green Giant*), ½ cup | 60 |
| baby, in cheese sauce (*Stokely Singles*), 4 oz. | 70 |
| cauliflower and red peppers (*Birds Eye* Farm Fresh), 4 oz. | 30 |
| corn and red peppers (*Birds Eye* Farm Fresh), 4 oz. | 60 |
| fanfare (*Green Giant Valley Combinations*), ½ cup | 70 |
| green beans, pearl onions, and red peppers (*Birds Eye* Farm Fresh), 4 oz. | 35 |
| red peppers, bamboo shoots, and straw mushrooms (*Birds Eye* Farm Fresh), 4 oz. | 30 |
| rotini, in cheese sauce (*Green Giant* One Serving), 5.5 oz. | 120 |

**Brown gravy:**

| | |
|---|---|
| canned, regular or w/onion (*Heinz*), 2 oz. or ¼ cup | 25 |
| canned (*McCormick/Schilling*), ⅓ cup | 30 |
| mix, prepared: | |
| (*French's*), ¼ cup | 20 |
| (*Lawry's*), 1 cup | 94 |
| (*McCormick/Schilling*), ¼ cup | 23 |
| (*McCormick/Schilling* Lite), ¼ cup | 10 |
| (*Pillsbury*), ¼ cup | 15 |

**Brownie,** 1 piece:

| | |
|---|---|
| fudge (*Little Debbie*), 2 oz. | 240 |
| fudge nut (*Awrey's* Sheet Cake), 1.25 oz. | 150 |
| fudge nut, iced (*Awrey's* Sheet Cake), 2.5 oz. | 300 |
| fudge walnut (*Tastykake*), 3 oz. | 335 |
| frozen, chocolate (*Weight Watchers*), ⅓ pkg. | 100 |
| frozen, chocolate chip, double (*Nestlé* Toll House Ready to Bake), 1.4 oz. | 150 |
| frozen, hot fudge (*Pepperidge Farm* Newport), 3.25 oz. | 400 |
| mix, prepared: | |
| (*Duncan Hines Gourmet Truffle*) | 280 |
| (*Duncan Hines Gourmet Turtle*) | 240 |
| (*Estee*), 2″ square | 50 |
| caramel fudge chunk (*Pillsbury*), 2″ square | 170 |
| caramel swirl (*Betty Crocker*) | 120 |
| chocolate, German (*Betty Crocker*) | 160 |

| FOOD AND MEASURE | CALORIES |
|---|---|
| *Brownie, mix, prepared, continued* | |
| chocolate, milk (*Duncan Hines*) | 160 |
| chocolate chip (*Betty Crocker*) | 140 |
| frosted (*Betty Crocker*) | 160 |
| frosted (*Betty Crocker MicroRave*) | 180 |
| fudge (*Betty Crocker/Betty Crocker MicroRave*) | 150 |
| fudge (*Betty Crocker* Family Size) | 140 |
| fudge (*Betty Crocker* Supreme) | 120 |
| fudge (*Duncan Hines*) | 160 |
| fudge (*Pillsbury* Microwave) | 190 |
| fudge, chewy (*Duncan Hines*) | 130 |
| fudge, deluxe (*Pillsbury*), 2″ square | 150 |
| fudge, double (*Pillsbury*), 2″ square | 160 |
| fudge, peanut butter (*Duncan Hines*) | 150 |
| fudge, triple, chunky (*Pillsbury*), 2″ square | 170 |
| rocky road, fudge (*Pillsbury*), 2″ square | 170 |
| walnut (*Betty Crocker*) | 140 |
| walnut (*Betty Crocker MicroRave*) | 160 |
| white, Vienna (*Duncan Hines*) | 240 |

**Browning sauce:**

| | |
|---|---|
| (*Gravymaster*), 1 tsp. | 12 |

**Brussels sprouts:**

| | |
|---|---|
| fresh, raw, ½ cup | 19 |
| fresh, boiled, drained, ½ cup | 30 |
| frozen: | |
| (*Birds Eye*), 3.3 oz. | 35 |
| (*Green Giant* Polybag), ½ cup | 25 |
| (*Seabrook*), 3.3 oz. | 35 |
| (*Southern*), 3.5 oz. | 37 |
| (*Stokely Singles*), 3 oz. | 35 |
| baby (*Seabrook*), 3.3 oz. | 40 |
| in butter sauce (*Green Giant*), ½ cup | 40 |
| in butter sauce (*Stokely Singles*), 4 oz. | 50 |
| w/cheese sauce, baby (*Birds Eye* Combinations), 4.5 oz. | 130 |
| w/cauliflower and carrots (*Birds Eye* Farm Fresh), 4 oz. | 40 |

**Buckwheat:**

| | |
|---|---|
| whole-grain, 1 oz. | 97 |
| flour, see "Flour" | |
| groats, brown or white (*Arrowhead Mills*), 2 oz. | 190 |

| FOOD AND MEASURE | CALORIES |
|---|---|
| **Bulgur** (see also "Tabbouleh mix"): | |
| dry, 1 oz. | 97 |
| cooked, 1 cup | 152 |
| **Bun, sweet,** 1 piece: | |
| cinnamon, frozen (*Rich's Ever Fresh*), 2.5 oz. | 293 |
| honey, glazed (*Hostess Breakfast Bake Shop*) | 360 |
| honey, glazed (*Tastykake*), 3.25 oz. | 362 |
| honey, iced (*Hostess Breakfast Bake Shop*) | 430 |
| honey, iced (*Tastykake*), 3.25 oz. | 348 |
| honey, mini, frozen (*Rich's Ever Fresh*), 1.36 oz. | 133 |
| **Burbot,** meat only: | |
| raw, 4 oz. | 103 |
| **Burdock root:** | |
| raw, pieces, ½ cup | 43 |
| boiled, drained, 1" pieces, ½ cup | 55 |
| ***Burger King,*** 1 serving: | |
| breakfast, 1 serving: | |
| bagel | 272 |
| bagel, w/cream cheese | 370 |
| bagel sandwich, w/egg and cheese | 407 |
| bagel sandwich, w/bacon, egg, and cheese | 453 |
| bagel sandwich, w/ham, egg, and cheese | 438 |
| bagel sandwich, w/sausage, egg, and cheese | 626 |
| biscuit | 332 |
| biscuit, w/bacon | 378 |
| biscuit, w/bacon and egg | 467 |
| biscuit, w/sausage | 478 |
| biscuit, w/sausage and egg | 568 |
| croissant | 180 |
| *Croissan'wich*, w/egg and cheese | 315 |
| *Croissan'wich*, w/bacon, egg, and cheese | 361 |
| *Croissan'wich*, w/ham, egg, and cheese | 346 |
| *Croissan'wich*, w/sausage, egg, and cheese | 534 |
| danish, apple cinnamon | 390 |
| danish, cheese | 406 |
| danish, cinnamon raisin | 449 |
| French toast sticks | 538 |

| FOOD AND MEASURE | CALORIES |
|---|---|
| *Burger King, breakfast, continued* | |
| mini muffins, blueberry | 292 |
| mini muffins, lemon poppyseed | 318 |
| mini muffins, raisin oat bran | 291 |
| scrambled egg platter | 549 |
| scrambled egg platter, w/bacon | 610 |
| scrambled egg platter, w/sausage | 768 |
| sandwiches and burgers: | |
| bacon double cheeseburger | 515 |
| bacon double cheeseburger deluxe | 592 |
| barbecue bacon double cheeseburger | 536 |
| BK Broiler chicken | 379 |
| *Burger Buddies* | 349 |
| cheeseburger | 318 |
| cheesburger, double | 483 |
| cheeseburger deluxe | 390 |
| chicken sandwich | 685 |
| hamburger | 272 |
| mushroom Swiss double cheeseburger | 473 |
| Ocean Catch fish filet | 495 |
| *Whopper* | 614 |
| *Whopper*, w/cheese | 706 |
| *Whopper*, double | 844 |
| *Whopper*, double, w/cheese | 935 |
| tenders, chicken, 6 pieces | 236 |
| salad, chef | 178 |
| salad, chicken, chunky | 142 |
| salad, garden | 95 |
| salad, side | 25 |
| dressing, *Newman's Own*, 1 pkt.: | |
| bleu cheese dressing | 300 |
| French or Thousand Island dressing | 290 |
| Italian dressing, reduced calorie | 170 |
| olive oil and vinegar dressing | 310 |
| ranch dressing | 350 |
| dipping sauces: | |
| barbecue dipping sauce | 36 |
| *Burger King A.M. Express* dip | 84 |
| honey dipping sauce | 91 |
| ranch dipping sauce | 171 |
| sweet & sour sauce | 45 |

| FOOD AND MEASURE | CALORIES |
|---|---|
| side dishes: | |
| french fries, medium | 372 |
| onion rings, 3.4 oz. | 339 |
| tater tenders, 2.5 oz. | 213 |
| apple pie | 311 |

## "Burger," vegetarian:

| | |
|---|---|
| canned (*Worthington Vegetarian Burger*), ½ cup | 150 |
| frozen (*Morningstar Farms Grillers*), 2.25-oz. patty | 180 |
| frozen (*Worthington FriPats*), 2.25-oz. piece | 180 |
| mix, prepared, except as noted: | |
| (*Love Natural Foods Loveburger*), 4-oz. burger | 245 |
| (*Nature's Burger* Original), 3-oz. burger[1] | 152 |
| (*Worthington Granburger*), 6 tbsp. mix | 110 |
| barbecue (*Nature's Burger*), 3-oz. burger[1] | 117 |
| pizza (*Nature's Burger*), 3-oz. burger[1] | 121 |
| w/tofu (*Fantastic Foods*), 3.4-oz. burger[1] | 133 |

## **Burrito,** frozen:

| | |
|---|---|
| (*Hormel* Burrito Grande), 5.5 oz. | 380 |
| beef: | |
| (*Hormel*), 1 piece | 205 |
| and bean (*Patio*), 5-oz. pkg. | 370 |
| and bean (*Patio Britos*), 3.63 oz. | 250 |
| and bean green chili (*Patio*), 5-oz. pkg. | 330 |
| and bean red chili (*Patio*), 5-oz. pkg. | 340 |
| nacho (*Patio Britos*), 3.63 oz. | 270 |
| cheese (*Hormel*), 1 piece | 210 |
| cheese, nacho (*Patio Britos*), 3.63 oz. | 250 |
| chicken, spicy (*Patio Britos*), 3.63 oz. | 250 |
| chicken and rice (*Hormel*), 1 piece | 200 |
| chili, green (*Patio Britos*), 3.63 oz. | 250 |
| chili, hot (*Hormel*), 1 piece | 240 |
| chili, red (*Patio Britos*), 3.63 oz. | 240 |
| red hot (*Patio*), 5-oz. pkg. | 360 |

## **Burrito dinner,** frozen:

| | |
|---|---|
| (*Patio*), 12 oz. | 517 |
| beef and bean (*Old El Paso* Festive Dinners), 11 oz. | 470 |

[1]Does not include value for oil or fat used in cooking.

| FOOD AND MEASURE | CALORIES |
|---|---|
| **Burrito entree,** frozen: | |
| bean and cheese (*Old El Paso*), 1 pkg. | 330 |
| beef and bean, hot (*Old El Paso*), 1 pkg. | 310 |
| beef and bean, medium (*Old El Paso*), 1 pkg. | 330 |
| beef and bean, mild (*Old El Paso*), 1 pkg. | 320 |
| chicken (*Weight Watchers*), 7.62 oz. | 330 |
| **Burrito filling mix:** | |
| bean (*Del Monte*), ½ cup | 110 |
| **Burrito seasoning mix:** | |
| (*Lawry's*), 1 pkg. | 132 |
| (*Old El Paso*), ⅛ pkg. | 17 |
| **Butter,** salted or unsalted: | |
| regular, 1 stick or 4 oz. | 813 |
| regular, 1 tbsp. | 100 |
| regular, 1 tsp. | 34 |
| whipped, 1 tbsp. | 67 |
| whipped, 1 tsp. | 23 |
| **Butterbur:** | |
| fresh, boiled, drained, 4 oz. | 9 |
| canned, chopped, ½ cup | 2 |
| **Butterfish,** meat only: | |
| raw, 4 oz. | 165 |
| **Buttermilk,** see "Milk" | |
| **Butternut,** shelled: | |
| dried, 1 oz. | 174 |
| **Butterscotch baking chips:** | |
| (*Nestlé* Toll House Morsels), 1 oz. | 150 |

# C

| FOOD AND MEASURE | CALORIES |
|---|---|

## Cabbage:

| | |
|---|---|
| raw, untrimmed, 1 lb. | 86 |
| raw, shredded, ½ cup | 8 |
| boiled, drained, shredded, ½ cup | 16 |

## Cabbage, Chinese:

| | |
|---|---|
| bok choy, raw, untrimmed, 1 lb. | 52 |
| bok choy, raw, shredded, ½ cup | 5 |
| bok choy, boiled, drained, shredded, ½ cup | 10 |
| pe-tsai, raw, untrimmed, 1 lb. | 68 |
| pe-tsai, raw, shredded, ½ cup | 6 |
| pe-tsai, boiled, drained, shredded, ½ cup | 8 |

## Cabbage, red:

| | |
|---|---|
| raw, untrimmed, 1 lb. | 100 |
| raw, shredded, ½ cup | 10 |
| boiled, drained, shredded, ½ cup | 16 |

## Cabbage, savoy:

| | |
|---|---|
| raw, untrimmed, 1 lb. | 100 |
| raw, shredded, ½ cup | 10 |
| boiled, drained, shredded, ½ cup | 18 |

## Cabbage, entree, frozen:

| | |
|---|---|
| stuffed, w/meat (*Lean Cuisine*), 10.75 oz. | 220 |

## Cake:

| | |
|---|---|
| apple streusel (*Awrey's*), 2″ × 2″ piece | 160 |
| banana, iced (*Awrey's*), 2″ × 2″ piece | 140 |
| Black Forest torte (*Awrey's*), 1⁄14 cake | 350 |
| carrot, layer, cream cheese-iced (*Awrey's*), 1⁄12 cake | 390 |
| carrot supreme, iced (*Awrey's*), 2″ × 2″ piece | 210 |
| chocolate: | |
| (*Awrey's*), .8-oz. piece | 70 |
| double, iced (*Awrey's*), 2″ × 2″ piece | 130 |

| FOOD AND MEASURE | CALORIES |
|---|---|
| *Cake, chocolate, continued* | |
| double, two-layer (*Awrey's*), 1/12 cake | 250 |
| double, three-layer (*Awrey's*), 1/12 cake | 310 |
| double, torte (*Awrey's*), 1/14 cake | 340 |
| German, iced (*Awrey's*), 2″ × 2″ piece | 160 |
| German, three-layer (*Awrey's*), 1/12 cake | 350 |
| milk, yellow, two-layer (*Awrey's*), 1/12 cake | 290 |
| white iced, two-layer (*Awrey's*), 1/12 cake | 270 |
| coconut, butter cream (*Awrey's*), 2″ × 2″ piece | 160 |
| coconut, yellow, three-layer (*Awrey's*), 1/12 cake | 350 |
| coffee, caramel nut (*Awrey's*), 1/12 cake | 140 |
| devil's food, white-iced (*Awrey's*), 2″ × 2″ piece | 150 |
| lemon or orange, three layer (*Awrey's*), 1/12 cake | 320 |
| lemon, yellow, two-layer (*Awrey's*), 1/12 cake | 290 |
| Neapolitan or peanut butter, torte (*Awrey's*), 1/14 cake | 380 |
| orange, frosty, iced (*Awrey's*), 2″ × 2″ piece | 150 |
| pistachio, torte (*Awrey's*), 1/14 cake | 370 |
| pound (*Drake's*), 1/10 cake, approx. 1.1 oz. | 110 |
| pound, golden (*Awrey's*), 1/14 loaf | 130 |
| raisin spice, iced (*Awrey's*), 2″ × 2″ piece | 160 |
| raspberry nut (*Awrey's*), 1/16 cake | 310 |
| sponge (*Awrey's*), 2″ × 2″ piece | 80 |
| strawberry supreme, torte (*Awrey's*), 1/14 cake | 270 |
| walnut, torte (*Awrey's*), 1/14 cake | 320 |
| yellow (*Awrey's*), .9-oz. piece | 80 |
| yellow, white-iced (*Awrey's*), 2″ × 2″ piece | 150 |

## **Cake,** frozen:

| FOOD AND MEASURE | CALORIES |
|---|---|
| banana, single layer, iced (*Sara Lee*), 1/8 cake | 170 |
| Black Forest, two-layer (*Sara Lee*), 1/8 cake | 190 |
| Boston creme (*Pepperidge Farm* Supreme), 2 7/8 oz. | 290 |
| Boston creme pie (*Weight Watchers*), 3 oz. | 160 |
| carrot (*Weight Watchers*), 3 oz. | 170 |
| carrot, single layer, iced (*Sara Lee*), 1/8 cake | 250 |
| carrot, w/cream cheese icing (*Pepperidge Farm*), 1.5 oz. | 150 |
| cheesecake: | |
| (*Weight Watchers*), 3.9 oz. | 210 |
| brownie (*Weight Watchers*), 3.5 oz. | 200 |
| cream (*Sara Lee* Original), 1/6 cake | 230 |
| cream, cherry (*Sara Lee* Original), 1/6 cake | 243 |
| cream, strawberry (*Sara Lee* Original), 1/6 cake | 222 |

| FOOD AND MEASURE | CALORIES |
|---|---|
| French (*Sara Lee* Classics), ⅛ cake | 250 |
| strawberry (*Weight Watchers*), 3.9 oz. | 180 |
| strawberry, French (*Sara Lee*), ⅛ cake | 240 |
| cherries and cream (*Weight Watchers*), 3 oz. | 190 |
| chocolate: | |
| (*Pepperidge Farm* Supreme), 2⅞ oz. | 300 |
| (*Sara Lee Free & Light*), ⅛ cake | 110 |
| (*Weight Watchers*), 2.5 oz. | 180 |
| double, three-layer (*Sara Lee*), ⅛ cake | 220 |
| fudge, double (*Weight Watchers*), 2.75 oz. | 200 |
| fudge, layer (*Pepperidge Farm*), 1⅝ oz. | 180 |
| fudge, stripe, layer (*Pepperidge Farm*), 1⅝ oz. | 170 |
| German (*Weight Watchers*), 2.5 oz. | 200 |
| German, layer (*Pepperidge Farm*), 1⅝ oz. | 180 |
| mousse (*Sara Lee* Classics), ⅛ cake | 260 |
| coconut, layer (*Pepperidge Farm*), 1⅝ oz. | 180 |
| coffee, cheese (*Sara Lee* All Butter), ⅛ cake | 210 |
| coffee, cinnamon streusel (*Weight Watchers*), 2.25 oz. | 190 |
| coffee, pecan or streusel (*Sara Lee* All Butter), ⅛ cake | 160 |
| devil's food or golden layer (*Pepperidge Farm*), 1⅝ oz. | 180 |
| lemon coconut (*Pepperidge Farm* Supreme), 3 oz. | 280 |
| lemon creme (*Pepperidge Farm* Supreme), 1⅝ oz. | 170 |
| pineapple cream (*Pepperidge Farm* Supreme), 2 oz. | 190 |
| pound: | |
| (*Pepperidge Farm* Old Fashioned Cholesterol Free), 1 oz. | 110 |
| (*Sara Lee Free & Light*), ⅒ cake | 70 |
| all butter (*Sara Lee* Original), ⅒ cake | 130 |
| all butter (*Sara Lee* Family Size Original), 1/15 cake | 130 |
| strawberry cream (*Pepperidge Farm* Supreme), 2 oz. | 190 |
| strawberry shortcake (*Sara Lee*), ⅛ cake | 190 |
| strawberry stripe, layer (*Pepperidge Farm*), 1⅝ oz. | 160 |
| vanilla, layer (*Pepperidge Farm*), 1⅝ oz. | 190 |

## **Cake, snack,** 1 piece, except as noted:

| FOOD AND MEASURE | CALORIES |
|---|---|
| apple bar, baked (*Sunbelt*), 1.31 oz. | 130 |
| apple delight (*Little Debbie*), 1.25 oz. | 140 |
| apple spice (*Hostess* Light) | 130 |
| apple spice (*Little Debbie*), 2.2 oz. | 270 |
| banana (*Hostess Suzy Q's*) | 240 |
| banana (*Hostess Twinkies*) | 150 |
| banana (*Tastykake Creamie*), 1.5 oz. | 165 |

| FOOD AND MEASURE | CALORIES |
|---|---|
| *Cake, snack, continued* | |
| banana slices (*Little Debbie*), 3 oz. | 340 |
| butterscotch (*Tastykake Krimpets*), 1 oz. | 103 |
| cherry cordial (*Little Debbie*), 1.3 oz. | 170 |
| chocolate: | |
| (*Hostess Choco Bliss*) | 200 |
| (*Hostess Choco-Diles*) | 240 |
| (*Hostess Ding Dongs*) | 170 |
| (*Hostess Ho Hos*) | 120 |
| (*Hostess Suzy Q's*) | 250 |
| (*Little Debbie*), 3 oz. | 390 |
| (*Little Debbie Choco-Cake*), 2.7 oz. | 330 |
| (*Tastykake* Creamie), 1.5 oz. | 168 |
| (*Tastykake* Juniors), 3.3 oz. | 341 |
| (*Tastykake* Kandy Kakes), .7 oz. | 78 |
| cream-filled (*Drake's Devil Dog*) | 160 |
| cream-filled (*Drake's Ring Ding*) | 180 |
| fudge crispy (*Little Debbie*), 2.08 oz. | 260 |
| fudge round (*Little Debbie*), 2.75 oz. | 330 |
| mint, cream-filled (*Drake's Ring Ding*) | 190 |
| roll, cream-filled (*Drake's Yodel*) | 150 |
| roll, Swiss, cream-filled (*Drake's*) | 170 |
| slices (*Little Debbie*), 3 oz. | 320 |
| twins (*Little Debbie*), 2.2 oz. | 240 |
| w/vanilla pudding (*Hostess* Light) | 130 |
| chocolate chip (*Little Debbie*), 2.4 oz. | 320 |
| coconut (*Tastykake* Juniors), 3.3 oz. | 296 |
| coconut (*Tastykake* Kandy Kakes), .7 oz. | 78 |
| coconut, round (*Little Debbie*), 1.13 oz. | 150 |
| coconut covered (*Hostess Sno Balls*) | 150 |
| coconut crunch (*Little Debbie*), 2 oz. | 320 |
| coffee: | |
| (*Drake's Jr.*) | 140 |
| (*Drake's* Small) | 220 |
| (*Little Debbie*), 2.1 oz. | 250 |
| (*Tastykake* Koffee Kake Juniors), 2.5 oz. | 261 |
| cinnamon crumb (*Drake's*) | 150 |
| cream-filled (*Tastykake Koffee Kake*), 1 oz. | 110 |
| crumb cake (*Hostess*) | 120 |
| crumb cake (*Hostess* Light) | 80 |

| FOOD AND MEASURE | CALORIES |
|---|---|
| cupcake: | |
| butter cream, cream-filled (*Tastykake*), 1.1 oz. | 118 |
| chocolate (*Hostess*) | 180 |
| chocolate (*Tastykake*), 1.1 oz. | 100 |
| chocolate (*Tastykake* Royale), 1.6 oz. | 171 |
| chocolate, cream-filled (*Drake's Yankee Doodle*) | 100 |
| chocolate, creme-filled (*Hostess* Light) | 130 |
| chocolate, cream-filled (*Tastykake*), 1.1 oz. | 118 |
| chocolate, cream-filled (*Tastykake Krimpets*), 1.2 oz. | 124 |
| chocolate or vanilla, cream-filled (*Tastykake* Tastylite), 1.1 oz. | 100 |
| creme (*Tastykake* Kreme Kup), .9 oz. | 86 |
| golden, cream-filled (*Drake's Sunny Doodle*) | 100 |
| orange (*Hostess*) | 160 |
| dessert cup (*Hostess*) | 90 |
| dessert cup (*Little Debbie*), .79 oz. | 80 |
| devil's food (*Little Debbie* Devil Cremes), 2.5 oz. | 300 |
| devil's food (*Little Debbie* Devil Squares), 2.2 oz. | 270 |
| donut, see "Donut" | |
| (*Drake's Funny Bone*) | 150 |
| (*Drake's Zoinks*) | 130 |
| fancy (*Little Debbie*), 2.6 oz. | 340 |
| fig (*Little Debbie Figaroos*), 1.5 oz. | 160 |
| golden cremes (*Little Debbie*), 2.5 oz. | 270 |
| honey, glazed (*Hostess*) | 370 |
| honey, iced (*Hostess*) | 410 |
| (*Hostess Li'l Angels*) | 90 |
| (*Hostess O's*) | 220 |
| (*Hostess Tiger Tail*) | 240 |
| (*Hostess Twinkies*) | 150 |
| (*Hostess Twinkies* Light) | 110 |
| jelly (*Tastykake Krimpets*), 1 oz. | 85 |
| jelly roll (*Little Debbie*), 2.2 oz. | 250 |
| lemon (*Tastykake* Juniors), 3.3 oz. | 306 |
| lemon stix (*Little Debbie*), 1.5 oz. | 220 |
| (*Little Debbie Caravella*), 1.2 oz. | 200 |
| (*Little Debbie* Doodle Dandies), 2.5 oz. | 320 |
| (*Little Debbie* Star Crunch), 1.08 oz. | 150 |
| marshmallow supreme (*Little Debbie*), 1.25 oz. | 150 |
| orange (*Tastykake* Juniors), 3.3 oz. | 337 |
| peanut butter (*Tastykake* Kandy Kakes), .7 oz. | 87 |
| peanut butter bar (*Little Debbie*), 2.5 oz. | 370 |

| FOOD AND MEASURE | CALORIES |
|---|---|
| *Cake, snack, continued* | |
| peanut butter-jelly sandwich (*Little Debbie*), 1.13 oz. | 150 |
| pecan twins (*Little Debbie*), 2 oz. | 220 |
| pecan twists (*Tastykake*), 1 oz. | 109 |
| pie, see "Pie, snack" | |
| strawberry (*Tastykake Krimpets*), 1 oz. | 101 |
| strawberry (*Twinkies* Fruit'N Creme), 1.5 oz. | 140 |
| Swiss roll (*Little Debbie*), 2.25 oz. | 280 |
| (*Tastykake* Tasty Twist), .1 oz. | 18 |
| vanilla (*Little Debbie*), 3 oz. | 390 |
| vanilla (*Tastykake* Creamie), 1.5 oz. | 184 |
| vanilla, cream-filled (*Tastykake Krimpets*), 1.1 oz. | 116 |

**Cake, snack,** frozen, 1 piece or serving:

| | |
|---|---|
| apple crisp (*Sara Lee* Lights), 3 oz. | 150 |
| Black Forest (*Sara Lee* Lights), 3.6 oz. | 170 |
| Boston cream pie (*Pepperidge Farm* Hyannis), 3.25 oz. | 230 |
| carrot (*Pepperidge Farm* Classic), 2.5 oz. | 260 |
| carrot (*Sara Lee* Deluxe), 1.8 oz. | 180 |
| carrot (*Sara Lee* Lights), 2.5 oz. | 170 |
| cheesecake, classic (*Sara Lee*), 2 oz. | 200 |
| cheesecake, French, plain or strawberry (*Sara Lee* Lights) | 150 |
| cheesecake, strawberry (*Pepperidge Farm* Manhattan), 4.25 oz. | 300 |
| chocolate: | |
| double (*Pepperidge Farm*), 2.25 oz. | 250 |
| double (*Sara Lee* Lights), 2.5 oz. | 150 |
| fudge (*Sara Lee*), 1.6 oz. | 190 |
| German (*Pepperidge Farm* Classic), 2.25 oz. | 250 |
| mousse (*Pepperidge Farm* Dessert Lights), 2.5 oz. | 190 |
| mousse (*Sara Lee*), 3. oz. | 180 |
| mousse (*Sara Lee* Lights), 3 oz. | 170 |
| coconut (*Pepperidge Farm* Classic), 2.25 oz. | 230 |
| coffee, apple cinnamon (Sara Lee Individually Wrapped) | 290 |
| coffee, butter streusel (*Sara Lee* Individually Wrapped) | 230 |
| coffee, pecan (*Sara Lee* Individually Wrapped) | 280 |
| donut, see "Donut" | |
| lemon cream (*Sara Lee* Lights), 3.25 oz. | 180 |
| lemon supreme (*Pepperidge Farm* Dessert Lights), 2.75 oz. | 170 |
| pound, all butter (*Sara Lee*), 1.6 oz. | 200 |
| strawberry shortcake (*Pepperidge Farm* Dessert Lights), 3 oz. | 170 |
| vanilla fudge swirl (*Pepperidge Farm* Classic), 2.25 oz. | 250 |

| FOOD AND MEASURE | CALORIES |
|---|---|
| **Cake mix**[1], 1/12 cake, except as noted: | |
| all varieties (*Estee*), 1/10 cake | 100 |
| angel food (*Betty Crocker* traditional), 1/12 mix, dry | 130 |
| angel food (*Duncan Hines*) | 140 |
| angel food, all varieties, except traditional (*Betty Crocker*), 1/12 mix, dry | 150 |
| apple cinnamon (*Betty Crocker SuperMoist*) | 250 |
| apple streusel (*Betty Crocker MicroRave*), 1/6 cake | 240 |
| banana (*Pillsbury Plus*) | 250 |
| Black Forest cherry (*Pillsbury Bundt*), 1/16 cake | 240 |
| Black Forest mousse (*Duncan Hines Tiarra*) | 260 |
| Boston cream (*Betty Crocker* Classic), 1/8 cake | 270 |
| Boston cream (*Pillsbury Bundt*), 1/16 cake | 270 |
| butter, chocolate (*Betty Crocker SuperMoist*) | 270 |
| butter, yellow (*Betty Crocker SuperMoist*) | 260 |
| butter brickle or pecan (*Betty Crocker SuperMoist*) | 250 |
| butter recipe (*Pillsbury Plus*) | 260 |
| butter recipe, golden (*Duncan Hines*) | 270 |
| carrot (*Betty Crocker SuperMoist*) | 250 |
| carrot (*Dromedary*) | 232 |
| carrot 'n spice (*Pillsbury Plus*) | 260 |
| cheesecake (*Jell-O/Jell-O* New York Style No Bake), 1/8 cake | 280 |
| cheesecake, lemon (*Jell-O* No Bake), 1/8 cake | 270 |
| cheesecake, lite (*Royal No-Bake*), 1/8 cake | 210 |
| cheesecake, real (*Royal No-Bake*), 1/8 cake | 280 |
| cherries and cream (*Duncan Hines Tiarra*) | 250 |
| cherry chip (*Betty Crocker SuperMoist*) | 190 |
| chocolate: | |
| (*Pillsbury Microwave*), 1/8 cake | 210 |
| dark or German (*Pillsbury Plus*) | 250 |
| double supreme (*Pillsbury* Microwave), 1/8 cake | 330 |
| fudge (*Betty Crocker SuperMoist*) | 260 |
| fudge (*Duncan Hines* Butter Recipe) | 270 |
| fudge (*Pillsbury Bundt Tunnel of Fudge*), 1/16 cake | 260 |
| fudge (*Pillsbury Bundt Tunnel of Fudge* Microwave), 1/8 cake | 290 |
| fudge, dark Dutch (*Duncan Hines*) | 280 |
| fudge, marble (*Duncan Hines*) | 260 |
| fudge, marble (*Pillsbury Plus*) | 270 |
| fudge, w/vanilla frosting (*Betty Crocker MicroRave*), 1/6 cake | 310 |

[1]Prepared according to basic package directions, except as noted.

| FOOD AND MEASURE | CALORIES |
|---|---|
| *Cake mix, chocolate, continued* | |
| German (*Betty Crocker SuperMoist*) | 260 |
| German, w/coconut pecan frosting (*Betty Crocker MicroRave*), ⅙ cake | 320 |
| milk (*Betty Crocker SuperMoist*) | 260 |
| mousse (*Duncan Hines Tiarra*) | 270 |
| pudding (*Betty Crocker* Classic), ⅙ cake | 230 |
| Swiss (*Duncan Hines*) | 280 |
| w/frosting (*Pillsbury* Microwave), ⅛ cake | 300 |
| chocolate chip (*Betty Crocker SuperMoist*) | 280 |
| chocolate chip (*Pillsbury Plus*) | 270 |
| chocolate chocolate chip (*Betty Crocker SuperMoist*) | 260 |
| chocolate macaroon (*Pillsbury Bundt*), 1/16 cake | 240 |
| cinnamon (*Streusel Swirl*), 1/16 cake | 260 |
| cinnamon (*Streusel Swirl* Microwave), ⅛ cake | 240 |
| cinnamon, pecan (*Betty Crocker MicroRave*), ⅙ cake | 290 |
| coffee (*Aunt Jemima* Easy), 1 serving | 156 |
| coffee, apple cinnamon (*Pillsbury*), ⅛ cake | 240 |
| devil's food: | |
| (*Betty Crocker SuperMoist*) | 260 |
| (*Duncan Hines*) | 280 |
| (*Pillsbury Plus*) | 270 |
| w/chocolate frosting (*Betty Crocker MicroRave*), ⅙ cake | 310 |
| gingerbread (*Dromedary*), 2″ × 2″ square or 3 tbsp. dry | 100 |
| lemon: | |
| (*Betty Crocker SuperMoist*) | 260 |
| (*Duncan Hines* Supreme) | 260 |
| (*Pillsbury Bundt Tunnel of Lemon*), 1/16 cake | 270 |
| (*Pillsbury* Microwave), ⅛ cake | 220 |
| (*Pillsbury Plus*) | 250 |
| (*Streusel Swirl*), 1/16 cake | 270 |
| chiffon (*Betty Crocker* Classic) | 200 |
| double supreme (*Pillsbury* Microwave), ⅛ cake | 300 |
| w/lemon frosting (*Betty Crocker MicroRave*), ⅙ cake | 300 |
| w/lemon frosting (*Pillsbury* Microwave), ⅛ cake | 300 |
| pudding (*Betty Crocker* Classic), ⅙ cake | 230 |
| marble (*Betty Crocker SuperMoist*) | 250 |
| pineapple (*Duncan Hines* Supreme) | 260 |
| pineapple cream (*Pillsbury Bundt*), 1/16 cake | 260 |
| pineapple upside-down (*Betty Crocker* Classic), 1/9 cake | 250 |
| pound (*Dromedary*), ½″ slice | 150 |

| FOOD AND MEASURE | CALORIES |
|---|---|
| pound (*Martha White*), 1/10 cake | 120 |
| pound, golden (*Betty Crocker* Classic) | 200 |
| rainbow chip (*Betty Crocker SuperMoist*) | 250 |
| sour cream, chocolate (*Betty Crocker SuperMoist*) | 260 |
| sour cream, white (*Betty Crocker SuperMoist*) | 180 |
| spice (*Betty Crocker SuperMoist*) | 260 |
| spice (*Duncan Hines*) | 260 |
| strawberry (*Duncan Hines* Supreme) | 260 |
| strawberry (*Pillsbury Plus*) | 260 |
| vanilla, French (*Duncan Hines*) | 260 |
| vanilla, golden (*Betty Crocker SuperMoist*) | 280 |
| vanilla, golden, w/rainbow chip frosting (*Betty Crocker MicroRave*), 1/6 cake | 320 |
| white (*Betty Crocker SuperMoist*) | 240 |
| white (*Duncan Hines*) | 250 |
| white (*Pillsbury Plus*) | 240 |
| yellow: | |
| (*Betty Crocker SuperMoist*) | 260 |
| (*Duncan Hines*) | 260 |
| (*Pillsbury* Microwave), 1/8 cake | 220 |
| (*Pillsbury Plus*) | 260 |
| w/chocolate frosting (*Betty Crocker MicroRave*), 1/6 cake | 300 |
| w/chocolate frosting (*Pillsbury* Microwave), 1/8 cake | 300 |

**Calves liver,** see "Liver"

**Candy:**

| FOOD AND MEASURE | CALORIES |
|---|---|
| almond, candy-coated (*Brach's* Jordan Almonds), 1 oz. | 120 |
| (*Baby Ruth*), 1 oz. | 130 |
| bridge mix (*Brach's*), 1 oz. | 130 |
| (*Butterfinger*), 1 oz. | 130 |
| butterscotch (*Brach's* Disks), 1 oz. | 110 |
| butterscotch (*Callard & Bowser*), 1 oz. | 115 |
| butterscotch (*Featherweight*), 1 piece | 25 |
| candy corn (*Heide*), 1 piece | 9 |
| candy corn, Indian or three color (*Brach's*), 1 oz. | 100 |
| caramel: | |
| (*Brach's* Milk Maid), 1 oz. | 110 |
| (*Featherweight*), 1 piece | 30 |
| (*Kraft*), 1 piece | 30 |
| (*Sugar Babies* Regular/Tidbits), 1 5/8-oz. pkg. | 180 |

| FOOD AND MEASURE | CALORIES |
|---|---|
| *Candy, caramel, continued* | |
| (*Sugar Daddy*), 1⅜-oz. pop | 150 |
| chocolate (*Brach's* Milk Maid), 1 oz. | 110 |
| chocolate, vanilla (*Estee*), 1 piece | 20 |
| chocolate-coated (*Pom Poms*), 1 oz. | 100 |
| chocolate-coated, w/cookies (*Twix*), 2-oz. piece | 140 |
| milk chocolate-coated (*Rolo*), 1.93 oz. or 8 pieces | 270 |
| cherry (*Heide* Jersey Cherries), 1 piece | 13 |
| cherry, chocolate-coated (*Brach's*), 1 oz. | 110 |
| chocolate: | |
| (*Brach's* Jots), 1 oz. | 130 |
| almond (*Estee*), 2 squares | 60 |
| almond (*Featherweight*), 1 section | 90 |
| w/almonds (*Hershey's Golden Almond/Solitaires*), 1.6 oz. | 260 |
| w/almonds, roasted (*Cadbury*), 1 oz. | 150 |
| assorted, wrapped (*Brach's*), 1 oz. | 110 |
| babies (*Heide*), 1 piece | 12 |
| candy-coated (*M&M's*), 1.69 oz. | 250 |
| candy-coated, w/peanuts (*M&M's*), 1.74 oz. | 250 |
| w/caramel (*Caramello*), 1.6 oz. | 220 |
| cream (*Callard & Bowser*), 1 oz. | 120 |
| crunch (*Estee*), 2 squares | 45 |
| crunch (*Featherweight*), 1 section | 80 |
| dark, deluxe (*Estee*), 2 squares | 60 |
| dark, sweet (*Hershey's Special Dark*), 1.45 oz. | 220 |
| w/fruit and nuts or krisps and honey (*Cadbury*), 1 oz. | 150 |
| fruit & nut (*Estee*), 2 squares | 60 |
| milk (*Brach's* Stars), 1 oz. | 150 |
| milk (*Cadbury Dairy Milk*), 1 oz. | 150 |
| milk (*Estee*), 2 squares | 60 |
| milk (*Featherweight*), 1 section | 80 |
| milk (*Hershey's*), 1.55 oz. | 240 |
| milk (*Hershey's Kisses*), 1.46 oz. or 9 pieces | 220 |
| milk (*Nabisco* Stars), 1 oz. | 160 |
| milk (*Nestlé*), 1.45 oz. | 220 |
| milk, w/almonds (*Hershey's*), 1.45 oz. | 230 |
| milk, w/almonds (*Nestlé*), 1.45 oz. | 230 |
| milk, creamy (*Hershey's Symphony*), 1.75 oz., 5 sections. | 270 |
| milk, creamy, w/almonds and toffee chips (*Hershey's Symphony*), 1.75 oz. | 280 |
| milk, w/crisps (*Krackel*), 1.55 oz. | 230 |

| FOOD AND MEASURE | CALORIES |
|---|---|
| milk, w/crisps (*Nestlé Crunch*), 1.4 oz. | 210 |
| milk, w/crisps and peanuts (*Nestlé 100 Grand*), 1.5 oz. | 200 |
| milk, w/fruit and nuts (*Chunky*), 1.4 oz. | 210 |
| milk, w/peanuts (*Brach's* Peanut Clusters), 1 oz. | 150 |
| milk, w/peanuts (*Mr. Goodbar*), 1.75 oz. | 290 |
| mint or peanut (*Estee*), 2 squares | 60 |
| white, w/almonds (*Nestlé Alpine*), 1.25 oz. | 210 |
| chocolate chips, see "Chocolate, baking" | |
| cinnamon disks, hearts, or Imperial (*Brach's*), 1 oz. | 110 |
| coconut, chocolate-coated (*Bounty*), 1.05 oz. | 150 |
| coconut, chocolate-coated (*Mounds*), 1.9 oz. | 260 |
| coconut, chocolate-coated (*Sunbelt Macaroo*), 2 oz. | 288 |
| coconut, chocolate-coated, w/almonds (*Almond Joy*), 1.76 oz. | 250 |
| coconut, Neapolitan (*Brach's*), 1 oz. | 120 |
| eggs, creme (*Cadbury*), 1.37 oz. | 190 |
| eggs, creme, mini (*Cadbury*), 1 oz. | 140 |
| eggs, malted milk, chocolate (*Brach's*), 1 oz. | 130 |
| eggs, pastel (*Brach's* Fiesta), 1 oz. | 120 |
| (*Estee-ets*), 5 pieces | 35 |
| filled, assorted (*Brach's*), 1 oz. | 110 |
| fruit-flavored, all flavors: | |
| (*Brach's* Fruit Bunch), 1 oz. | 90 |
| (*Skittles*), 2.3 oz. | 265 |
| chews (*Bonkers!*), 1 piece | 20 |
| chews (*Rascals*), 1 piece | 4 |
| chews (*Starburst*), 2.07 oz. | 240 |
| drops (*Featherweight*), ⅓ oz. | 30 |
| fudge (*Kraft* Fudgies), 1 piece | 35 |
| fudge, all varieties (*Woodys*), 1 oz. | 120 |
| gum, 1 piece, except as noted: | |
| (*Beech-Nut*) | 10 |
| (*Big Red*) | 10 |
| (*Care*Free*) | 8 |
| (*Chewels*) | 8 |
| (*Clorets* Stick) | 9 |
| (*Dentyne*) | 6 |
| (*Dentyne* Sugarless) | 5 |
| (*Doublemint/Wrigley's Spearmint*) | 10 |
| (*Extra*) | 8 |
| (*Freedent*) | 10 |
| (*Freshen-Up*) | 13 |

| FOOD AND MEASURE | CALORIES |
|---|---|
| *Candy, gum, continued* | |
| (*Juicy Fruit*) | 10 |
| bubble (*Bubble Yum*) | 25 |
| bubble (*Bubble Yum* Sugarless) | 20 |
| bubble (*Bubblicious*) | 25 |
| bubble (*Bubblicious* Sugarless) | 5 |
| bubble (*Care*Free*) | 10 |
| bubble (*Extra*) | 7 |
| bubble (*Hubba Bubba*) | 23 |
| bubble (*Hubba Bubba* Original Sugar Free) | 14 |
| bubble, grape (*Hubba Bubba* Sugar Free) | 13 |
| candy-coated (*Beechies*) | 6 |
| candy-coated (*Chiclets*) | 6 |
| candy-coated (*Chiclets* Tiny), 1 pkg. | 8 |
| candy-coated (*Clorets*) | 6 |
| gum drops, see "jellied and gummed," below | |
| halvah (*Fantastic Foods*), 1.5-oz. bar | 232 |
| hard (*Estee*), 2 pieces | 25 |
| hard, all flavors (*Life Savers*), 1 piece | 8 |
| hard, fruit-flavored drops (*Heide*), 1 piece | 11 |
| hard, sour balls (*Brach's*), 1 oz. | 110 |
| (*Heath Bits'O Brickle*), 3 oz. | 448 |
| (*Heath* Soft'n Crunchy Bar), 2 pieces | 190 |
| (*Heide* Red Hot Dollars), 1 piece | 9 |
| honey (*Bit-O-Honey*), 1.7 oz. | 200 |
| (*Hot Tamales*), 1 piece | 9 |
| jellied and gummed (see also specific listings): | |
| (*Brach's* Gummi Bears/Jujube/Rainbow Bears/Worms), 1 oz. | 100 |
| (*Heide* Fish), 1 piece | 21 |
| (*Heide* Jujubes), 1 piece | 3 |
| (*Heide* Mexican Hats), 1 piece | 10 |
| beans (*Brach's*), 1 oz. | 100 |
| beans, large (*Heide*), 1 piece | 9 |
| cinnamon (*Brach's* Cinnamon Bears), 1 oz. | 80 |
| eggs (*Brach's/Brach's* Tiny), 1 oz. | 100 |
| eggs (*Just Born* Petite), 1 piece | 4 |
| eggs (*Rodda*), 1 piece | 7 |
| eggs, speckled (*Brach's*), 1 oz. | 110 |
| fruit-flavored (*Jujyfruits*), 1 oz. or 11 pieces | 100 |
| gum drops (*Estee*), 4 pieces | 25 |
| gummi bears (*Estee*), 4 pieces | 20 |

| FOOD AND MEASURE | CALORIES |
|---|---|
| gummi bears (*Heide*), 1 piece | 3 |
| hearts, red (*Brach's*), 1 oz. | 100 |
| juicy (*Callard & Bowser*), 1 oz. | 90 |
| spearmint leaves (*Brach's*), 1 oz. | 100 |
| (*Jolly Joes*), 1 piece | 9 |
| lemon drops (*Brach's*), 1 oz. | 110 |
| licorice: | |
| (*Brach's* Red Laces/Twists/Twin Twists), 1 oz. | 100 |
| (*Pearson's Licorice Nip*), 1 oz. | 120 |
| candy-coated (*Good & Fruity/Good & Plenty*), 1 oz. | 106 |
| cherry (*Y&S Bites/Nibs*), 1 oz. | 100 |
| drops (*Diamond*), 1 piece | 14 |
| strawberry (*Y&S Twizzlers*), 1 oz. | 100 |
| lollipop: | |
| all flavors (*Brach's Pops*), 1 oz. | 110 |
| all flavors (*Estee*), 1 piece | 25 |
| all flavors (*Life Savers*), 1 piece | 45 |
| all flavors, except chocolate (*Tootsie Pop*), 1 oz. | 111 |
| chocolate (*Tootsie Pop*), 1 oz. | 110 |
| malted milk balls, chocolate-coated (*Brach's*), 1 oz. | 130 |
| (*Mars*), 1.76-oz. bar | 240 |
| marshmallow (see also specific listings): | |
| (*Brach's* Perkys Circus Peanuts), 1 oz. | 100 |
| (*Campfire*), 2 large or 24 mini pieces | 40 |
| (*Funmallows*), 1 piece | 30 |
| (*Kraft* Jet-Puffed), 1 piece | 25 |
| coconut, toasted (*Just Born*), 1 piece | 30 |
| miniature (*Funmallows/Kraft*), 10 pieces | 18 |
| (*Mike & Ikes*), 1 piece | 9 |
| (*Milky Way*), 2.15-oz. bar | 280 |
| (*Milky Way* Dark), 1.76-oz. bar | 220 |
| mint (see also specific listings): | |
| (*Brach's* Coolers/Kentucky Mint/Starlight), 1 oz. | 110 |
| (*Brach's* Creme de Menthe), 1 oz. | 150 |
| (*Brach's* Jots/Pearls), 1 oz. | 120 |
| (*Certs* Sugar Free), 1 piece | 6 |
| (*Featherweight* Cool Blue), 1 piece | 25 |
| (*Mint Meltaway*), .33-oz. piece | 50 |
| all flavors (*Breath Savers*), 1 piece | 8 |
| assorted (*Brach's* Dessert Mints), 1 oz. | 110 |
| butter or party (*Kraft*), 1 piece | 8 |

| FOOD AND MEASURE | CALORIES |
|---|---|
| *Candy, mint, continued* | |
| clear (*Clorets*), 1 piece | 8 |
| mini (*Certs* Sugar Free), 1 piece | 1 |
| parfait (*Brach's*), 1 oz. | 150 |
| pressed (*Clorets*), 1 piece | 6 |
| chocolate-coated (*Junior Mints*), 1 oz. or 12 pieces | 120 |
| chocolate-coated (*York Peppermint Pattie*), 1.5 oz. | 180 |
| dark chocolate-coated (*After Eight*), 1 piece | 35 |
| (*Munch*), 1.42-oz. bar | 220 |
| (*Necco Sky Bar*), 1.5-oz. bar | 196 |
| nonpareils (*Nestlé Sno-Caps*), 1 oz. | 140 |
| nonpareils, dark chocolate (*Brach's*), 1 oz. | 140 |
| nougat, chocolate-coated (*Charleston Chew!*), 1 oz. | 120 |
| nougat, jelly (*Brach's*), 1 oz. | 100 |
| nougat, kisses (*Brach's*), 1 oz. | 110 |
| nut (*Brach's* Nut Goodies), 1 oz. | 130 |
| (*Oh Henry!*), 2 oz. | 280 |
| orange (*Brach's* Orangettes), 1 oz. | 100 |
| orange sticks, chocolate-coated (*Brach's*), 1 oz. | 110 |
| peanut: | |
| (*Brach's* Jots), 1 oz. | 140 |
| butter toffee (*Flavor House*), 1 oz. | 150 |
| chocolate-coated (*Brach's*), 1 oz. | 150 |
| chocolate-coated (*Brach's* Small), 1 oz. | 140 |
| chocolate-coated (*Goobers*), 1⅜ oz. | 220 |
| chocolate-coated (*Nabisco*), 1 oz. | 160 |
| filled (*Brach's*), 1 oz. | 110 |
| French burnt (*Brach's*), 1 oz. | 130 |
| peanut brittle (*Estee*), ¼ oz. | 35 |
| peanut brittle (*Kraft*), 1 oz. | 130 |
| peanut butter: | |
| (*PB Max*), 1.48 oz. | 240 |
| candy-coated (*Reese's Pieces*), 1.85 oz. | 260 |
| chocolate-coated, w/cookies (*Twix*), 1.77-oz. bar | 130 |
| cup (*Estee*), 1 piece | 40 |
| cup, chocolate-coated (*Reese's*), 1.8 oz. | 280 |
| kisses (*Brach's*), 1 oz. | 110 |
| peanut caramel cluster (*Brach's*), 1 oz. | 150 |
| peanut parfait (*Brach's*), 1 oz. | 160 |
| peppermint kisses (*Brach's*), 1 oz. | 100 |
| peppermint swirls (*Featherweight*), 1 piece | 20 |

| FOOD AND MEASURE | CALORIES |
|---|---|
| popcorn, caramel-coated (*Estee*), 1-oz. bag | 140 |
| popcorn, caramel-coated (*Orville Redenbacher*), 2½ cups | 240 |
| popcorn, caramel-coated, w/peanuts (*Cracker Jack*), 1 oz. | 120 |
| raisins, chocolate-coated (*Brach's*), 1 oz. | 130 |
| raisins, chocolate-coated (*Estee*), 10 pieces | 30 |
| raisins, chocolate-coated (*Nabisco*), 1 oz. | 130 |
| raisins, chocolate-coated (*Raisinets*), 1⅜ oz. | 180 |
| ribbon, crimp (*Brach's*), 1 oz. | 110 |
| rock candy (*Brach's* Cut Rock), 1 oz. | 110 |
| (*Snickers*), 2.07-oz. bar | 280 |
| spice (*Brach's* Spicettes), 1 oz. | 100 |
| straws, mint-filled (*Brach's*), 1 oz. | 110 |
| taffy, all flavors (*Brach's* Salt Water Taffy), 1 oz. | 100 |
| (*3 Musketeers*), 2.13-oz. bar | 260 |
| toffee: | |
| (*Brach's*), 1 oz. | 110 |
| (*Callard & Bowser*), 1 oz. | 135 |
| (*Skor*), 1.4 oz. | 220 |
| English (*Bits 'O Heath*), 3.5 oz. | 520 |
| English (*Heath* Bar), 2 pieces | 180 |
| (*Tootsie Roll*), 1 oz. | 112 |
| wafer, assorted (*Necco*), 2.02-oz. roll | 225 |
| wafer bar, chocolate-coated (*Kit Kat*), 1.63 oz. | 250 |

**Cane syrup:**

| | |
|---|---|
| 1 tbsp. | 52 |

**Cannellini beans,** see "Beans, kidney, white"

**Cannelloni entree,** frozen:

| | |
|---|---|
| beef and pork, w/Mornay sauce (*Lean Cuisine*), 9⅝ oz. | 260 |
| cheese (*Dining Lite*), 9 oz. | 310 |
| cheese, w/tomato sauce (*Lean Cuisine*), 9⅛ oz. | 260 |
| Florentine (*Celentano*), 12 oz. | 350 |

**Canola oil,** see "Oil"

**Cantaloupe,** fresh:

| | |
|---|---|
| ½ of 5"-diam. melon | 94 |
| cubed, ½ cup | 29 |

**Capers:**

| | |
|---|---|
| (*Crosse & Blackwell*), 1 tbsp. | 6 |

| FOOD AND MEASURE | CALORIES |
|---|---|
| **Capocollo:** | |
| (*Hormel*), 1 oz. | 80 |
| **Carambola:** | |
| 1 medium, 4.7 oz. | 42 |
| cubed, ½ cup | 23 |
| **Caramel danish:** | |
| w/nuts, refrigerated (*Pillsbury*) | 160 |
| **Caraway seed:** | |
| 1 tsp. | 7 |
| **Cardamom:** | |
| ground, 1 tsp. | 6 |
| seed (*Spice Islands*), 1 tsp. | 6 |
| **Cardoon:** | |
| raw, shredded, ½ cup | 18 |
| boiled, drained, 4 oz. | 25 |
| **Carissa** (natal plum): | |
| 1 medium, .8 oz. | 12 |
| sliced, ½ cup | 46 |
| ***Carl's Jr.,*** 1 serving: | |
| breakfast: | |
| bacon, 2 strips, .4 oz. | 50 |
| eggs, scrambled, 2.4 oz. | 120 |
| English muffin, w/margarine, 2 oz. | 180 |
| French toast dips, w/out syrup, 4.7 oz. | 480 |
| hash brown nuggets, 3 oz. | 170 |
| hot cakes, w/margarine, w/out syrup, 5.5 oz. | 360 |
| sausage, 1 patty, .5 oz. | 190 |
| *Sunrise Sandwich*, w/bacon, 4.5 oz. | 370 |
| *Sunrise Sandwich*, w/sausage, 6.1 oz. | 500 |
| sandwiches: | |
| *California Roast Beef 'n Swiss*, 7.4 oz. | 360 |
| *Charbroiler BBQ Chicken Sandwich*, 6.3 oz. | 320 |
| *Charbroiler Chicken Club Sandwich*, 8.3 oz. | 510 |
| *Country Fried Steak* Sandwich, 7.2 oz. | 610 |
| *Double Western Bacon Cheeseburger*, 7.5 oz. | 890 |

| FOOD AND MEASURE | CALORIES |
| --- | --- |
| *Famous Star Hamburger*, 8.1 oz. | 590 |
| fish fillet, 7.9 oz. | 550 |
| *Happy Star* hamburger, 3 oz. | 220 |
| *Old Time Star* hamburger, 5.9 oz. | 400 |
| *Super Star* hamburger, 10.6 oz. | 770 |
| *Western Bacon Cheeseburger*, 7.5 oz. | 630 |
| potatoes: | |
| bacon and cheese, 14.1 oz. | 650 |
| broccoli and cheese, 14 oz. | 470 |
| cheese, 14.2 oz. | 350 |
| *Fiesta*, 15.2 oz. | 550 |
| Lite, 9.8 oz. | 250 |
| sour cream and chive, 10.4 oz. | 350 |
| salad-to-go: | |
| chef, 10.7 oz. | 180 |
| chicken, 10.9 oz. | 206 |
| garden, 4.1 oz. | 46 |
| taco, 14.3 oz. | 356 |
| salad dressing, 1 oz.: | |
| blue cheese | 151 |
| French, reduced calorie | 38 |
| house | 110 |
| Italian | 120 |
| Thousand Island | 110 |
| side dishes: | |
| french fries, regular, 6 oz. | 360 |
| onion rings, 3.2 oz. | 310 |
| zucchini, 4.3 oz. | 300 |
| soups: | |
| Boston clam chowder, 6.6 oz. | 140 |
| broccoli, cream of, 6.6 oz. | 140 |
| chicken noodle, old fashioned, 6.6 oz. | 80 |
| *Lumber Jack Mix* vegetable, 6.6 oz. | 70 |
| bakery products: | |
| blueberry muffin, 3.5 oz. | 256 |
| bran muffin, 4 oz. | 220 |
| brownie, fudge, 4.5 oz. | 597 |
| chocolate chip cookie, 2.5 oz. | 327 |
| cinnamon roll, 4 oz. | 459 |
| danish (varieties), 4 oz. | 519 |
| shakes, regular, 11.6 oz. | 353 |

| FOOD AND MEASURE | CALORIES |
|---|---|

**Carob flavor drink mix:**

powder, 3 tsp. .......... 45
beverage, 1 cup whole milk and 3 tsp. powder .......... 195

**Carp,** meat only:

raw, 4 oz. .......... 145
baked, broiled, or microwaved, 4 oz. .......... 184

**Carrot:**

fresh, raw, 1 medium, 7½" long × 1⅛" diam. .......... 31
fresh, raw, shredded, ½ cup .......... 24
fresh, boiled, drained, sliced, ½ cup .......... 35
canned, ½ cup, except as noted:
  (*Stokely* Regular/No Salt or Sugar Added) .......... 35
  all cuts (*Allens*) .......... 30
  all cuts (*Del Monte*) .......... 30
  all cuts (*S&W* Fancy/*S&W Nutradiet*) .......... 30
  sliced (*Featherweight*) .......... 30
frozen:
  (*Birds Eye* Deluxe Parisienne), 2.6 oz. .......... 30
  (*Seabrook*), 3.3 oz. .......... 40
  baby (*Green Giant Harvest Fresh*), ½ cup .......... 18
  whole (*Southern*), 3.5 oz. .......... 42
  whole, baby (*Birds Eye* Deluxe), 3.3 oz. .......... 40
  whole, baby (*Stokely Singles*), 3 oz. .......... 35
  sliced (*Birds Eye*), 3.2 oz. .......... 35
  baby, w/sweet peas and onions (*Birds Eye* Deluxe), 3.3 oz. .......... 50

**Carrot chips:**

(*Hain* Regular/No Salt Added), 1 oz. .......... 150
barbecue (*Hain*), 1 oz. .......... 140

**Carrot juice:**

(*Hain*), 6 fl. oz. .......... 80

**Casaba:**

1/10 of 7¾" melon, 2" slice .......... 43
cubed, ½ cup .......... 23

**Cashew:**

dry-roasted (*Planters* Regular/Unsalted), 1 oz. .......... 160
dry-roasted, whole (*Guys*), 1 oz. .......... 170

| FOOD AND MEASURE | CALORIES |
|---|---|
| honey-roasted, plain or w/peanuts (*Planters*), 1 oz. | 170 |
| oil-roasted (*Flavor House*), 1 oz. | 180 |
| oil-roasted (*Planters*/*Planters* Fancy), 1 oz. | 170 |
| **Cashew butter:** | |
| (*Westbrae Natural*), 2 tbsp. | 190 |
| raw (*Hain*), 2 tbsp. | 190 |
| raw (*Hain* Unsalted), 2 tbsp. | 210 |
| toasted (*Hain*), 2 tbsp. | 210 |
| **Cassava:** | |
| raw, trimmed, 4 oz. | 136 |
| **Catfish,** channel, meat only: | |
| raw, 4 oz. | 132 |
| breaded w/cornmeal, egg, and milk, fried, 4 oz. | 260 |
| **Catjang:** | |
| raw, ½ cup | 288 |
| boiled, ½ cup | 100 |
| **Catsup:** | |
| (*Del Monte* Regular/No Salt Added), ¼ cup | 60 |
| (*Estee*), 1 tbsp. | 6 |
| (*Featherweight*), 1 tbsp. | 6 |
| (*Hain* Natural Regular/No Salt Added), 1 tbsp. | 16 |
| (*Heinz*), 1 tbsp. | 16 |
| (*Heinz* Lite), 1 tbsp. | 8 |
| (*Hunt's*), 1 tbsp. | 15 |
| (*Hunt's* No Salt Added), 1 tbsp. | 20 |
| (*Smucker's*), 1 tsp. | 8 |
| (*Stokely*), 1 tbsp. | 20 |
| (*Weight Watchers*), 2 tsp. | 8 |
| hot (*Heinz*), 1 tbsp. | 16 |
| w/onions (*Heinz*), 1 tbsp. | 19 |
| **Cauliflower:** | |
| fresh, raw, 3 flowerets, approx. 5 oz. | 13 |
| fresh, raw, 1″ pieces, ½ cup | 12 |
| fresh, boiled, drained, 1″ pieces, ½ cup | 15 |
| frozen: | |
| (*Birds Eye*), 3.3 oz. | 25 |

| FOOD AND MEASURE | CALORIES |
|---|---|

*Cauliflower, frozen, continued*

(*Seabrook*), 3.3 oz. .......... 25
(*Southern*), 3.5 oz. .......... 26
(*Stokely Singles*), 3 oz. .......... 20
cuts (*Green Giant*), ½ cup .......... 12
in cheddar cheese sauce (*The Budget Gourmet*), 5 oz. .......... 110
in cheese sauce (*Birds Eye* Combinations), 5 oz. .......... 130
in cheese sauce (*Green Giant*), 5.5 oz. .......... 80
in cheese sauce (*Stokely Singles*), 4 oz. .......... 70
in cheese flavor sauce (*Green Giant*), ½ cup .......... 60

**Cauliflower, combinations,** frozen:

broccoli and carrots, in cheese sauce (*Freezer Queen* Family Side Dishes), 5 oz. .......... 60
carrots, baby whole, and snow pea pods (*Birds Eye* Farm Fresh), 4 oz. .......... 40
zucchini, carrots, and red peppers (*Birds Eye* Farm Fresh), 4 oz. .......... 30

**Cavatelli,** frozen:

(*Celentano*), 3.2 oz. .......... 250

**Caviar,** granular:

black and red, 1 oz. .......... 71
black and red, 1 tbsp. .......... 40

**Celeriac:**

raw, untrimmed, 1 lb. .......... 154
raw, trimmed, ½ cup .......... 31
boiled, drained, 4 oz. .......... 28

**Celery:**

raw, 1 stalk, 7½″ long × 1¼″ diam. .......... 6
raw, diced, ½ cup .......... 10
boiled, drained, diced, ½ cup .......... 13

**Celery, dried,** seasoning:

flakes (*Tone's*), 1 tsp. .......... 9
salt (*Tone's*), 1 tsp. .......... 6
seed, 1 tsp. .......... 8

**Cellophane noodles,** see "Noodle, Chinese"

| FOOD AND MEASURE | CALORIES |
|---|---|

**Celtus:**

raw, trimmed, 1 oz. . . . . . 6

**Cereal, cooking,** uncooked (see also specific grains):

bran (*H-O Brand* Super Bran), ⅓ cup dry . . . . . . 110
farina, see "wheat," below
multigrain, four grain (*Arrowhead Mills*), 1 oz. . . . . . 94
multigrain, seven grain (*Arrowhead Mills*), 1 oz. . . . . . 100
multigrain, w/apple cinnamon (*Roman Meal*), ⅓ cup dry . . . . . . 112
oat bran:
(*Arrowhead Mills*), 1 oz. . . . . . 110
(*Quaker/Mother's*), ⅓ cup dry or ⅔ cup cooked . . . . . . 92
(*3-Minute Brand* Regular or Instant), 1 oz. . . . . . 90
(*Wholesome 'N Hearty*), 1 oz. . . . . . 100
apple cinnamon (*Wholesome 'N Hearty* Instant), 1 pkt. . . . . . 130
honey (*Wholesome 'N Hearty* Instant), 1 pkt. . . . . . 110
raisins and spice (*Health Valley* Natural), 1 oz. . . . . . 110
oatmeal and oats:
(*Arrowhead Mills* Instant), 1 oz. . . . . . 100
(*H-O Brand* Gourmet), ⅓ cup dry . . . . . . 100
(*H-O Brand* Instant), 1 pkt. . . . . . 110
(*H-O Brand* Quick/Instant, box), ½ cup dry . . . . . . 130
(*Instant Quaker*), 1 pkt. . . . . . 94
(*Maypo* 30 Second), 1 oz. . . . . . 100
(*Quaker* Quick/Old Fashioned), ⅓ cup dry . . . . . . 99
(*Quaker Extra*), 1 pkt. . . . . . 95
(*3-Minute Brand* Quick or Old Fashioned), 1 oz. . . . . . 100
(*Total* Instant), 1.2 oz. . . . . . 110
(*Total* Quick), 1 oz. . . . . . 90
apple and cinnamon (*H-O Brand* Instant), 1 pkt. . . . . . 130
apple and cinnamon (*Instant Quaker*), 1 pkt. . . . . . 118
apple and cinnamon (*Oatmeal Swirlers*), 1 pkt. . . . . . 160
apple and cinnamon (*Total* Instant), 1.5 oz. . . . . . 150
apple, date, and almond (*Arrowhead Mills* Instant), 1 oz. . . . . . 130
apples and spice (*Quaker Extra*), 1 pkt. . . . . . 133
cherry (*Oatmeal Swirlers*), 1 pkt. . . . . . 150
chocolate, milk (*Oatmeal Swirlers*), 1 pkt. . . . . . 170
cinnamon raisin (*Total* Instant), 1.8 oz. . . . . . 170
cinnamon and spice (*Instant Quaker*), 1 pkt. . . . . . 164
cinnamon spice (*Oatmeal Swirlers*), 1 pkt. . . . . . 160

| FOOD AND MEASURE | CALORIES |
|---|---|
| *Cereal, cooking, oatmeal and oats, continued* | |
| w/fiber (*H-O Brand* Instant), 1 pkt. | 110 |
| w/fiber (*H-O Brand* Instant, Box), ⅓ cup dry | 100 |
| w/fiber, apple, and bran (*H-O Brand* Instant), 1 pkt. | 130 |
| w/fiber, raisin, and bran (*H-O Brand* Instant), 1 pkt. | 150 |
| maple flavored (*Maypo* Vermont Style), 1 oz. | 105 |
| maple brown sugar (*H-O Brand* Instant), 1 pkt. | 160 |
| maple brown sugar (*Instant Quaker*), 1 pkt. | 152 |
| maple brown sugar (*Oatmeal Swirlers*), 1 pkt. | 160 |
| maple brown sugar (*Total* Instant), 1.6 oz. | 160 |
| w/oat bran (*3-Minute Brand* Quick), 1 oz. | 100 |
| peaches and cream (*Instant Quaker*), 1 pkt. | 129 |
| raisin (*3-Minute Brand*), 1 oz. | 100 |
| raisin and cinnamon (*Quaker Extra*), 1 pkt. | 129 |
| raisin, date, and walnut (*Instant Quaker*), 1 pkt. | 141 |
| raisin, w/oat bran (*3-Minute Brand*), 1 oz. | 100 |
| raisin and spice (*H-O Brand* Instant), 1 pkt. | 150 |
| raisin and spice (*Instant Quaker*), 1 pkt. | 149 |
| strawberry (*Oatmeal Swirlers*), 1 pkt. | 150 |
| strawberries and cream (*Instant Quaker*), 1 pkt. | 129 |
| sweet 'n mellow (*H-O Brand* Instant), 1 pkt. | 150 |
| w/wheat, dates, raisins, almonds (*Roman Meal*), 1.3 oz. | 140 |
| w/wheat, honey, coconut, almonds (*Roman Meal*), 1.3 oz. | 150 |
| w/wheat, rye, bran, and flax (*Roman Meal*), 1.2 oz. | 116 |
| rye, cream of (*Roman Meal*), 1.3 oz. | 110 |
| wheat: | |
| (*Arrowhead Mills* Bear Mush), 1 oz. | 100 |
| (*Cream of Wheat* Instant/Quick), 1 oz. | 100 |
| (*Mix'n Eat Cream of Wheat* Instant, Original), 1 pkt. | 100 |
| (*Wheat Hearts*), 1 oz. or ¾ cup cooked | 110 |
| (*Wheatena*), 1 oz. | 100 |
| apple or brown sugar cinnamon (*Mix'n Eat Cream of Wheat* Instant), 1 pkt. | 130 |
| cracked (*Arrowhead Mills*), 2 oz. | 180 |
| farina (*H-O Brand* Instant), 1 pkt. | 110 |
| farina, cream (*H-O Brand*), 3 tbsp. | 120 |
| w/rye, bran, and flax (*Roman Meal*), 1 oz. | 80 |
| whole (*Quaker/Mother's* Hot Natural), ⅓ cup dry | 92 |
| wheat and barley (*Maltex*), 1 oz. | 105 |

| FOOD AND MEASURE | CALORIES |
|---|---|
| **Cereal, ready-to-eat,** 1 oz., except as noted: | |
| amaranth, flakes or w/banana (*Health Valley*) | 100 |
| amaranth, w/raisins (*Health Valley Amaranth Crunch*) | 110 |
| bran (see also "oat bran," below): | |
| (*All Bran*) | 70 |
| (*Arrowhead Mills* Bran Flakes) | 100 |
| (*Bran Buds*) | 70 |
| (*Bran Chex*) | 90 |
| (*Kellogg's 40%+ Bran Flakes/Kellogg's Heartwise*) | 90 |
| (*Nabisco 100% Bran*) | 70 |
| (*Post* Natural Bran Flakes) | 90 |
| (*Quaker Crunchy Bran*) | 89 |
| apple spice or cinnamon (*Ralston Bran News*) | 100 |
| extra fiber (*All Bran*) | 50 |
| w/fruit (*Fruitful Bran*), 1.3 oz. | 110 |
| w/fruit and nuts (*Mueslix*), 1.4 oz. | 140 |
| w/raisins (*Health Valley* Flakes) | 100 |
| w/raisins (*Health Valley* 100% Natural) | 70 |
| w/raisins (*Kellogg's* Raisin Bran), 1.4 oz. | 120 |
| w/raisins (*Post* Natural Raisin Bran), 1.4 oz. | 120 |
| w/raisins (*Total Raisin Bran*), 1.5 oz. | 140 |
| w/raisins and nuts (*Raisin Nut Bran*) | 110 |
| corn: | |
| (*Arrowhead Mills* Corn Flakes) | 110 |
| (*Arrowhead Mills* Puffed Corn), .5 oz. | 50 |
| (*Corn Chex*) | 110 |
| (*Corn Pops*) | 110 |
| (*Country* Corn Flakes) | 110 |
| (*Featherweight* Corn Flakes), 1¼ cup | 110 |
| (*Honeycomb*) | 110 |
| (*Kellogg's* Corn Flakes) | 100 |
| (*Kellogg's Frosted Flakes*) | 110 |
| (*Nutri•Grain*) | 100 |
| (*Post Toasties*) | 110 |
| (*Total Corn Flakes*) | 110 |
| chocolate flavor (*Cocoa Puffs*) | 110 |
| w/fruit (*Health Valley Fruit Lites*), .5 oz. | 45 |
| w/nuts and honey (*Nut & Honey Crunch*) | 110 |
| granola (see also "mixed grain and natural style," below): | |
| (*C.W. Post* Hearty) | 130 |

| FOOD AND MEASURE | CALORIES |
|---|---|
| *Cereal, ready-to-eat, granola, continued* | |
| w/almonds (*Sun Country* 100% Natural) | 130 |
| banana almond (*Sunbelt*) | 130 |
| fruit and nut (*Sunbelt*) | 120 |
| maple nut (*Arrowhead Mills*), 2 oz. | 250 |
| w/raisins (*Sun Country*) | 125 |
| w/raisins and dates (*Sun Country* 100% Natural) | 123 |
| millet (*Arrowhead Mills* Puffed Millet), .5 oz. | 50 |
| mixed grain and natural style: | |
| (*Almond Delight*) | 110 |
| (*Apple Jacks*) | 110 |
| (*Arrowhead Mills* Arrowhead Crunch) | 120 |
| (*Arrowhead Mills* Nature O's) | 110 |
| (*Cinnamon Toast Crunch*) | 120 |
| (*Crispix*) | 110 |
| (*Crunchy Nut Oh!s*) | 127 |
| (*Double Chex*) | 100 |
| (*Familia* Champion), 2 oz. | 200 |
| (*Familia* Crunchy) | 116 |
| (*Familia* No Added Sugar), 2 oz. | 206 |
| (*Fiber One*) | 60 |
| (*Froot Loops*) | 110 |
| (*Golden Grahams*) | 110 |
| (*Grape Nuts*) | 110 |
| (*Grape Nuts* Flakes) | 100 |
| (*Health Valley Healthy O's/Fiber 7* Flakes) | 100 |
| (*Heartland*) | 130 |
| (*Honey Graham Chex*) | 110 |
| (*Honey Graham Oh!s*) | 122 |
| (*Just Right*) | 100 |
| (*Kaboom*) | 110 |
| (*King Vitaman*) | 110 |
| (*Kix*) | 110 |
| (*Nutri•Grain* Nuggets) | 100 |
| (*Product 19*) | 100 |
| (*Quaker* 100% Natural) | 127 |
| (*Special K*) | 110 |
| (*Sunflakes Multi-Grain*) | 100 |
| (*Trix*) | 110 |
| all varieties (*Fruit & Fibre*), 1.25 oz. | 120 |
| w/almonds (*Honey Bunches of Oats*) | 120 |

| FOOD AND MEASURE | CALORIES |
|---|---|
| w/almonds and raisins (*Nutri•Grain*), 1.4 oz. | 140 |
| almond-date or apple (*Health Valley Healthy Crunch*) | 100 |
| apple and cinnamon (*Quaker* 100% Natural) | 126 |
| w/apples and raisins (*Apple Raisin Crisp*), 1.3 oz. | 130 |
| w/bananas and Hawaiian fruit (*Health Valley Sprouts 7*) | 90 |
| chocolate chip (*Cookie-Crisp*) | 110 |
| cinnamon and raisin (*Nature Valley* 100% Natural) | 120 |
| coconut (*Heartland*) | 130 |
| w/fruit (*Health Valley Fruit & Fitness*), 2 oz. | 190 |
| w/fruit and nuts (*Just Right*), 1.3 oz. | 140 |
| w/fruit and nuts (*Mueslix* Five Grain), 1.45 oz. | 140 |
| w/fruit and nuts (*Nature Valley* 100% Natural) | 130 |
| honey roasted (*Honey Bunches of Oats*) | 110 |
| w/raisins (*Grape Nuts*) | 100 |
| w/raisins (*Health Valley Sprouts 7*) | 90 |
| w/raisins (*Heartland*) | 130 |
| w/raisins and almonds (*Nutrific*), 1.5 oz. | 140 |
| raisins and dates (*Quaker* 100% Natural) | 123 |
| raisins, dates, and almonds (*Ralston Muesli*), 1.45 oz. | 140 |
| raisins, peaches, and pecans (*Ralston Muesli*), 1.45 oz. | 150 |
| raisins, walnuts, and cranberries (*Ralston Fruit Muesli*), 1.45 oz. | 150 |
| vanilla wafer (*Cookie-Crisp*) | 110 |
| oat: | |
| (*Alpha-Bits*) | 110 |
| (*Apple Cinnamon Cheerios*) | 110 |
| (*Cheerios*) | 110 |
| (Cinnamon *Life*) | 101 |
| (*General Mills* Oatmeal Crisp) | 110 |
| (*General Mills* Toasted Oat) | 130 |
| (*Honey Nut Cheerios*) | 110 |
| (*Life*) | 101 |
| (*Oat Chex*) | 100 |
| (*Post* Oat Flakes) | 110 |
| (*Quaker Oat Squares*) | 105 |
| w/marshmallow (*Lucky Charms*) | 110 |
| w/raisins (*General Mills* Oatmeal Raisin Crisp) | 110 |
| oat bran: | |
| (*Arrowhead Mills* Oat Bran Flakes) | 110 |
| (*Common Sense*) | 100 |
| (*Craklin' Oat Bran*) | 110 |

| FOOD AND MEASURE | CALORIES |
|---|---|
| *Cereal, ready-to-eat, oat bran, continued* | |
| (*Health Valley* Flakes) | 100 |
| (*Health Valley Oat Bran O's*) | 90 |
| almond crunch or raisin nut (*Health Valley Real*) | 110 |
| fruit, Hawaiian (*Health Valley Real*) | 130 |
| w/raisins (*Common Sense*), 1.3 oz. | 120 |
| w/raisins (*General Mills Raisin Oat Bran*), 1.5 oz. | 150 |
| w/raisins (*Raisin Oat Bran Options*), 1.45 oz. | 130 |
| rice: | |
| (*Arrowhead Mills* Puffed Rice), .5 oz. | 50 |
| (*Health Valley Lites* Puffed Rice), .5 oz. | 50 |
| (*Kellogg's Frosted Krispies*) | 110 |
| (*Kellogg's Rice Krispies*) | 110 |
| (*Quaker* Puffed Rice), .5 oz. or 1 cup | 54 |
| (*Rice Chex*) | 110 |
| chocolate flavor (*Cocoa Krispies*) | 110 |
| w/fruit (*Health Valley Fruit Lites*), .5 oz. | 45 |
| w/marshmallow bits (*Fruity Marshmallow Krispies*), 1.3 oz. | 140 |
| rice bran (*Health Valley Rice Bran O's*) | 110 |
| rice bran, w/almonds and dates (*Health Valley*) | 110 |
| wheat: | |
| (*Arrowhead Mills* Puffed Wheat), .5 oz. | 50 |
| (*Arrowhead Mills* Wheat Flakes) | 110 |
| (*Clusters*) | 110 |
| (*Health Valley Lites* Puffed Wheat), .5 oz. | 50 |
| (*Honey Smacks*) | 110 |
| (*Nutri•Grain*) | 100 |
| (*Quaker* Puffed Wheat), .5 oz. | 50 |
| (*Total*) | 100 |
| (*Wheat Chex*) | 100 |
| (*Wheaties*) | 100 |
| apple-cinnamon filled (*Kellogg's Apple Cinnamon Squares*) | 90 |
| blueberry filled (*Kellogg's Blueberry Squares*) | 90 |
| brown sugar, nut, and honey filled (*Nut & Honey Crunch* Biscuits) | 100 |
| w/fruit (*Health Valley Fruit Lites*), .5 oz. | 45 |
| honey sweetened puffs (*Super Golden Crisp*) | 110 |
| raisin filled (*Kellogg's Raisin Squares*) | 90 |
| w/raisins (*Crispy Wheats'N Raisins*) | 100 |
| w/raisins (*Nutri•Grain*), 1.4 oz. | 130 |
| raspberry filled (*Fruit Wheats*) | 90 |
| strawberry filled (*Kellogg's Strawberry Squares*) | 90 |

| FOOD AND MEASURE | CALORIES |
|---|---|
| wheat, shredded: | |
| (*Frosted Mini-Wheats*), 4 biscuits | 100 |
| (*Nabisco*), 1 piece | 80 |
| (*Nutri•Grain*) | 90 |
| (*Quaker*), 2 biscuits | 132 |
| (*S.W. Graham*) | 100 |
| bite size (*Frosted Mini-Wheats*) | 100 |
| w/bran (*Nabisco Shredded Wheat 'n Bran*) | 90 |
| mini (*Nabisco* Spoon Size) | 90 |

**Cereal beverage,** see "Coffee, substitute"

**Cervelat,** see "Thuringer cervelat" and "Summer sausage"

**Champagne,** see "Wine"

**Chayote:**

| | |
|---|---|
| raw, 1 medium, 5¾" × 2⅞" | 49 |
| boiled, drained, 1" pieces, ½ cup | 19 |

**Cheddarwurst:**

| | |
|---|---|
| (*Hillshire Farm* Bun Size), 2 oz. | 200 |
| (*Hillshire Farm* Links), 2 oz. | 190 |

**Cheese,** 1 oz., except as noted:

| | |
|---|---|
| all varieties, reduced fat (*Kraft Light Naturals*) | 80 |
| American, processed: | |
| (*Borden*) | 110 |
| (*Dorman's*/*Dorman's* Loaf Low Sodium) | 110 |
| (*Kraft* Deluxe) | 110 |
| (*Land O'Lakes*) | 110 |
| hot pepper (*Sargento*) | 110 |
| sharp (*Old English*) | 110 |
| asiago, wheel (*Frigo*) | 110 |
| babybel (*Laughing Cow*) | 91 |
| babybel, mini (*Laughing Cow*), ¾ oz. | 74 |
| (*Bel Paese* Domestic Traditional) | 101 |
| (*Bel Paese* Imported) | 90 |
| (*Bel Paese* Lite) | 76 |
| (*Bel Paese* Medallion Process) | 71 |
| blue (*Dorman's* Danablu 50%) | 100 |
| blue (*Dorman's* Danablu 60%) | 108 |
| blue (*Kraft*) | 100 |

| FOOD AND MEASURE | CALORIES |
|---|---|
| *Cheese, continued* | |
| blue (*Sargento*) | 100 |
| blue castello or saga (*Dorman's* 70%) | 134 |
| bonbel (*Laughing Cow*) | 100 |
| bonbel, mini (*Laughing Cow*), ¾ oz. | 74 |
| bonbino (*Laughing Cow*) | 103 |
| brick (*Dorman's*) | 110 |
| brick (*Kraft*) | 110 |
| brick (*Land O'Lakes*) | 110 |
| Brie (*Dorman's*) | 81 |
| Brie (*Sargento*) | 100 |
| Cajun (*Sargento*) | 110 |
| caljack (*Churney*) | 100 |
| Camembert (*Dorman's* 45%) | 82 |
| Camembert (*Dorman's* 50%) | 89 |
| Camembert (*Sargento*) | 90 |
| cheddar: | |
| (*Alpine Lace* Cheddar Flavored) | 100 |
| (*Dorman's*) | 110 |
| (*Dorman's* Chedda-Delite) | 90 |
| (*Kraft*) | 110 |
| (*Land O'Lakes*) | 110 |
| (*Laughing Cow*) | 110 |
| (*Sargento/Sargento* New York) | 110 |
| all varieties (*Weight Watchers* Natural) | 80 |
| reduced fat (*Dorman's* Low Sodium) | 80 |
| Vermont (*Churny*) | 110 |
| cheddar jack (*Dorman's* Chedda-Jack) | 90 |
| colby: | |
| (*Alpine Lace Colby-Lo*) | 80 |
| (*Dorman's*) | 110 |
| (*Kraft*) | 110 |
| (*Land O'Lakes*) | 110 |
| (*Sargento*) | 110 |
| (*Weight Watcher's* Natural) | 80 |
| colby jack (*Sargento*) | 110 |
| cottage, ½ cup, except as noted: | |
| (*Bison* 4% fat) | 120 |
| (*Borden* 4% fat Regular/Unsalted) | 120 |
| (*Breakstones*), 4 oz. | 110 |
| (*Crowley* 4% fat) | 120 |

| FOOD AND MEASURE | CALORIES |
|---|---|
| (*Friendship* California Style 4%) | 120 |
| dry curd, unsalted (*Borden*) | 80 |
| lowfat 2% (*Breakstones*) 4 oz. | 90 |
| lowfat 2% (*Weight Watchers*) | 100 |
| lowfat 1½% (*Lite-Line*) | 90 |
| lowfat 1% (*Bison*) | 90 |
| lowfat 1% (*Crowley* Regular/No Salt Added) | 90 |
| lowfat 1% (*Friendship* Regular/No Salt Added) | 90 |
| lowfat 1% (*Weight Watchers*) | 90 |
| lowfat, calcium fortified, 1% (*Crowley*) | 90 |
| lowfat, lactose reduced, 1% (*Friendship*) | 90 |
| nonfat (*Knudsen*), 4 oz. | 70 |
| chive (*Boston*) | 120 |
| garden salad (*Bison*) | 110 |
| w/peaches or pineapple (*Crowley* 4% fat) | 140 |
| w/pineapple (*Bison*) | 140 |
| w/pineapple (*Friendship* 4%) | 140 |
| w/pineapple, lowfat 1% (*Crowley*) | 110 |
| w/pineapple, lowfat 1% (*Friendship*) | 110 |
| pot style, large curd, lowfat 2% (*Friendship*) | 100 |
| cream cheese: | |
| (*Crowley*) | 110 |
| (*Dorman's* 65%) | 90 |
| (*Dorman's* 70%) | 102 |
| (*Philadelphia Brand*) | 100 |
| w/chives or pimiento (*Philadelphia Brand*) | 90 |
| soft (*Friendship*) | 103 |
| soft (*Philadelphia Brand*) | 100 |
| soft, all flavors, except w/chives and onion or w/herb and garlic (*Philadelphia Brand*) | 90 |
| soft, w/chives and onion or w/herb and garlic (*Philadelphia Brand*) | 100 |
| whipped (*Philadelphia Brand*) | 100 |
| whipped, all flavors (*Philadelphia Brand*) | 90 |
| danbo (*Dorman's* 20%) | 62 |
| danbo (*Dorman's* 45%) | 98 |
| (*Dorman's* Crema Dania 70%) | 134 |
| Edam (*Dorman's*) | 100 |
| Edam (*Dorman's* 45%) | 91 |
| Edam (*Kraft*) | 90 |
| Edam (*Land O'Lakes*) | 100 |

| FOOD AND MEASURE | CALORIES |
|---|---|
| *Cheese, continued* | |
| Edam (*Sargento*) | 100 |
| farmer (*Friendship*), ½ cup | 160 |
| farmer (*Sargento*) | 100 |
| feta (*Churny* Natural) | 75 |
| feta (*Dorman's* 45%) | 91 |
| feta (*Sargento*) | 80 |
| fontina (*Sargento*) | 110 |
| gjetost (*Sargento*) | 130 |
| Gouda: | |
| (*Dorman's*) | 100 |
| (*Kraft*) | 110 |
| (*Land O'Lakes*) | 100 |
| (*Laughing Cow*) | 110 |
| (*Sargento*) | 100 |
| mini (*Laughing Cow*), ¾ oz. | 80 |
| grated (*Polly-O*) | 130 |
| Havarti (*Casino*) | 120 |
| Havarti (*Dorman's* 45%) | 91 |
| Havarti (*Dorman's* 60%) | 118 |
| Havarti (*Sargento*) | 120 |
| Italian-style grated (*Sargento*) | 110 |
| Jarlsberg (*Norseland Jarlsberg*) | 97 |
| (*Laughing Cow* Reduced mini), ¾ oz. | 45 |
| Limburger (*Sargento*) | 90 |
| Limburger, natural (*Mohawk Valley* Little Gem) | 90 |
| mascarpone (*Galbani* Imported) | 128 |
| Monterey Jack: | |
| (*Alpine Lace Monti-Jack-Lo*) | 80 |
| (*Dorman's*) | 100 |
| (*Land O'Lakes*) | 110 |
| (*Sargento*) | 110 |
| (*Weight Watchers* Natural) | 80 |
| all varieties (*Axelrod*) | 100 |
| w/caraway seeds (*Kraft*) | 100 |
| w/peppers, mild (*Casino*) | 110 |
| plain or w/jalapeño peppers (*Kraft*) | 100 |
| reduced fat (*Dorman's* Low Sodium) | 80 |
| mozzarella: | |
| (*Dorman's*) | 90 |
| (*Polly-O Lite*) | 70 |

| FOOD AND MEASURE | CALORIES |
|---|---|
| (*Weight Watchers* Natural) | 70 |
| fresh (*Polly-O Fior di Latte*) | 80 |
| shredded (*Weight Watchers*) | 80 |
| whole milk (*Crowley*) | 90 |
| whole milk (*Polly-O*) | 90 |
| whole milk (*Sargento*) | 90 |
| part skim (*Crowley*) | 70 |
| part skim (*Polly-O*) | 80 |
| part skim, low moisture (*Alpine Lace*) | 70 |
| part skim, low moisture (*Kraft*) | 80 |
| part skim, low moisture (*Land O'Lakes*) | 80 |
| part skim, low moisture (*Sargento*) | 80 |
| part skim, w/jalapeño pepper (*Kraft*) | 80 |
| low moisture (*Casino*) | 90 |
| part skim or reduced fat (*Dorman's* Low Sodium) | 80 |
| Muenster: | |
| (*Alpine Lace*) | 100 |
| (*Dorman's* Regular/Low Sodium) | 110 |
| (*Dorman's* 50%) | 100 |
| (*Land O'Lakes*) | 100 |
| reduced fat (*Dorman's* Low Sodium) | 80 |
| red rind (*Sargento*) | 100 |
| Neufchâtel, light (*Philadelphia Brand*) | 80 |
| Parmesan: | |
| (*Kraft*) | 100 |
| fresh (*Sargento*) | 110 |
| grated (*Kraft*) | 130 |
| grated (*Polly-O*) | 130 |
| grated (*Progresso*), 1 tbsp. | 23 |
| grated (*Sargento*) | 130 |
| Reggiano (*Galbani* Imported) | 105 |
| Parmesan and Romano, grated (*Sargento*) | 110 |
| pimiento, processed (*Kraft Deluxe*) | 100 |
| pot cheese (*Sargento*) | 25 |
| Primavera (*Bel Paese* Lite) | 68 |
| provolone: | |
| (*Alpine Lace Provo-Lo*) | 70 |
| (*Dorman's* Regular/Low Sodium) | 90 |
| (*Kraft*) | 100 |
| (*Land O'Lakes*) | 100 |
| (*Sargento*) | 100 |

| FOOD AND MEASURE | CALORIES |
|---|---|
| *Cheese, provolone, continued* | |
| queso blanco (*Sargento*) | 100 |
| queso de papa (*Sargento*) | 110 |
| ricotta: | |
| (*Polly-O* Lite), 2 oz. | 80 |
| (*Sargento*) | 40 |
| (*Sargento* Lite) | 23 |
| whole milk (*Crowley*), 2 oz. | 100 |
| whole milk (*Polly-O*), 2 oz. | 100 |
| part skim (*Crowley*), 2 oz. | 80 |
| part skim (*Polly-O*), 2 oz. | 90 |
| part skim (*Sargento*) | 30 |
| low fat (*Frigo*) | 20 |
| Romano: | |
| (*Kraft* Natural) | 110 |
| (*Sargento*) | 110 |
| grated (*Kraft*) | 130 |
| grated (*Polly-O*) | 130 |
| grated (*Progresso*), 1 tbsp. | 23 |
| slim jack (*Dorman's*) | 90 |
| smoked (*Sargento* Smokestick) | 100 |
| string (*Polly-O*), 1-oz. stick | 90 |
| string, low moisture (*Kraft*) | 80 |
| string, regular or smoked (*Sargento*) | 80 |
| Swiss: | |
| (*Alpine Lace Swiss-Lo*) | 100 |
| (*Casino*) | 110 |
| (*Dorman's* Regular/No Salt Added) | 100 |
| (*Dorman's* Reduced Fat) | 90 |
| (*Kraft* Light Naturals) | 90 |
| (*Kraft* 75% Very Low Sodium) | 110 |
| (*Land O'Lakes*) | 110 |
| (*Sargento*/*Sargento* Finland) | 110 |
| (*Weight Watchers* Natural) | 90 |
| processed (*Borden*) | 100 |
| processed (*Kraft* Deluxe) | 90 |
| regular or aged (*Kraft*) | 110 |
| smoked (*Dorman's*) | 100 |
| taco (*Sargento*) | 110 |
| taco, shredded (*Kraft*) | 110 |
| taleggio (*Tal-Fino* Brand Imported) | 89 |

| FOOD AND MEASURE | CALORIES |
|---|---|
| Tilsit (*Sargento*) | 100 |
| tybo (*Dorman's* 45%) | 98 |
| tybo, red wax (*Sargento*) | 100 |
| **Cheese, substitute and imitation,** 1 oz.: | |
| all varieties (*Churny* Delicia) | 80 |
| all varieties except creamed (*Weight Watchers*) | 50 |
| American (*Golden Image*) | 90 |
| cheddar, imitation (*Sargento*) | 90 |
| cheddar, mild, imitation (*Golden Image*) | 110 |
| cheddar, shredded (*Fisher Ched-O-Mate*) | 90 |
| cheese food (*Cheeztwin*) | 90 |
| cheese food (*Fisher Sandwich-Mate*) | 90 |
| cheese food (*Lite-Line* Low Cholesterol) | 90 |
| colby (*Dorman's* LoChol) | 90 |
| colby, imitation (*Golden Image*) | 110 |
| creamed cheese (*Weight Watchers*) | 35 |
| mozzarella, imitation (*Sargento*) | 80 |
| mozzarella, shredded (*Fisher Pizza-Mate*) | 90 |
| Muenster or Swiss (*Dorman's* LoChol) | 100 |
| (*Nucoa Heart Beat*) | 50 |
| **Cheese blintz,** frozen: | |
| (*King Kold*), 2.5-oz. piece | 113 |
| (*King Kold* No Salt Added), 2.5-oz. piece | 96 |
| **Cheese danish,** 1 piece: | |
| (*Awrey's* Round), 4.5 oz. | 420 |
| (*Awrey's* Square), 2.5 oz. | 210 |
| miniature (*Awrey's*), 1.7 oz. | 170 |
| frozen (*Pepperidge Farm*), 2.25 oz. | 240 |
| frozen (*Sara Lee* Individual), 1.3 oz. | 130 |
| **Cheese dip:** | |
| jalapeño (*Kraft* Premium), 2 tbsp. | 50 |
| nacho (*Kraft* Premium), 2 tbsp. | 55 |
| nacho (*Price's*), 1 oz. | 80 |
| **Cheese food,** 1 oz.: | |
| all varieties: | |
| (*Velveeta*) | 100 |
| cold pack (*Wispride*) | 100 |

| FOOD AND MEASURE | CALORIES |
|---|---|
| *Cheese food, all varieties, continued* | |
| except port wine and sharp cheddar (*Cracker Barrel*) | 90 |
| except salami (*Land O'Lakes*) | 90 |
| except sharp (*Kraft* Singles) | 90 |
| American: | |
| (*Borden* Singles) | 90 |
| (*Borden* Slices) | 100 |
| grated (*Kraft*) | 130 |
| sharp (*Borden* Singles) | 90 |
| w/bacon (*Kraft Cheez'N Bacon*) | 90 |
| w/garlic or jalapeño pepper (*Kraft*) | 90 |
| (*Nippy*) | 90 |
| salami (*Land O'Lakes*) | 100 |
| sharp (*Kraft* Singles) | 100 |
| sharp cheddar or port wine (*Cracker Barrel*) | 100 |

**Cheese nut ball or log,** 1 oz.:

| | |
|---|---|
| ball or log, all varieties, except sharp cheddar ball (*Cracker Barrel*) | 90 |
| ball, sharp cheddar (*Cracker Barrel*) | 100 |
| log, sharp cheddar or port wine (*Sargento*) | 100 |
| log, Swiss almond (*Sargento*) | 90 |

**Cheese pastry pocket:**

| | |
|---|---|
| (*Tastykake*), 3 oz. | 332 |

**Cheese product,** processed, 1 oz.:

| | |
|---|---|
| all varieties (*Light N' Lively* Singles) | 70 |
| all varieties (*Lite-Line*) | 50 |
| all varieties (*Spreadery* Cheese Snack) | 70 |
| all varieties, except nonfat (*Kraft Free* Singles) | 70 |
| American flavor (*Alpine Lace*) | 90 |
| American flavor (*Borden* Light) | 70 |
| American flavor (*Harvest Moon*) | 70 |
| American flavor (*Lite-Line* Reduced Sodium/Sodium Lite) | 70 |
| cream cheese, light (*Philadelphia Brand*) | 60 |
| nonfat (*Kraft Free* Singles) | 45 |
| sandwich slices (*Lunch Wagon*) | 90 |

**Cheese sauce** (see also "Welsh rarebit"):

| | |
|---|---|
| aged (*White House*), 3.5 oz. | 213 |
| cheddar or nacho (*Lucky Leaf/Musselman's*), 4 oz. | 220 |
| four cheese (*Contadina Fresh*), 6 oz. | 470 |

| FOOD AND MEASURE | CALORIES |
|---|---|
| jalapeño (*White House*), 3.5 oz. | 193 |
| nacho (*White House*), 3.5 oz. | 193 |
| mix (*McCormick/Schilling*), ¼ pkg. | 35 |
| mix, nacho (*McCormick/Schilling*), ¼ pkg. | 42 |
| mix, prepared w/whole milk (*French's*), ¼ cup | 80 |

**Cheese spreads,** 1 oz.:

| | |
|---|---|
| all varieties (*Cheez Whiz*) | 80 |
| all varieties (*Squeeze-A-Snak*) | 80 |
| all varieties (*Weight Watchers* Cup), 1 oz. or 2 tbsp. | 70 |
| American, processed (*Kraft*) | 80 |
| American, processed, sharp or pimiento (*Sargento* Cracker Snacks) | 110 |
| w/bacon (*Kraft*) | 80 |
| blue (*Roka*) | 70 |
| brick (*Sargento* Cracker Snacks) | 100 |
| cream cheese, see "Cheese" | |
| w/jalapeño pepper (*Kraft*) | 70 |
| w/jalapeño pepper, loaf (*Kraft*) | 80 |
| (*Land O'Lakes* Golden Velvet) | 80 |
| Limburger (*Mohawk Valley*) | 70 |
| Mexican or pimiento (*Velveeta*) | 80 |
| (*Micro Melt*) | 80 |
| olives and pimiento (*Kraft*) | 60 |
| pimiento or pineapple (*Kraft*) | 70 |
| sharp (*Old English*) | 80 |
| Swiss (*Sargento* Cracker Snacks) | 100 |
| (*Velveeta*) | 80 |
| (*Velveeta* Slices) | 90 |

**Cheese sticks,** frozen, breaded, 3 oz.:

| | |
|---|---|
| cheddar (*Farm Rich*) | 300 |
| hot pepper (*Farm Rich*) | 260 |
| mozzarella (*Farm Rich*) | 240 |
| provolone (*Farm Rich*) | 270 |

**Cheeseburger,** frozen:

| | |
|---|---|
| (*MicroMagic*), 4.75 oz. | 450 |

**Cheesecake,** see "Cake"

| FOOD AND MEASURE | CALORIES |
|---|---|
| **Cherimoya:** | |
| 1 medium, 1.9 lb. | 515 |
| **Cherries supreme,** frozen: | |
| (*Pepperidge Farm* Dessert Lights), 3¼ oz. | 170 |
| **Cherry:** | |
| fresh, sour, red, pitted, ½ cup | 39 |
| fresh, sour, red, w/pits, ½ cup | 26 |
| fresh, sweet, whole, ½ cup | 52 |
| fresh, sweet, 10 medium | 49 |
| canned, sour, red: | |
| pitted (*White House*), 3.5 oz. | 43 |
| tart (*Lucky Leaf/Musselman's*), 4 oz. | 50 |
| in water (*Stokely*), ½ cup | 45 |
| in light syrup, ½ cup | 94 |
| in heavy syrup, ½ cup | 116 |
| canned, sweet: | |
| (*Mott's* Cherry Fruit Pak), 3.75 oz. | 72 |
| dark, w/pits or pitted (*Del Monte*), ½ cup | 90 |
| light, w/pits (*Del Monte*), ½ cup | 100 |
| in water, ½ cup | 57 |
| in juice, ½ cup | 68 |
| in light syrup, ½ cup | 85 |
| in heavy syrup, ½ cup | 107 |
| frozen, sour, red, unsweetened, ½ cup | 36 |
| frozen, sweet, sweetened, ½ cup | 116 |
| **Cherry cobbler,** frozen: | |
| (*Pet-Ritz*), ⅙ pkg. | 280 |
| (*Stilwell*), 4 oz. | 250 |
| **Cherry fruit concentrate:** | |
| black (*Hain*), 1 oz. or 2 tbsp. | 70 |
| **Cherry fruit roll:** | |
| (*Flavor Tree*), 1 piece | 75 |
| **Cherry juice:** | |
| black (*Smucker's* Naturally 100%), 8 fl. oz. | 130 |
| blend (*Dole Pure & Light* Mountain Cherry), 6 fl. oz. | 87 |
| blend (*Libby's Juicy Juice*), 6 fl. oz. | 90 |

| FOOD AND MEASURE | CALORIES |
|---|---|

**Cherry juice cocktail:**

(*Welch's Orchard*), 6 fl. oz. . . . . . . . . . . . . . . . . . . . . . . . . . . . . . . 180

**Cherry juice drink:**

(*Hi-C*), 8.45 fl. oz. . . . . . . . . . . . . . . . . . . . . . . . . . . . . . . . . . . 141
(*Hi-C*), 6 fl. oz. . . . . . . . . . . . . . . . . . . . . . . . . . . . . . . . . . . . . 100
(*Kool-Aid Koolers*), 8.45 fl. oz. . . . . . . . . . . . . . . . . . . . . . . . . . . 140
(*Tang* Fruit Box), 8.45 fl. oz. . . . . . . . . . . . . . . . . . . . . . . . . . . . . 120

**Cherry pastry pocket:**

(*Tastykake*), 3 oz. . . . . . . . . . . . . . . . . . . . . . . . . . . . . . . . . . . 325

**Cherry pie,** see "Pie"

**Cherry turnover,** 1 piece:

frozen (*Pepperidge Farm*) . . . . . . . . . . . . . . . . . . . . . . . . . . . . . . 310
refrigerated (*Pillsbury*) . . . . . . . . . . . . . . . . . . . . . . . . . . . . . . . . 170

**Chervil,** dried:

1 tsp. . . . . . . . . . . . . . . . . . . . . . . . . . . . . . . . . . . . . . . . . . . . . . 1

**Chestnuts,** shelled:

Chinese, raw, 1 oz. . . . . . . . . . . . . . . . . . . . . . . . . . . . . . . . . . . 64
Chinese, boiled or steamed, 1 oz. . . . . . . . . . . . . . . . . . . . . . . . . . 44
Chinese, dried, 1 oz. . . . . . . . . . . . . . . . . . . . . . . . . . . . . . . . . . 103
Chinese, roasted, 1 oz. . . . . . . . . . . . . . . . . . . . . . . . . . . . . . . . . 68
European, raw, peeled, 1 oz. . . . . . . . . . . . . . . . . . . . . . . . . . . . . 56
European, boiled or steamed, 1 oz. . . . . . . . . . . . . . . . . . . . . . . . . 37
European, dried, peeled, 1 oz. . . . . . . . . . . . . . . . . . . . . . . . . . . . 105
European, roasted, peeled, 1 oz. . . . . . . . . . . . . . . . . . . . . . . . . . 70
Japanese, raw, 1 oz. . . . . . . . . . . . . . . . . . . . . . . . . . . . . . . . . . 44
Japanese, boiled or steamed, 1 oz. . . . . . . . . . . . . . . . . . . . . . . . . 16
Japanese, dried, 1 oz. . . . . . . . . . . . . . . . . . . . . . . . . . . . . . . . . 102
Japanese, roasted, 1 oz. . . . . . . . . . . . . . . . . . . . . . . . . . . . . . . . 57

**Chewing gum,** see "Candy"

**Chicken, boneless and luncheon meat:**

bologna, see "Chicken bologna"
breast:
(*Longacre* Premium), 1 oz. . . . . . . . . . . . . . . . . . . . . . . . . . . . . . 45
(*Mr. Turkey*), 1 oz. . . . . . . . . . . . . . . . . . . . . . . . . . . . . . . . . . . 32

| FOOD AND MEASURE | CALORIES |
|---|---|
| *Chicken, boneless and luncheon meat, breast, continued* | |
| hickory smoked (*Louis Rich*), 1 oz. | 30 |
| oven-roasted (*Louis Rich* Deluxe), 1 oz. | 30 |
| oven-roasted (*Louis Rich* Thin Sliced), .4-oz. slice | 12 |
| oven-roasted (*Oscar Mayer*), 1 oz. | 29 |
| roast (*Oscar Mayer* Thin Sliced), .4-oz. slice | 13 |
| smoked (*Eckrich Lite*), 1 oz. | 30 |
| smoked (*Hillshire Farm* Deli Select), 1 oz. | 31 |
| smoked (*Oscar Mayer*), 1 oz. | 25 |
| ham, see "Chicken ham" | |
| roll (*Pilgrim's Pride*), 1 oz. | 35 |
| roll, sliced (*Longacre*), 1 oz. | 60 |
| white meat, oven-roasted (*Louis Rich*), 1 oz. | 35 |

**Chicken, broiler or fryer,** fresh:

| FOOD AND MEASURE | CALORIES |
|---|---|
| fried, flour coated, meat w/skin: | |
| dark meat, 4 oz. | 323 |
| light meat, 4 oz. | 279 |
| back, 4 oz. | 375 |
| breast, 4 oz. | 252 |
| drumstick, 4 oz. | 278 |
| leg, 4 oz. | 285 |
| neck, 4 oz. | 376 |
| thigh, 4 oz. | 297 |
| wing, 4 oz. | 364 |
| fried, flour coated, skin only, 1 oz. | 142 |
| roasted: | |
| meat w/skin, ½ chicken, 10.5 oz. (15.8 oz. w/bone) | 715 |
| meat w/skin, 4 oz. | 271 |
| meat only, 4 oz. | 215 |
| meat only, chopped or diced, 1 cup not packed | 266 |
| skin only, 1 oz. | 129 |
| dark meat w/skin, 4 oz. | 287 |
| dark meat only, 4 oz. | 232 |
| light meat w/skin, 4 oz. | 252 |
| light meat only, 4 oz. | 196 |
| back, meat w/skin, 4 oz. | 340 |
| back, meat only, 4 oz. | 271 |
| breast, meat w/skin, 4 oz. | 223 |
| breast, meat only, 4 oz. | 187 |
| drumstick, meat w/skin, 4 oz. | 245 |

| FOOD AND MEASURE | CALORIES |
|---|---|
| drumstick, meat only, 4 oz. | 195 |
| leg, meat w/skin, 4 oz. | 265 |
| leg, meat only, 4 oz. | 217 |
| thigh, meat w/skin, 4 oz. | 280 |
| thigh, meat only, 4 oz. | 237 |
| wing, meat w/skin, 4 oz. | 329 |
| wing, meat only, 4 oz. | 230 |

**Chicken,** canned:

| | |
|---|---|
| chunk: | |
| (*Featherweight*), 3 oz. | 90 |
| breast (*Hormel*), 6.75 oz. | 350 |
| dark (*Hormel*), 6.75 oz. | 327 |
| style (*Swanson* Mixin' Chicken), 2.5 oz. | 130 |
| white and dark (*Hormel*), 6.75 oz. | 340 |
| white and dark, unsalted (*Hormel*), 6.75 oz. | 330 |
| loaf (*Hormel*), 2 oz. | 130 |
| white, or white and dark (*Swanson*), 2.5 oz. | 100 |

**Chicken, capon,** fresh, meat w/skin:

| | |
|---|---|
| roasted, ½ capon, 1.4 lbs. (2 lbs. w/bone) | 1,457 |
| roasted, 4 oz. | 260 |

**Chicken, roaster,** fresh, roasted:

| | |
|---|---|
| meat w/skin, ½ chicken, 1 lb. (1.5 lbs. w/bone) | 1,071 |
| meat w/skin, 4 oz. | 253 |
| meat only, 4 oz. | 189 |
| meat only, chopped or diced, 1 cup not packed | 233 |
| dark meat only, 4 oz. | 202 |
| light meat only, 4 oz. | 174 |

**Chicken, stewing,** fresh, stewed:

| | |
|---|---|
| meat w/skin, ½ chicken, 9.2 oz. (13.5 oz. w/bone) | 744 |
| meat w/skin, 4 oz. | 323 |
| meat only, 4 oz. | 269 |
| meat only, chopped or diced, 1 cup not packed | 332 |
| dark meat only, 4 oz. | 293 |
| light meat only, 4 oz. | 242 |

**"Chicken," vegetarian:**

| | |
|---|---|
| canned (*Worthington FriChik*), 2 pieces or 3.2 oz. | 180 |
| canned, sliced, drained (*Worthington*), 2 slices | 90 |
| canned, diced, drained (*Worthington*), ¼ cup | 90 |

| FOOD AND MEASURE | CALORIES |
|---|---|

*"Chicken," vegetarian, continued*

frozen:

(*Worthington Crispy Chik*), 3 oz. .............................. 280
diced (*Worthington* Meatless Chicken), ½ cup ................ 190
nuggets, homestyle (*Morningstar Farms Country Crisps*), 3 oz. .. 250
nuggets, zesty (*Morningstar Farms Country Crisps*), 3 oz. ....... 280
patty (*Morningstar Farms Country Crisps*), 2.5-oz. patty ......... 220
patty (*Worthington Crispy Chik*), 2.5-oz. patty .................. 220
pie (*Worthington*), 8-oz. pie ..................................... 380
roll (*Worthington* Meatless Chicken), 2.5 oz. .................... 150
slices (*Worthington* Meatless Chicken), 2 slices ................ 130
sticks (*Worthington Chik Stiks),* 1 piece ........................ 110

## Chicken bologna:

(*Health Valley*), 1 slice ........................................... 85

## Chicken dinner, frozen:

à la king (*Armour Classics Lite*), 11.25 oz. ........................ 290
à la king (*Le Menu*), 10.25 oz. ................................... 330
barbecue-style (*Stouffer's Dinner Supreme*), 10.5 oz. ............. 390
boneless (*Swanson Hungry Man*), 17.75 oz. ........................ 700
breast, baked, w/gravy (*Stouffer's Dinner Supreme*), 10 oz. ....... 300
breast, glazed (*Le Menu* LightStyle), 10 oz. ....................... 230
breast, Marsala (*Armour Classics Lite*), 10.5 oz. ................. 250
Burgundy (*Armour Classics Lite*), 10 oz. ........................... 210
cacciatore (*The Budget Gourmet*), 11 oz. ........................... 300
casserole (*Pillsbury Microwave Classic*), 1 pkg. ................... 400
and cheese, casserole (*Pillsbury Microwave Classic*), 1 pkg. ...... 480
cordon bleu (*Le Menu*), 11 oz. ...................................... 460
and dumplings (*Banquet*), 10 oz. .................................... 430
fettuccine (*Armour Classics*), 11 oz. ............................... 260
Florentine (*Stouffer's Dinner Supreme*), 11 oz. .................... 430
fried:

(*Banquet*), 10 oz. ............................................... 400
(*Banquet Extra Helping*), 16 oz. ................................. 570
(*Stouffer's Dinner Supreme*), 10⅝ oz. ........................... 450
barbecue flavored (*Swanson*), 10 oz. ............................ 540
dark meat (*Swanson*), 9.75 oz. ................................... 560
dark meat (*Swanson Hungry Man*), 1 pkg. ......................... 860
white meat (*Banquet Extra Helping*), 16 oz. ..................... 570

| FOOD AND MEASURE | CALORIES |
|---|---|
| white meat (*Swanson*), 10.25 oz. | 550 |
| white meat (*Swanson Hungry Man*), 1 pkg. | 870 |
| glazed (*Armour Classics*), 10.75 oz. | 300 |
| herb roasted (*Healthy Choice*), 11 oz. | 260 |
| herb roasted (*Le Menu* LightStyle), 10 oz. | 240 |
| mesquite (*Armour Classics*), 9.5 oz. | 370 |
| mesquite (*Healthy Choice*), 10.5 oz. | 310 |
| Mexicana (*The Budget Gourmet*), 12.8 oz. | 510 |
| and noodles (*Armour Classics*), 11 oz. | 230 |
| nuggets: | |
| (*Swanson*), 8.75 oz. | 470 |
| w/barbecue sauce (*Banquet Extra Helping*), 10 oz. | 640 |
| platter (*Freezer Queen*), 6 oz. | 410 |
| w/sweet and sour sauce (*Banquet Extra Helping*), 10 oz. | 650 |
| Oriental (*Armour Classics Lite*), 10 oz. | 180 |
| Oriental (*Healthy Choice*), 11.25 oz. | 220 |
| parmigiana (*Armour Classics*), 11.5 oz. | 370 |
| parmigiana (*Healthy Choice*), 11.5 oz. | 280 |
| parmigiana (*Le Menu*), 11.75 oz. | 410 |
| parmigiana (*Stouffer's Dinner Supreme*), 11.5 oz. | 360 |
| and pasta divan (*Healthy Choice*), 11.5 oz. | 310 |
| pattie platter (*Freezer Queen*), 7.5 oz. | 360 |
| roast (*The Budget Gourmet*), 11.2 oz. | 280 |
| w/supreme sauce (*Stouffer's Dinner Supreme*), 11⅜ oz. | 360 |
| sweet and sour (*Armour Classics Lite*), 11 oz. | 240 |
| sweet and sour (*Healthy Choice*), 11.5 oz. | 280 |
| sweet and sour (*Le Menu*), 11.25 oz. | 400 |
| teriyaki (*The Budget Gourmet*), 12 oz. | 360 |
| in wine sauce (*Le Menu*), 10 oz. | 280 |
| w/wine and mushroom sauce (*Armour Classics*), 10.75 oz. | 280 |

**Chicken entree,** canned (see also "Chicken entree, packaged"):

| | |
|---|---|
| à la king (*Swanson*), 5.25 oz. | 190 |
| chow mein (*La Choy* Bi-Pack), ¾ cup | 80 |
| and dumplings (*Featherweight*), 7.5 oz. | 160 |
| and dumplings (*Luck's*), 7.25 oz. | 240 |
| and dumplings (*Swanson*), 7.5 oz. | 220 |
| Oriental (*La Choy* Bi-Pack), ¾ cup | 240 |
| stew (*Swanson*), 7⅝ oz. | 160 |
| stew, w/dumplings (*Heinz*), 7.5 oz. | 210 |
| stew, w/wild rice (*Featherweight*), 7.5 oz. | 140 |

| FOOD AND MEASURE | CALORIES |
|---|---|

**Chicken entree,** frozen:

à la king:
(*Banquet Cookin' Bags*), 4 oz. . . . . . . . . 110
(*Dining Lite*), 9 oz. . . . . . . . . 240
(*Freezer Queen Cook-In-Pouch*), 4 oz. . . . . . . . . 70
(*Le Menu* LightStyle), 8.25 oz. . . . . . . . . 240
(*Weight Watchers*), 9 oz. . . . . . . . . 240
w/rice (*Freezer Queen* Single Serve), 9 oz. . . . . . . . . 270
w/rice (*Stouffer's*), 9.5 oz. . . . . . . . . 290
w/seasoned rice (*Le Menu* LightStyle), 8.25 oz. . . . . . . . . 240
almond, w/rice, vegetables (*La Choy Fresh & Lite*), 9.75 oz. . . . . . . . . 270
à l'orange (*Healthy Choice*), 9 oz. . . . . . . . . 260
à l'orange (*Tyson Gourmet Selection*), 9.5 oz. . . . . . . . . 300
à l'orange, w/almond rice (*Lean Cuisine*), 8 oz. . . . . . . . . 260
au gratin (*The Budget Gourmet* Slim Selects), 9.1 oz. . . . . . . . . 260
and beef luau (*Tyson Gourmet Selection*), 10.5 oz. . . . . . . . . 330
breast, boneless:
barbecue marinated (*Tyson*), 3.75 oz. . . . . . . . . 120
butter garlic-marinated (*Tyson*), 3.75 oz. . . . . . . . . 160
chunks (*Tyson*), 3 oz. . . . . . . . . 240
fillets (*Pilgrim's Pride*), 3 oz. . . . . . . . . 195
fillets (*Tyson*), 3 oz. . . . . . . . . 190
in herb cream sauce (*Lean Cuisine*), 9.5 oz. . . . . . . . . 260
herb-roasted, w/rice and vegetables (*Le Menu* LightStyle), 7.75 oz. . . . . . . . . 260
Italian-marinated (*Tyson*), 3.75 oz. . . . . . . . . 130
lemon pepper-marinated (*Tyson*), 3.75 oz. . . . . . . . . 120
Marsala, w/vegetables (*Lean Cuisine*), 8⅛ oz. . . . . . . . . 190
Parmesan (*Lean Cuisine*), 10 oz. . . . . . . . . 260
patties, see "patties," below
tenders (*Banquet* Chicken Hot Bites), 2.25 oz. . . . . . . . . 150
tenders (*Banquet* Chicken Hot Bites Microwave), 4 oz. . . . . . . . . 260
tenders (*Pilgrim's Pride*), 3 oz. . . . . . . . . 181
tenders, Southern fried (*Banquet* Chicken Hot Bites), 2.25 oz. . . . 160
tenders, Southern fried (*Tyson*), 3 oz. . . . . . . . . 220
teriyaki-marinated (*Tyson*), 3.75 oz. . . . . . . . . 130
and broccoli (*Green Giant* Entrees), 9.5 oz. . . . . . . . . 340
cacciatore (*Freezer Queen* Single Serve), 9 oz. . . . . . . . . 270
cacciatore (*Swanson* Homestyle Recipe), 10.95 oz. . . . . . . . . 260
cacciatore, w/vermicelli (*Lean Cuisine*), 10⅞ oz. . . . . . . . . 250

| FOOD AND MEASURE | CALORIES |
|---|---|
| Cajun style (*Pilgrim's Pride*), 3-oz. portion | 241 |
| cashew, in sauce, w/rice (*Stouffer's*), 9.5 oz. | 380 |
| w/cheddar, boneless (*Tyson* Chick'n Cheddar), 2.6 oz. | 220 |
| chow mein: | |
| (*Chun King*), 13 oz. | 370 |
| (*Dining Lite*), 9 oz. | 180 |
| (*Healthy Choice*), 8.5 oz. | 220 |
| w/out noodles (*Stouffer's*), 8 oz. | 130 |
| w/rice (*Lean Cuisine*), 11.25 oz. | 250 |
| chunks: | |
| (*Country Pride*), 3 oz. | 240 |
| (*Tyson* Chick'n Chunks), 2.6 oz. | 220 |
| Southern-fried (*Country Pride*), 3 oz. | 280 |
| Southern-fried (*Tyson* Chick'n Chunks), 2.6 oz. | 220 |
| cordon bleu (*Swift International*), 6 oz. | 360 |
| cordon bleu (*Weight Watchers*), 8 oz. | 220 |
| creamed (*Stouffer's*), 6.5 oz. | 300 |
| croquettes, breaded, gravy and (*Freezer Queen Family Suppers*), 7 oz. | 240 |
| diced (*Tyson*), 3 oz. | 150 |
| Dijon (*Le Menu* LightStyle), 8.5 oz. | 240 |
| Dijon (*Tyson Gourmet Selection*), 8.5 oz. | 310 |
| divan (*Stouffer's*), 8.5 oz. | 320 |
| drumsnackers (*Banquet* Chicken Hot Bites), 2.63 oz. | 220 |
| drumsnackers (*Banquet* Platters), 7 oz. | 430 |
| drumsters (*Pilgrim's Pride*), 3 oz. | 200 |
| and dumplings (*Banquet Family Entrees*), 7 oz. | 280 |
| and egg noodles, w/broccoli (*The Budget Gourmet*), 10 oz. | 450 |
| empress (*Le Menu* LightStyle), 8.25 oz. | 210 |
| enchilada, see "Enchilada entree, frozen" | |
| escalloped, and noodles (*Stouffer's*), 10 oz. | 420 |
| fajita, see "Fajita entree" | |
| w/fettuccine (*The Budget Gourmet*), 10 oz. | 400 |
| fettuccine (*Weight Watchers*), 8.25 oz. | 280 |
| fiesta (*Healthy Choice*), 8.5 oz. | 250 |
| Français (*Tyson Gourmet Selection*), 9.5 oz. | 280 |
| French recipe (*The Budget Gourmet* Slim Selects), 10 oz. | 260 |
| fried: | |
| (*Banquet*/*Banquet* Hot'n Spicy), 6.4 oz. | 330 |
| (*Pilgrim's Pride*), 3-oz. portion | 255 |
| (*Swanson* Homestyle Recipe), 7-oz. portion | 390 |

| FOOD AND MEASURE | CALORIES |
|---|---|
| *Chicken entree, frozen, fried, continued* | |
| (*Swanson* 1 lb. Take-Out Pre-Fried), 3.25 oz. | 270 |
| breast portions (*Banquet*), 5.75 oz. | 220 |
| breast portions (*Swanson* Plump & Juicy), 4.5-oz. portion | 360 |
| thighs and drumsticks (*Banquet*), 6.25 oz. | 250 |
| white meat (*Banquet* Platter), 9 oz. | 430 |
| white meat, hot'n spicy (*Banquet* Platter), 9 oz. | 430 |
| glazed (*Dining Lite*), 9 oz. | 220 |
| glazed (*Healthy Choice*), 8.5 oz. | 220 |
| glazed, w/vegetable rice (*Lean Cuisine*), 8.5 oz. | 270 |
| herb-roasted (*Le Menu* LightStyle), 7.75 oz. | 260 |
| hot'n spicy (*Banquet* Snack'n), 3.75 oz. | 140 |
| imperial (*Chun King*), 13 oz. | 300 |
| imperial (*Weight Watchers*), 9.25 oz. | 240 |
| imperial, w/rice (*La Choy Fresh & Lite*), 11 oz. | 260 |
| Italiano, w/fettuccine, vegetables (*Right Course*), 9⅝ oz. | 280 |
| Kiev (*Swift International*), 6 oz. | 420 |
| Kiev (*Tyson Gourmet Selection*), 9.25 oz. | 520 |
| Kiev (*Weight Watchers*), 7 oz. | 230 |
| Mandarin (*The Budget Gourmet* Slim Selects), 10 oz. | 290 |
| Marsala (*The Budget Gourmet*), 10 oz. | 250 |
| Marsala (*Tyson Gourmet Selection*), 10.5 oz. | 300 |
| mesquite (*Tyson Gourmet Selection*), 9.5 oz. | 320 |
| nibbles (*Swanson* Homestyle Recipe), 4.25 oz. | 340 |
| nibbles (*Swanson* Plump & Juicy), 3.25-oz. portion | 300 |
| and noodles (*Dining Lite*), 9 oz. | 240 |
| and noodles, homestyle (*Stouffer's*), 10 oz. | 310 |
| and noodles, homestyle (*Weight Watchers*), 9 oz. | 240 |
| nuggets: | |
| (*Banquet* Chicken Hot Bites), 2.63 oz. | 210 |
| (*Banquet* Platters), 6.4 oz. | 430 |
| (*Country Pride*), 3 oz. | 250 |
| (*Freezer Queen Deluxe Family Suppers*), 3 oz. | 270 |
| (*Pilgrim's Pride*), 3 oz. | 202 |
| (*Swanson* Plump & Juicy), 3 oz. | 230 |
| (*Tyson* Microwave), 3.5 oz. | 220 |
| (*Weight Watchers*), 5.9 oz. | 270 |
| breast, Southern-fried, w/barbecue sauce (*Banquet* Microwave Chicken Hot Bites), 4.5 oz. | 370 |
| w/cheddar (*Banquet* Chicken Hot Bites), 2.63 oz. | 250 |
| hot'n spicy (*Banquet* Chicken Hot Bites), 2.63 oz. | 250 |

| FOOD AND MEASURE | CALORIES |
|---|---|
| hot'n spicy, w/barbecue sauce (*Banquet* Microwave Chicken Hot Bites), 4.5 oz. | 360 |
| Southern-fried (*Banquet* Chicken Hot Bites), 2.63 oz. | 220 |
| Southern-fried, w/barbecue sauce (*Banquet* Microwave Chicken Hot Bites), 4.5 oz. | 370 |
| w/sweet and sour sauce (*Banquet* Microwave Chicken Hot Bites), 4.5 oz. | 360 |
| Oriental (*Lean Cuisine*), 9⅜ oz. | 230 |
| Oriental (*Tyson Gourmet Selection*), 10.25 oz. | 270 |
| Oriental, spicy (*La Choy Fresh & Lite*), 9.75 oz. | 270 |
| parmigiana (*Celentano*), 9 oz. | 330 |
| parmigiana (*Tyson Gourmet Selection*), 11.25 oz. | 380 |
| patties: | |
| (*Banquet* Platters), 7.5 oz. | 380 |
| (*Country Pride*), 3 oz. | 250 |
| (*Pilgrim's Pride*), 3 oz. | 205 |
| (*Tyson*), 2.6 oz. | 220 |
| (*Tyson* Thick & Crispy), 2.6 oz. | 220 |
| breast (*Banquet* Chicken Hot Bites), 2.63 oz. | 210 |
| breast, w/bun (*Banquet* Microwave Chicken Hot Bites), 4 oz. | 310 |
| breast, Southern-fried (*Country Pride*), 3 oz. | 240 |
| breast, Southern-fried (*Banquet* Chicken Hot Bites), 2.63 oz. | 210 |
| breast, Southern-fried (*Tyson*), 2.6 oz. | 220 |
| breast, Southern-fried, w/biscuit (*Banquet* Microwave Chicken Hot Bites), 4 oz. | 320 |
| Southern-fried (*Weight Watchers*), 6.5 oz. | 320 |
| piccata (*Tyson Gourmet Selection*), 9 oz. | 240 |
| pie: | |
| (*Banquet*), 7 oz. | 550 |
| (*Banquet* Supreme Microwave), 7 oz. | 430 |
| (*Morton*), 7 oz. | 420 |
| (*Stouffer's*), 10 oz. | 530 |
| (*Swanson* Homestyle Recipe), 8 oz. | 410 |
| (*Swanson* Pot Pie), 7 oz. | 380 |
| (*Swanson Hungry Man*), 16 oz. | 630 |
| primavera (*Celentano*), 11.5 oz. | 270 |
| primavera, and vegetable (*Banquet Cookin' Bags*), 4 oz. | 100 |
| primavera, and vegetable (*Banquet Family Entrees*), 7 oz. | 140 |
| sesame (*Right Course*), 10 oz. | 320 |
| sliced, gravy and (*Freezer Queen Cook-In-Pouch*), 5 oz. | 80 |
| steaks, chicken-fried (*Pilgrim's Pride*), 3 oz. | 183 |

| FOOD AND MEASURE | CALORIES |
|---|---|
| *Chicken entree, frozen, continued* | |
| sticks (*Banquet* Chicken Hot Bites), 2.63 oz. | 220 |
| sticks (*Country Pride*), 3 oz. | 240 |
| sweet and sour: | |
| (*Banquet Cookin' Bags*), 4 oz. | 130 |
| (*Tyson Gourmet Selection*), 11 oz. | 420 |
| w/rice (*The Budget Gourmet*), 10 oz. | 350 |
| w/rice (*Freezer Queen* Single Serve), 9 oz. | 300 |
| w/rice and vegetables (*La Choy Fresh & Lite*), 10 oz. | 260 |
| tenders (*Weight Watchers*), 10.19 oz. | 250 |
| tenderloins, in barbecue sauce (*Right Course*), 8.75 oz. | 270 |
| tenderloins, in peanut sauce (*Right Course*), 9.25 oz. | 330 |
| tenders (*Tyson* Microwave), 3.5 oz. | 230 |
| thighs and drumsticks (*Swanson*), 3.25 oz. | 290 |
| and vegetables, w/vermicelli (*Lean Cuisine*), 11.75 oz. | 270 |
| walnut, crunchy (*Chun King*), 13 oz. | 310 |
| wings (*Pilgrim's Pride* Wing Zappers), 3-oz. portion | 187 |
| wings, all varieties (*Tyson Flyers*), 3.5 oz. or 6–7 wings | 220 |
| wings, Southern-fried (*Pilgrim's Pride*), 3-oz. portion | 228 |

**Chicken entree,** packaged, 1 serving:

| | |
|---|---|
| Acapulco (*Hormel Top Shelf*) | 390 |
| breast of, glazed (*Hormel Top Shelf*) | 210 |
| sweet and sour (*Hormel Top Shelf*) | 270 |

**Chicken fat:**

| | |
|---|---|
| 1 oz. | 178 |

**Chicken frankfurter:**

| | |
|---|---|
| (*Health Valley* Weiners), 1 link | 96 |
| (*Longacre*), 1 oz. | 63 |
| batter-wrapped (*Tyson* Corn Dogs) 3.5 oz. | 280 |

**Chicken giblets:**

| | |
|---|---|
| broiler-fryer, simmered, 4 oz. | 178 |
| roaster, simmered, 4 oz. | 187 |
| capon, simmered, 4 oz. | 186 |

**Chicken gizzard:**

| | |
|---|---|
| broiler-fryer, simmered, 4 oz. | 172 |

| FOOD AND MEASURE | CALORIES |
|---|---|
| **Chicken gravy:** | |
| canned (*Franco-American*), 2 oz. | 45 |
| canned (*Heinz*), 2 oz. or ¼ cup | 35 |
| canned, w/chicken (*Hormel Great Beginnings*), 5 oz. | 147 |
| canned, giblet (*Franco-American*), 2 oz. | 30 |
| mix, prepared: | |
| (*French's* Gravy for Chicken), ¼ cup | 25 |
| (*Lawry's*), 1 cup | 99 |
| (*McCormick/Schilling*), ¼ cup | 22 |
| (*McCormick/Schilling* Lite), ¼ cup | 12 |
| **Chicken ham:** | |
| (*Pilgrim's Pride*), 1-oz. slice | 35 |
| **Chicken pie,** see "Chicken entree, frozen" | |
| **Chicken salad:** | |
| (*Longacre*), 1 oz. | 64 |
| (*Longacre* Saladfest), 1 oz. | 47 |
| **Chicken sandwich,** frozen: | |
| (*MicroMagic*), 4.5 oz. | 390 |
| barbecue (*Tyson* Microwave), 4 oz. | 230 |
| breast (*Tyson* Microwave), 3.5 oz. | 275 |
| mini (*Tyson* Microwave), 3.5 oz. | 230 |
| pocket (*Lean Pockets* Supreme), 1 pkg. | 280 |
| pocket, 'n cheddar (*Hot Pockets*), 5 oz. | 310 |
| pocket, Oriental (*Lean Pockets*), 1 pkg. | 250 |
| pocket, Parmesan (*Lean Pockets*), 1 pkg. | 270 |
| **Chicken sauce mix,** 1 pkg.: | |
| cacciatore (*McCormick/Schilling* Sauce Blends) | 132 |
| creole (*McCormick/Schilling* Sauce Blends) | 140 |
| curry (*McCormick/Schilling* Sauce Blends) | 152 |
| Dijon (*McCormick/Schilling* Sauce Blends) | 151 |
| Italian marinade (*McCormick/Schilling* Sauce Blends) | 120 |
| mesquite marinade (*McCormick/Schilling* Sauce Blends) | 132 |
| stir fry (*McCormick/Schilling* Sauce Blends) | 124 |
| sweet and sour (*McCormick/Schilling* Sauce Blends) | 204 |
| teriyaki (*McCormick/Schilling* Sauce Blends) | 172 |

| FOOD AND MEASURE | CALORIES |
|---|---|
| **Chicken seasoning and coating mix:** | |
| (*Featherweight*), ¼ pkg. | 18 |
| (*Golden Dipt*), 1 oz. | 90 |
| (*McCormick/Schilling* Bag'n Season), 1 pkg. | 177 |
| (*Shake'n Bake*), ¼ pouch | 80 |
| (*Shake'n Bake Oven Fry* Extra Crispy), ¼ pouch | 110 |
| barbecue (*Shake'n Bake*), ¼ pouch | 90 |
| homestyle (*Shake'n Bake Oven Fry*), ¼ pouch | 80 |
| **Chicken spread,** canned: | |
| (*Hormel*), ½ oz. | 30 |
| chunky (*Underwood* Light), 2⅛ oz. | 80 |
| chunky or smoky flavored (*Underwood*), 2⅛ oz. | 150 |
| **Chick-peas:** | |
| raw (*Arrowhead Mills*), 2 oz. | 200 |
| boiled, ½ cup | 134 |
| canned: | |
| (*Allens*), ½ cup | 110 |
| (*Old El Paso*), ½ cup | 190 |
| (*Progresso*), ½ cup | 110 |
| (*S&W/Nutradiet*), ½ cup | 100 |
| large (*S&W* Lite 50% Less Salt), ½ cup | 110 |
| **Chicory, witloof:** | |
| 1 head, 5–7" long, 2.1 oz. | 8 |
| trimmed, ½ cup | 7 |
| **Chicory greens:** | |
| untrimmed, 1 lb. | 87 |
| trimmed, chopped, ½ cup | 21 |
| **Chicory root:** | |
| 1 medium, 2.6 oz. | 44 |
| 1" pieces, ½ cup | 33 |
| **Chili,** canned: | |
| (*Chef Boyardee* Chili Mac), 7.5 oz. | 230 |
| (*Heinz* Chili Con Carne), 7.75 oz. | 350 |
| (*Heinz* Chili Mac), 7.5 oz. | 250 |
| (*Old El Paso*), 1 cup | 162 |

| FOOD AND MEASURE | CALORIES |
|---|---|
| w/beans: | |
| (*Dennison's,* 15 oz.), 7.5 oz. | 310 |
| (*Dennison's* Cook-Off), 7.5 oz. | 340 |
| (*Estee*), 7.5 oz. | 370 |
| (*Featherweight*), 7.5 oz. | 280 |
| (*Hormel,* 15 oz.), 7.5 oz. | 310 |
| (*Hormel Micro-Cup*), 7.5 oz. | 250 |
| (*Libby's,* 15 oz.), 7.5 oz. | 270 |
| (*Old El Paso*), 1 cup | 217 |
| (*Van Camp's*), 1 cup | 350 |
| (*Wolf* Brand), 1 scant cup | 350 |
| beef (*Chef Boyardee*), 7.5 oz. | 330 |
| chunky or hot (*Dennison's*), 7.5 oz. | 310 |
| extra spicy (*Wolf* Brand), 1 scant cup | 330 |
| hot (*Gebhardt*), 4 oz. | 189 |
| hot (*Heinz*), 7.75 oz. | 330 |
| hot (*Hormel,* 15 oz.), 7.5 oz. | 310 |
| w/out beans: | |
| (*Dennison's,* 15 oz.), 7.5 oz. | 300 |
| (*Hormel,* 15 oz.), 7.5 oz. | 370 |
| (*Libby's*), 7.5 oz. | 390 |
| (*Van Camp's*), 1 cup | 410 |
| (*Wolf* Brand), 1 cup | 390 |
| (*Wolf* Brand Chili-Mac), 1 scant cup | 320 |
| extra spicy (*Wolf* Brand), 1 scant cup | 360 |
| w/franks (*Van Camp's Chilee Weenee*), 1 cup | 310 |
| hot (*Hormel,* 15 oz.), 7.5 oz. | 370 |
| w/chicken, spicy (*Hain*), 7.5 oz. | 130 |
| vegetarian: | |
| w/out beans (*Gebhardt*), 4 oz. | 220 |
| w/lentils or beans (*Health Valley*), 4 oz. | 130 |
| spicy (*Hain*), 7.5 oz. | 160 |
| spicy (*Hain* Reduced Sodium), 7.5 oz. | 170 |
| spicy (*Natural Touch*), ⅔ cup | 230 |
| tempeh, spicy (*Hain*), 7.5 oz. | 160 |

## Chili dip:

| | |
|---|---|
| (*La Victoria*), 1 tbsp. | 6 |

| FOOD AND MEASURE | CALORIES |
|---|---|
| **Chili entree,** frozen: | |
| con carne (*Swanson* Homestyle Recipe), 8.25 oz. | 270 |
| con carne, w/beans (*Stouffer's*), 8.75 oz. | 260 |
| vegetarian (*Right Course*), 9.75 oz. | 280 |
| **Chili entree,** packaged: | |
| con carne suprema (*Hormel Top Shelf*), 1 serving | 320 |
| **Chili mix:** | |
| (*Gebhardt Chili Quik*), 1.5-oz. pkt. | 82 |
| w/beans, vegetarian, prepared (*Fantastic Foods*), ½ cup | 104 |
| **Chili pepper,** see "Pepper, chili, hot" | |
| **Chili powder:** | |
| (*Gebhardt*), 1 tsp. | 6 |
| hot or mild (*Tone's*), 1 tsp. | 8 |
| **Chili sauce:** | |
| (*Heinz*), 1 tbsp. | 17 |
| (*S&W Chili Makin's*), ½ cup | 100 |
| green, mild (*El Molino*), 2 tbsp. | 10 |
| hot dog (*Gebhardt*), 2 tbsp. | 20 |
| hot dog (*Wolf* Brand), 1.25 oz., approx. ⅙ cup | 40 |
| tomato (*Del Monte*), ¼ cup | 70 |
| **Chili seasoning mix:** | |
| (*Lawry's* Seasoning Blends), 1 pkg. | 143 |
| (*McCormick/Schilling*), ¼ pkg. | 27 |
| (*Old El Paso*), ⅕ pkg. | 21 |
| (*Tio Sancho*), 1.23 oz. | 109 |
| all varieties (*Hain*), ¼ pkg. | 30 |
| **Chimichanga,** frozen: | |
| beef (*Old El Paso*), 1 piece | 370 |
| chicken (*Old El Paso*), 1 piece | 360 |
| **Chimichanga dinner,** frozen: | |
| beef (*Old El Paso* Festive Dinners), 11 oz. | 540 |
| beef and cheese (*Old El Paso* Festive Dinners), 11 oz. | 510 |

| FOOD AND MEASURE | CALORIES |
| --- | --- |

**Chimichanga entree,** frozen:

| | |
| --- | --- |
| bean and cheese, or beef (*Old El Paso*), 1 pkg. | 380 |
| beef and pork (*Old El Paso*), 1 pkg. | 340 |
| chicken (*Old El Paso*), 1 pkg. | 370 |

**Chives:**

| | |
| --- | --- |
| fresh or freeze-dried, chopped, 1 tbsp. | 1 |

**Chocolate,** see "Candy"

**Chocolate, baking:**

| | |
| --- | --- |
| bars, 1 oz.: | |
| all varieties (*Baker's/Baker's German*) | 140 |
| semisweet (*Hershey's* Premium) | 140 |
| semisweet (*Nestlé*) | 160 |
| unsweetened (*Hershey's*) | 190 |
| unsweetened (*Nestlé*) | 180 |
| white (*Nestlé* Premier) | 160 |
| chips, ¼ cup, except as noted: | |
| all varieties (*Nestlé* Toll House Morsels), 1 oz. | 150 |
| milk (*Baker's*), 1 oz. | 140 |
| milk (*Baker's* Big Chip) | 240 |
| milk (*Hershey's*), 1 oz. | 150 |
| mint (*Hershey's*) | 230 |
| semisweet (*Baker's* Big Chip) | 220 |
| semisweet, regular or chocolate flavor (*Baker's*) | 200 |
| semisweet, regular or mini (*Hershey's*) | 220 |
| vanilla (white), milk (*Hershey's*) | 240 |
| chunks or pieces, 1 oz.: | |
| milk (*Hershey's* Chunks) | 160 |
| milk or semisweet (*Nestlé* Toll House *Treasures*) | 150 |
| semisweet (*Hershey's* Chunks) | 140 |
| white (*Nestlé* Toll House Premier Treasures) | 160 |
| premelted, unsweetened (*Nestlé Choco Bake*), 1 oz. | 190 |

**Chocolate drink,** see "Milk beverages"

**Chocolate milk,** see "Milk, chocolate"

| FOOD AND MEASURE | CALORIES |
|---|---|
| **Chocolate mousse:** | |
| frozen (*Weight Watchers*), ½ pkg., 2.5 oz. | 170 |
| mix, all varieties: | |
| prepared w/whole milk (*Jell-O Rich & Luscious*), ½ cup | 150 |
| prepared w/skim milk (*Weight Watchers*), ½ cup | 60 |
| **Chocolate syrup:** | |
| (*Estee*), 1 tbsp. | 20 |
| (*Hershey's*), 1 oz. or 2 tbsp. | 80 |
| (*Nestlé Quik*), 1.22 oz., approx. 2 tbsp. | 100 |
| **Chocolate topping,** see "Toppings, dessert" | |
| **Chops, vegetarian,** canned: | |
| (*Worthington Choplets*), 2 slices or 3.25 oz. | 100 |
| **Chow mein,** see specific entree listings | |
| **Chow mein noodles,** see "Noodle, Chinese" | |
| **Chowder,** see "Soup" | |
| **Chrysanthemum garland:** | |
| raw, 1″ pieces, ½ cup | 2 |
| boiled, drained, 1″ pieces, ½ cup | 10 |
| **Chub,** see "Cisco" | |
| **Cilantro,** see "Coriander" | |
| **Cinnamon,** ground: | |
| 1 tsp. | 6 |
| **Cinnamon-raisin danish,** 1 piece: | |
| (*Awrey's* Square), 3 oz. | 290 |
| (*Awrey's* Miniature), 1.5 oz. | 160 |
| frozen (*Pepperidge Farm*), 2.25 oz. | 250 |
| frozen (*Sara Lee* Individual), 1.3 oz. | 150 |
| refrigerated, w/icing (*Pillsbury*) | 150 |
| **Cisco,** meat only: | |
| raw, 4 oz. | 112 |
| smoked, 1 oz. | 50 |

| FOOD AND MEASURE | CALORIES |
|---|---|
| **Citrus fruit juice drink:** | |
| (*Hi-C* Citrus Cooler), 6 fl. oz. | 95 |
| chilled or frozen, diluted (*Five Alive*), 6 fl. oz. | 87 |
| **Citrus punch:** | |
| chilled or frozen, diluted (*Minute Maid*), 6 fl. oz. | 93 |
| **Citrus salad:** | |
| (*Florigold*), 8 oz. | 120 |
| **Clam,** mixed species, meat only: | |
| fresh, raw, 1 lb. | 335 |
| fresh, raw, 9 large or 20 small, 6.3 oz. | 133 |
| fresh, boiled, poached, or steamed, 4 oz. | 168 |
| canned, chopped or minced: | |
| (*Gorton's*), ½ can | 70 |
| (*Progresso*), ½ cup | 70 |
| w/liquid (*Doxsee*), 6.5 oz. | 100 |
| w/liquid (*Orleans*), 6.5 oz. | 100 |
| **Clam chowder,** see "Soup" | |
| **Clam dip:** | |
| (*Kraft*), 2 tbsp. | 60 |
| (*Kraft* Premium), 2 tbsp. | 45 |
| **Clam dip,** 2 tbsp.: | |
| (*Breakstone's/Breakstone's* Gourmet Chesapeake) | 50 |
| (*Kraft*) | 60 |
| (*Kraft* Premium) | 45 |
| **Clam entree,** frozen: | |
| battered, fried (*Mrs. Paul's*), 2.5 oz. | 200 |
| strips, crunchy (*Gorton's* Microwave Specialty), 3.5 oz. | 330 |
| **Clam juice:** | |
| (*Doxsee*), 3 fl. oz. | 4 |
| (*Snow's*), 3 fl. oz. | 4 |
| **Clam sauce:** | |
| canned: | |
| red (*Buitoni*), approx. 5 oz. | 190 |
| red (*Ferrara*), 4 oz. | 70 |

| FOOD AND MEASURE | CALORIES |
|---|---|
| *Clam sauce, canned, continued* | |
| red (*Progresso*), ½ cup | 70 |
| white (*Ferrara*), 4 oz. | 80 |
| white (*Progresso*), ½ cup | 110 |
| white (*Progresso* Authentic Pasta Sauces), ½ cup | 130 |
| refrigerated, red (*Contadina Fresh*), 7.5 oz. | 120 |
| refrigerated, white (*Contadina Fresh*), 6 oz. | 290 |

**Cloves:**

| | |
|---|---|
| 1 tsp. | 7 |

**Cocktail sauce** (see also "Seafood sauce"):

| | |
|---|---|
| (*Del Monte*), ¼ cup | 70 |
| (*Estee*), 1 tbsp. | 10 |
| (*Great Impressions* Regular/Low Salt), 1 tbsp. | 21 |
| (*Great Impressions* Brandy Glow), 1 tbsp. | 68 |
| (*Sauceworks*), 1 tbsp. | 14 |
| (*Stokely*), 1 tbsp. | 18 |
| regular or extra hot (*Golden Dipt*), 1 tbsp. | 20 |
| seafood (*Heinz*), 1 tbsp. | 17 |

**Cocoa, powder:**

| | |
|---|---|
| (*Bensdorp*), 1 oz. | 130 |
| (*Hershey's*), 1 oz. or ⅓ cup | 120 |
| (*Hershey's* European), 1 oz. | 90 |
| (*Nestlé*), 1.5 oz. or ½ cup | 180 |

**Cocoa mix:**

| | |
|---|---|
| (*Carnation* 70-Calorie), 1 pkt. | 70 |
| (*Hills Bros*), 2 tbsp. | 110 |
| (*Hills Bros* Sugar Free), 3 tsp. | 60 |
| (*Swiss Miss* Lite), 1 pkt. | 70 |
| (*Swiss Miss* Sugar Free), 1 pkt. | 50 |
| all varieties (*Carnation*), 1 pkt. | 110 |
| all varieties (*Carnation* Sugar Free), 1 pkt. | 50 |
| all varieties (*Swiss Miss*), 1 oz. | 110 |
| chocolate, milk (*Swiss Miss* Sugar Free), 1 pkt. | 60 |
| chocolate, milk, and marshmallow (*Weight Watchers*), 1 pkt. | 60 |
| w/mini marshmallows (*Swiss Miss* Sugar Free), 1 pkt. | 50 |

| FOOD AND MEASURE | CALORIES |
|---|---|
| **Coconut,** mature kernel, meat only: | |
| fresh, 1 oz. | 100 |
| fresh, shredded or grated, 1 cup | 283 |
| dried, sweetened: | |
| flaked (*Baker's Angel Flake*), ⅓ cup | 120 |
| flaked, toasted (*Baker's Angel Flake*), ⅓ cup | 200 |
| flaked, canned (*Baker's Angel Flake*), ⅓ cup | 110 |
| shredded (*Baker's* Premium Shred), ⅓ cup | 140 |
| **Coconut cream:** | |
| canned, sweetened (*Coco Lopez*), 2 tbsp. | 120 |
| **Cod,** meat only: | |
| fresh, raw, 4 oz. | 93 |
| fresh, baked, broiled, or microwaved, 4 oz. | 119 |
| canned, w/liquid, 4 oz. | 119 |
| dried, salted, 1 oz. | 81 |
| frozen (*Booth*), 4 oz. | 89 |
| frozen (*Gorton's Fishmarket Fresh*), 5 oz. | 110 |
| frozen (*Van de Kamp's* Natural), 4 oz. | 90 |
| **Cod entree,** frozen: | |
| au gratin (*Booth*), 9.5 oz. | 280 |
| au gratin, w/broccoli (*Weight Watchers*), 9.25 oz. | 200 |
| breaded (*Van de Kamp's* Light), 1 piece | 250 |
| Florentine (*Booth*), 9.5 oz. | 244 |
| w/lemon butter sauce and rice (*Booth*), 9.5 oz. | 567 |
| w/mushroom sauce and rice (*Booth*), 9.5 oz. | 280 |
| nuggets, crunchy (*Frionor Bunch O'Crunch*), 8 pieces | 320 |
| oven-fried (*Weight Watchers*), 7.08 oz. | 240 |
| **Cod liver oil:** | |
| all varieties (*Hain*), 1 tbsp. | 120 |
| **Coffee,** prepared: | |
| (*Chock Full O'Nuts* Regular/Decaffeinated), 6 fl. oz. | 2 |
| instant, 8 fl. oz.: | |
| (*Nescafe/Nescafe Decaf*) | 4 |
| (*Nescafe* Classic/Brava/Silka) | 4 |
| w/chicory (*Nescafe* Mountain Blend/Regular/Decaf) | 6 |
| w/chicory (*Sunrise*) | 6 |
| freeze-dried, all varieties (*Taster's Choice*) | 4 |

| FOOD AND MEASURE | CALORIES |
|---|---|
| **Coffee, flavored,** prepared, 6 fl. oz.: | |
| all flavors, except café Français (*General Foods* International Sugar Free) | 30 |
| café Amaretto (*General Foods* International) | 50 |
| café Français (*General Foods* International) | 60 |
| café Français (*General Foods* International Sugar Free) | 35 |
| café Irish creme (*General Foods* International) | 50 |
| café Vienna (*General Foods* International) | 60 |
| café Vienna (*Hills Bros* Café Coffees) | 60 |
| chocolate, double Dutch (*General Foods* International) | 50 |
| chocolate mint, Dutch (*General Foods* International) | 50 |
| mocha (*General Foods* International Suisse Mocha) | 50 |
| mocha (*MJB*) | 52 |
| mocha, banana nut (*MJB* Sugar Free) | 39 |
| mocha, cherry or mint (*MJB*) | 53 |
| mocha, fudge (*MJB* Sugar Free) | 39 |
| mocha mint (*MJB* Sugar Free) | 37 |
| mocha, Swiss (*Hills Bros* Café Coffees) | 60 |
| mocha, Swiss (*Hills Bros* Café Coffees Sugar Free) | 40 |
| mocha, vanilla (*MJB* Sugar Free) | 39 |
| orange cappuccino (*General Foods* International) | 60 |
| orange Capri (*Hills Bros* Café Coffees) | 60 |
| **Coffee, substitute** (cereal grain beverage): | |
| (*Kaffree Roma*), 8 fl. oz. | 6 |
| (*Pero*), 1 serving, powder | 4 |
| (*Pionier*), 1 serving, powder | 6 |
| regular or coffee flavor (*Postum* Instant), 6 fl. oz. | 12 |
| **Coffee cake,** see "Cake" | |
| **Coffee liqueur:** | |
| 53 proof, 1 fl. oz. | 117 |
| cream, 34 proof, 1 fl. oz. | 102 |
| **Coleslaw dressing:** | |
| (*Miracle Whip*), 1 tbsp. | 70 |
| **Collards:** | |
| fresh, raw, chopped, ½ cup | 6 |
| fresh, boiled, drained, chopped, ½ cup | 17 |
| canned, chopped (*Allens*), ½ cup | 20 |

| FOOD AND MEASURE | CALORIES |
|---|---|
| canned, chopped, w/pork (*Luck's*), 7.5 oz. | 90 |
| frozen, chopped (*Seabrook*), 3.3 oz. | 25 |
| frozen, chopped (*Southern*), 3.5 oz. | 30 |

**Cookie,** 1 piece, except as noted:

| | |
|---|---|
| almond (*Stella D'Oro* Breakfast Treats) | 101 |
| almond (*Stella D'Oro* Chinese Dessert) | 169 |
| almond toast (*Stella D'Oro* Mandel) | 58 |
| almond-date (*Health Valley Fruit Jumbos*) | 70 |
| amaranth (*Health Valley Amaranth Cookies*) | 90 |
| animal crackers (*Barnum's*), 5 pieces, ½ oz. | 60 |
| animal crackers (*Keebler*), 5 pieces, approx. ½ oz. | 70 |
| anise (*Stella D'Oro* Anisette Sponge) | 51 |
| anise (*Stella D'Oro* Anisette Toast) | 46 |
| anise (*Stella D'Oro* Anisette Toast Jumbo) | 109 |
| apple bar (*Apple Newtons*) | 70 |
| apple bar, Dutch (*Stella D'Oro*) | 112 |
| apple pastry, dietetic (*Stella D'Oro*) | 86 |
| apple 'n' raisin (*Archway*) | 120 |
| apricot-almond (*Health Valley Fancy Fruit Chunks*) | 45 |
| apricot-raspberry (*Pepperidge Farm* Fruit Cookies) | 50 |
| apricot-raspberry (*Pepperidge Farm* Zurich) | 60 |
| arrowroot biscuit (*National*) | 20 |
| brownie chocolate nut (*Pepperidge Farm* Old Fashioned) | 55 |
| brownie cream sandwich (*Pepperidge Farm* Capri) | 80 |
| butter flavor (*Pepperidge Farm* Chessmen) | 45 |
| butter flavor, chocolate-coated (*Keebler E.L. Fudge*) | 40 |
| caramel patties (*FFV*) | 75 |
| (*Carr's Muesli*) | 84 |
| chocolate: | |
| (*Stella D'Oro Castelets*) | 64 |
| (*Stella D'Oro Margherite*) | 72 |
| chocolate walnut (*Pepperidge Farm* Beacon Hill) | 120 |
| creme wafer (*Featherweight*) | 20 |
| fudge (*Stella D'Oro* Swiss) | 68 |
| fudge mint (*Keebler Grasshopper*) | 35 |
| middles (*Nabisco*) | 80 |
| snaps (*Nabisco*), 4 pieces or ½ oz. | 70 |
| wafer (*Nabisco* Famous Wafers), ½ oz. or 2½ pieces | 70 |
| chocolate chip: | |
| (*Almost Home* Real Chocolate Chip) | 60 |

| FOOD AND MEASURE | CALORIES |
|---|---|
| *Cookie, chocolate chip, continued* | |
| (*Archway*) | 50 |
| (*Chips Ahoy!* Pure Chocolate Chip) | 50 |
| (*Drake's*) | 70 |
| (*Duncan Hines*) | 55 |
| (*Grandma's* Big Cookies) | 185 |
| (*Keebler Chips Deluxe/Keebler Soft Batch*) | 80 |
| (*Pepperidge Farm* Old Fashioned) | 50 |
| (*Tastykake* Soft'n Chewy) 1.4 oz. | 174 |
| bar (*Tastykake*) | 193 |
| w/candy-coated chocolate (*Keebler Rainbow Chips Deluxe*) | 80 |
| chewy (*Chips Ahoy!*) | 60 |
| chocolate (*Drake's*) | 65 |
| chocolate (*Tastykake* Soft'n Chewy), 1.4 oz. | 171 |
| chocolate walnut (*Chips Ahoy!* Selections) | 95 |
| w/chocolate middle (*Keebler Magic Middles*) | 80 |
| chunk (*Pepperidge Farm* Nantucket) | 120 |
| chunk pecan (*Chips Ahoy!* Selections) | 100 |
| chunk pecan (*Pepperidge Farm* Chesapeake) | 120 |
| chunk pecan (*Pepperidge Farm* Special Collection) | 70 |
| chunky or chocolate chunk (*Chips Ahoy!* Selections) | 90 |
| fudge (*Almost Home*) | 70 |
| fudge (*Grandma's* Big Cookies) | 175 |
| milk (*Duncan Hines*) | 55 |
| milk, macadamia (*Pepperidge Farm* Sausalito) | 120 |
| milk, macadamia (*Pepperidge Farm* Special Collection) | 70 |
| mini (*Chips Ahoy!*), 6 pieces | 70 |
| mint or walnut (*Keebler Soft Batch*) | 80 |
| snaps (*Nabisco*), 3 pieces, ½ oz. | 70 |
| sprinkled (*Chips Ahoy!*) | 50 |
| striped (*Chips Ahoy!*) | 90 |
| toffee (*Pepperidge Farm* Old Fashioned) | 50 |
| chocolate sandwich: | |
| (*Oreo*) | 50 |
| (*Oreo Big Stuf*) | 250 |
| (*Oreo Double Stuf*) | 70 |
| fudge-covered (*Oreo*) | 110 |
| fudge creme-filled (*Keebler* Chocolate Creme Sandwich) | 80 |
| fudge w/fudge creme filling (*Keebler E.L. Fudge*) | 70 |
| fudge w/peanut butter creme filling (*Keebler E.L. Fudge*) | 50 |
| white fudge-covered (*Oreo*) | 110 |

| FOOD AND MEASURE | CALORIES |
|---|---|
| chocolate-filled sandwich: | |
| (*Pepperidge Farm* Brussels) | 55 |
| (*Pepperidge Farm* Lido) | 90 |
| (*Pepperidge Farm* Milano/Orleans) | 60 |
| fudge creme (*Keebler E.L. Fudge*) | 60 |
| mint (*Pepperidge Farm* Brussels Mint) | 65 |
| mint or orange (*Pepperidge Farm* Milano) | 75 |
| chocolate peanut bar (*Ideal*) | 90 |
| cinnamon-raisin nut bar (*Cinnamon Raisin Nut Newtons*) | 60 |
| cinnamon-vanilla wafer (*Nabisco Nilla* Wafers), ½ oz. | 60 |
| coconut (*Drake's*) | 65 |
| coconut, chocolate-filled (*Pepperidge Farm* Tahiti) | 90 |
| coconut macaroon (*Stella D'Oro*) | 60 |
| coffee, filled (*Pepperidge Farm* Cappuccino) | 50 |
| date pecan (*Health Valley Fancy Fruit Chunks*) | 45 |
| date pecan (*Pepperidge Farm* Kitchen Hearth) | 55 |
| devil's food (*FFV* Trolley Cakes) | 60 |
| devil's food cakes (*Nabisco*) | 70 |
| egg biscuit: | |
| (*Stella D'Oro*) | 43 |
| (*Stella D'Oro Anginetti*) | 31 |
| (*Stella D'Oro* Jumbo) | 47 |
| dietetic (*Stella D'Oro* Kitchel) | 8 |
| Roman (*Stella D'Oro*) | 137 |
| sugared (*Stella D'Oro*) | 75 |
| (*FFV* T.C. Rounds/Tango) | 80 |
| fig bar (*Fig Newtons*) | 60 |
| fig bar (*Keebler*) | 60 |
| fig bar, vanilla or whole wheat (*FFV*) | 70 |
| fig pastry, dietetic (*Stella D'Oro*) | 89 |
| fruit (*Health Valley Fruit & Fitness*) | 40 |
| fruit slices (*Stella D'Oro*) | 60 |
| fruit, tropical (*Health Valley Fancy Fruit Chunks*) | 40 |
| fruit, tropical (*Health Valley Fruit Jumbos*) | 70 |
| fudge bar (*Tastykake*) | 205 |
| fudge bar, caramel and peanut (*Heyday*) | 110 |
| ginger (*Pepperidge Farm* Gingerman) | 35 |
| ginger boys (*FFV*), 1.25-oz. pkg. | 150 |
| gingersnaps (*Archway*, 80/pkg.) | 25 |
| gingersnaps (*Archway*, 54/pkg.) | 35 |
| gingersnaps (*FFV*) | 26 |

| FOOD AND MEASURE | CALORIES |
|---|---|
| *Cookie, continued* | |
| gingersnaps (*Nabisco* Old Fashioned) | 30 |
| graham cracker: | |
| (*Keebler*), 4 pieces, approx. ½ oz. | 70 |
| (*Nabisco*) | 30 |
| (*Regal*) | 70 |
| (*Rokeach*) | 15 |
| all varieties (*Honey Maid* Graham Bites), 11 pieces | 60 |
| all varieties (*Nabisco Teddy Grahams*), 11 pieces | 60 |
| all varieties, w/vanilla cream (*Nabisco Teddy Grahams Bearwich's*), 4 pieces | 70 |
| amaranth (*Health Valley*), 7 pieces | 110 |
| chocolate (*Keebler Thin Bits*), 12 pieces | 70 |
| chocolate (*Nabisco*) | 60 |
| cinnamon (*Keebler* Alpha Grahams), 6 pieces | 70 |
| cinnamon (*Keebler* Cinnamon Crisp), 4 pieces | 70 |
| cinnamon (*Keebler Thin Bits*), 12 pieces | 70 |
| cinnamon or honey (*Honey Maid*) | 30 |
| fudge-covererd (*Keebler* Deluxe) | 45 |
| w/fudge (*Nabisco Cookies'N Fudge*) | 45 |
| honey (*Keebler* Honey Grahams), 4 pieces | 70 |
| honey or oat bran (*Health Valley*), 7 pieces | 130 |
| wheat (*Carr's* Home Wheat Graham) | 74 |
| hazelnut (*Pepperidge Farm* Old Fashioned) | 55 |
| (*Health Valley The Great Wheat Free Cookie*), 4 pieces | 130 |
| honey, all varieties (*Health Valley Honey Jumbos*) | 70 |
| jelly tarts (*FFV*) | 60 |
| lemon nut crunch (*Pepperidge Farm* Old Fashioned) | 55 |
| marshmallow, chocolate cake (*Mallomars*) | 60 |
| marshmallow, chocolate cake (*Pinwheels*) | 130 |
| marshmallow, fudge cake (*Nabisco* Puffs) | 90 |
| marshmallow, fudge cake (*Nabisco* Twirls) | 140 |
| mint sandwich (*FFV*) | 80 |
| mint sandwich (*Mystic Mint*) | 90 |
| molasses (*Archway*) | 100 |
| molasses (*Grandma's* Old Time Big Cookies) | 160 |
| molasses (*Nabisco Pantry*) | 80 |
| molasses crisps (*Pepperidge Farm* Old Fashioned) | 35 |
| oat bran, fruit (*Health Valley Oat Bran Fruit Jumbos*) | 70 |
| oat bran, fruit and nut (*Health Valley*) | 55 |
| oat bran, raisin (*Awrey's*) | 100 |

| FOOD AND MEASURE | CALORIES |
|---|---|
| oat bran, raisin (*Health Valley Fancy Fruit Chunks*) | 45 |
| oatmeal: | |
| (*Archway*) | 110 |
| (*Archway* Ruth's Golden) | 120 |
| (*Drake's*) | 60 |
| (*FFV*) | 26 |
| (*Keebler* Old Fashioned) | 80 |
| apple-filled (*Archway*) | 90 |
| apple spice (*Grandma's* Big Cookies) | 165 |
| chocolate chunk (*Chips Ahoy!* Selections) | 95 |
| w/chocolate middle (*Keebler Magic Middles*) | 80 |
| date-filled (*Archway*) | 100 |
| iced (*Archway*) | 140 |
| Irish (*Pepperidge Farm* Old Fashioned) | 45 |
| milk chocolate (*Pepperidge Farm* Dakota) | 110 |
| oatmeal raisin: | |
| (*Almost Home*) | 70 |
| (*Duncan Hines*) | 55 |
| (*Keebler Soft Batch*) | 70 |
| (*Pepperidge Farm* Old Fashioned) | 55 |
| (*Pepperidge Farm* Santa Fe) | 100 |
| (*Tastykake* Soft'n Chewy), 2 pieces | 161 |
| bar (*Tastykake*) | 212 |
| oatmeal raisin or oatmeal raisin bran (*Archway*) | 100 |
| peach-apricot bar, vanilla or whole wheat (*FFV*) | 70 |
| peach-apricot pastry (*Stella D'Oro*) | 93 |
| peach-apricot pastry, dietetic (*Stella D'Oro*) | 87 |
| peanut (*Health Valley Fancy Peanut Chunks*) | 50 |
| peanut butter: | |
| (*Grandma's* Big Cookies) | 205 |
| chocolate chip (*Keebler Soft Batch*) | 80 |
| chocolate-filled (*Pepperidge Farm* Nassau) | 80 |
| cream-filled (*Pitter Patter*) | 90 |
| milk chocolate chunk (*Pepperidge Farm* Cheyenne) | 110 |
| nut (*Keebler Soft Batch*) | 80 |
| peanut butter sandwich (*FFV*) | 85 |
| peanut butter sandwich (*Nutter Butter*) | 70 |
| peanut creme patties (*Nutter Butter*) | 40 |
| pecan crunch (*Archway*) | 60 |
| praline pecan (*FFV*) | 40 |
| prune pastry, dietetic (*Stella D'Oro*) | 95 |

| FOOD AND MEASURE | CALORIES |
|---|---|
| *Cookie, continued* | |
| raisin (*Stella D'Oro* Golden Bars) | 109 |
| raisin, soft (*Grandma's* Big Cookies) | 160 |
| raisin bar, iced (*Keebler*) | 80 |
| raisin bran (*Pepperidge Farm* Kitchen Hearth) | 55 |
| raisin nut (*Health Valley Fruit Jumbos*) | 70 |
| raisin oatmeal (*Archway*) | 50 |
| raspberry bar (*Raspberry Newtons*) | 70 |
| raspberry-filled (*Pepperidge Farm* Chantilly) | 80 |
| raspberry-filled (*Pepperidge Farm* Linzer) | 120 |
| sesame (*Stella D'Oro Regina*) | 48 |
| sesame, dietetic (*Stella D'Oro Regina*) | 41 |
| shortbread: | |
| (*Lorna Doone*), 3 pieces or ½ oz. | 70 |
| (*Pepperidge Farm* Old Fashioned) | 75 |
| w/chocolate cream center (*Keebler Magic Middles*) | 80 |
| country (*FFV*) | 70 |
| fudge-striped (*Keebler* Fudge Stripes) | 50 |
| fudge-striped (*Nabisco Cookies'N Fudge*) | 60 |
| pecan (*Nabisco*) | 80 |
| pecan (*Pecan Sandies*) | 80 |
| pecan (*Pepperidge Farm* Old Fashioned) | 70 |
| vanilla (*Tastykake*), 4 pieces | 55 |
| spice drops (*Stella D'Oro* Pfeffernusse) | 35 |
| (*Stella D'Oro Angel Bars*) | 76 |
| (*Stella D'Oro Angel Wings*) | 74 |
| (*Stella D'Oro Angelica Goodies*) | 106 |
| (*Stella D'Oro Como Delight*) | 145 |
| strawberry bar (*Strawberry Newtons*) | 70 |
| strawberry-filled (*Pepperidge Farm* Fruit Cookies) | 50 |
| sugar (*Almost Home* Old Fashioned) | 70 |
| sugar (*Pepperidge Farm* Old Fashioned) | 50 |
| sugar wafer (*Biscos*), 4 pieces or ½ oz. | 70 |
| tea biscuit (*Social Tea*) | 20 |
| tofu (*Health Valley The Great Tofu Cookie*) | 45 |
| vanilla: | |
| (*Pepperidge Farm* Bordeaux/Pirouettes) | 35 |
| (*Stella D'Oro Castelets/Stella D'Oro Margherite*) | 72 |
| chocolate-coated (*Pepperidge Farm* Orleans) | 30 |
| chocolate nut-coated (*Pepperidge Farm* Geneva) | 65 |
| sugar wafer (*Tastykake*), 10 pieces | 34 |

| FOOD AND MEASURE | CALORIES |
|---|---|
| wafer (*Archway*) | 30 |
| wafer (*FFV*), 1 oz., approx. 8 pieces | 130 |
| wafer (*Nabisco Nilla* Wafers), ½ oz. | 60 |
| wafer, golden (*Keebler*) | 20 |
| vanilla creme sandwich (*Cameo*) | 70 |
| vanilla creme sandwich (*Keebler* French Vanilla Creme) | 80 |
| vanilla creme sandwich (*Nabisco Cookie Break*) | 50 |
| vanilla creme sandwich (*Nabisco Giggles*) | 60 |
| wafer, brown-edged (*Nabisco*), ½ oz. | 70 |
| wafer, creme, fudge-covered (*Keebler Fudge Sticks*) | 50 |
| wafer, fudge-striped (*Nabisco Cookies'N Fudge*) | 70 |
| waffle cremes (*Biscos*) | 35 |

**Cookie, ready-to-bake,** 2 pieces:

| | |
|---|---|
| all varieties, except oatmeal raisin (*Pillsbury*) | 140 |
| chocolate chip (*Nestlé* Toll House Ready To Bake) | 150 |
| chocolate chip, w/nuts (*Nestlé* Toll House Ready To Bake) | 160 |
| oatmeal raisin (*Nestlé* Toll House Ready To Bake) | 130 |
| oatmeal raisin (*Pillsbury*) | 120 |

**Cookie mix,** prepared, 2 pieces:

| | |
|---|---|
| all varieties, except peanut butter (*Duncan Hines*) | 130 |
| chocolate chip (*Betty Crocker Big Batch*) | 120 |
| peanut butter (*Duncan Hines*) | 140 |

**Coriander:**

| | |
|---|---|
| fresh, ¼ cup | 1 |
| dried, leaf, 1 tsp. | 2 |
| dried, seed (*Spice Islands*), 1 tsp. | 6 |

**Corn,** sweet:

| | |
|---|---|
| fresh, raw, kernels, ½ cup | 66 |
| fresh, boiled, drained, kernels, ½ cup | 89 |
| canned, kernel, ½ cup: | |
| (*Del Monte* Regular/No Salt Added Vacuum Pack) | 90 |
| (*Green Giant* Delicorn) | 80 |
| (*Green Giant/Green Giant Niblets* Vacuum Pack) | 80 |
| (*S&W/Nutradiet*) | 80 |
| (*Stokely/Stokely* Vacuum Pack) | 90 |
| golden (*Del Monte* No Salt Added) | 80 |
| golden (*Stokely* No Salt or Sugar Added) | 80 |

| FOOD AND MEASURE | CALORIES |
|---|---|
| *Corn, canned, continued* | |
| golden or white (*Del Monte*) | 70 |
| young tender (*S&W* Premium) | 90 |
| canned, cream-style, ½ cup: | |
| (*Green Giant*) | 100 |
| (*S&W/Nutradiet*) | 100 |
| (*S&W* Premium Homestyle No Starch Added) | 120 |
| (*S&W* Premium Homestyle Starch Added) | 105 |
| golden (*Del Monte* Regular/No Salt Added) | 80 |
| golden or white (*Stokely*) | 100 |
| white (*Del Monte*) | 90 |
| canned, w/peppers (*Green Giant Mexicorn*) | 80 |
| frozen, on cob: | |
| (*Birds Eye*), 1 ear | 120 |
| (*Birds Eye Big Ears*), 1 ear | 160 |
| (*Birds Eye Little Ears*), 2 ears | 130 |
| (*Green Giant* One Serving), 2 half ears | 120 |
| (*Green Giant Nibblers*), 1 ear | 120 |
| (*Green Giant Nibblers* Supersweet), 2 ears | 90 |
| (*Green Giant Niblet Ears* Supersweet), 1 ear | 90 |
| (*Ore-Ida*), 1 ear | 180 |
| (*Ore-Ida Mini-Gold*), 2 ears | 180 |
| (*Southern*), 5″ ear | 140 |
| baby (*Birds Eye* Deluxe), 2.6 oz. | 25 |
| frozen, kernel: | |
| (*Birds Eye* Sweet/Tender Sweet Deluxe), 3.3 oz. | 80 |
| (*Green Giant Harvest Fresh Niblets*), ½ cup | 80 |
| (*Green Giant Niblets*), ½ cup | 90 |
| (*Green Giant Niblets* Supersweet), ½ cup | 60 |
| cut (*Birds Eye* Portion Pack), 3 oz. | 70 |
| cut (*Southern*), 3.5 oz. | 98 |
| cut (*Stokely Singles*), 3 oz. | 75 |
| cut or white (*Seabrook*), 3.3 oz. | 80 |
| petite (*Birds Eye* Deluxe), 2.6 oz. | 70 |
| white (*Green Giant*), ½ cup | 90 |
| white, shoepeg (*Green Giant Harvest Fresh*), ½ cup | 90 |
| frozen, cream-style (*Green Giant*), ½ cup | 110 |
| frozen, in butter sauce: | |
| (*The Budget Gourmet* Side Dish), 5.5 oz. | 190 |
| (*Green Giant Niblets*), ½ cup | 100 |
| (*Green Giant Niblets* One Serving), 4.5 oz. | 120 |

| FOOD AND MEASURE | CALORIES |
|---|---|
| (*Stokely Singles*), 4 oz. | 110 |
| on cob (*Stokely Singles*), 1 ear | 70 |
| golden or white (*Green Giant*), ½ cup | 100 |
| tender sweet (*Birds Eye* Combinations), 3.3 oz. | 90 |
| frozen, in sauce (*The Budget Gourmet* Side Dish), 5.75 oz. | 140 |
| packaged, w/green beans, carrots, and pasta, in tomato sauce (*Green Giant Pantry Express*) | 80 |

**Corn, whole-grain:**

| | |
|---|---|
| blue or yellow (*Arrowhead Mills*), 2 oz. | 210 |

**Corn bran,** crude:

| | |
|---|---|
| 1 oz. | 64 |

**Corn cake:**

| | |
|---|---|
| (*Quaker* Grain Cakes), .32-oz. piece | 35 |

**Corn chips, puffs, and similar snacks:**

| | |
|---|---|
| (*Azteca* Unsalted) | 140 |
| (*Bachman*) | 160 |
| (*Bugles*) | 150 |
| (*Dipsy Doodles* Rippled Corn Chips) | 160 |
| (*Featherweight* Low Salt) | 170 |
| (*Fritos/Fritos* Dip Size) | 150 |
| (*Fritos Crisp'n Thin*) | 160 |
| (*Health Valley* Regular/No Salt Added) | 160 |
| (*Planters*) | 160 |
| (*Wise* Corn Chips or Crunchies) | 160 |
| (*Wise Corn Ridgies/Toasted Corn Spirals*) | 160 |
| all varieties (*Corn Snackers*), .5-oz. pkg. | 60 |
| barbecue flavor (*Bachman* BBQ) | 150 |
| barbecue flavor (*Fritos* Bar-B-Q) | 150 |
| blue (*Arrowhead Mills* Corn Curls Regular/Unsalted) | 120 |
| chili cheese (*Fritos*) | 160 |
| nacho cheese (*Wise Corn Spirals*) | 160 |
| ranch (*Fritos Wild'n Mild*) | 150 |
| tortilla, see "tortilla chips," below | |
| yellow corn (*Arrowhead Mills*), ¾ oz. | 90 |
| crisps and puffs, cheese-flavored: | |
| (*Chee•tos* Puffs/Puffed Balls) | 160 |
| (*Cheez Doodles* Baked Corn Puffs) | 150 |
| (*Cheez Doodles* Fried Corn Puffs) | 160 |

| FOOD AND MEASURE | CALORIES |
|---|---|
| *Corn chips, puffs, and similar snacks, crisps and puffs, continued* | |
| (*Featherweight* Cheese Curls Low Salt) | 150 |
| (*Jax* Baked) | 140 |
| (*Jax* Crunchy) | 160 |
| (*Planters* Cheez Balls/Curls) | 160 |
| (*Wise Cheez Waffies*) | 140 |
| cheddar cheese (*Health Valley*) | 160 |
| crunchy (*Chee•tos*) | 150 |
| crunchy (*Chee•tos* Light) | 140 |
| nacho cheese (*Bugles*) | 160 |
| tortilla chips: | |
| (*Buenitos Tortilla Chips* Regular/No Salt Added) | 150 |
| (*Featherweight* Round/Nacho Low Salt) | 150 |
| (*La Famous* Regular/No Salt Added) | 140 |
| (*Laura Scudder's* Restaurant Style Lightly Salted) | 140 |
| (*Old El Paso Nachips*) | 150 |
| (*Tostitos*) | 140 |
| all varieties (*Bachman* Regular/No Salt) | 140 |
| all varieties (*Doritos*) | 140 |
| all varieties (*Doritos* Light) | 120 |
| blue (*Bearitos* Organic) | 146 |
| blue (*Bearitos* Organic No Salt) | 137 |
| crispy (*Old El Paso*) | 150 |
| nacho (*Bravos* Rounds) | 150 |
| nacho (*Bravos* Strips) | 140 |
| nacho (*Laura Scudder's* Triangles) | 140 |
| nacho (*Tio Sancho*), ½ oz. | 70 |
| nacho, jalapeño flavor (*Bravos*) | 150 |
| nacho, jalapeño flavor (*Laura Scudder's* Strips) | 150 |
| nacho, sharp (*Tostitos*) | 150 |
| picante flavor (*Laura Scudder's* Restaurant Strips) | 150 |
| ranch (*Eagle*) | 140 |
| sesame (*Hain* Regular/No Salt Added) | 140 |
| sesame cheese or taco style (*Hain*) | 160 |
| yellow corn (*Bearitos* Organic) | 143 |
| yellow corn (*Bearitos* Organic No Salt) | 148 |

**Corn flake crumbs:**

| | |
|---|---|
| (*Kellogg's*), 1 oz. | 100 |

**Corn Flour,** see "Flour"

| FOOD AND MEASURE | CALORIES |
|---|---|
| **Corn fritter,** frozen: | |
| (*Mrs. Paul's*), 2 pieces | 240 |
| **Corn grits,** dry: | |
| (*Albers* Hominy Quick Grits), ¼ cup | 150 |
| (*Arrowhead Mills*), 2 oz. | 200 |
| enriched (*Quaker/Aunt Jemima* Regular/Quick), 3 tbsp. | 101 |
| instant, 1 pkt.: | |
| w/imitation bacon bits (*Quaker*) | 101 |
| w/real cheddar cheese flavor (*Quaker*) | 104 |
| w/imitation ham bits (*Quaker*) | 99 |
| white hominy product (*Quaker*) | 79 |
| **Corn nuggets,** frozen: | |
| breaded, fried (*Stilwell Quickkrisp*), 3 oz. | 210 |
| **Corn salad:** | |
| raw, 1 oz. or ½ cup | 6 |
| **Corn soufflé,** frozen: | |
| (*Stouffer's*), ⅓ of 12-oz. pkg. | 160 |
| **Corn syrup:** | |
| dark or light (*Karo*), 1 tbsp. | 60 |
| **Cornbread,** see "Bread, sweet, mix" and "Bread dough" | |
| **Cornish game hen,** frozen: | |
| (*Tyson*), 3.5 oz. | 240 |
| **Cornmeal** (see also "Polenta mix"): | |
| degermed, 1 cup | 506 |
| self-rising: | |
| bolted, 1 cup | 408 |
| bolted, w/wheat flour, 1 cup | 592 |
| degermed, 1 cup | 489 |
| white (*Aunt Jemima*), 1 oz. or ⅙ cup | 98 |
| white, enriched, bolted (*Aunt Jemima*), 1 oz. or ⅙ cup | 99 |
| white or yellow (*Albers*), 1 oz. | 100 |
| white or yellow, enriched (*Quaker/Aunt Jemima*), 1 oz. | 102 |
| whole-grain, all varieties (*Arrowhead Mills*), 2 oz. | 210 |
| mix, buttermilk, self-rising (*Aunt Jemima*), 3 tbsp. | 101 |
| mix, white, bolted (*Aunt Jemima*), 1 oz. or ⅙ cup | 99 |

| FOOD AND MEASURE | CALORIES |
|---|---|
| **Cornstarch:** | |
| (*Argo/Kingsford*), 1 tbsp. | 30 |
| **Cough drops:** | |
| (*Beech-Nut*), 1 piece | 10 |
| (*Halls* Cough Tablets), 1 piece | 15 |
| **Couscous:** | |
| dry, 1 oz. | 107 |
| cooked, 1 cup | 201 |
| mix (*Near East*), 1.25 oz. | 120 |
| mix, cooked, w/out added ingredients: | |
| (*Fantastic Foods*), ½ cup | 105 |
| pilaf (*Casbah*), ½ cup or 1 oz. dry | 100 |
| pilaf, savory (*Quick Pilaf*), ½ cup | 94 |
| whole wheat (*Fantastic Foods*), ½ cup | 94 |
| **Cowpeas:** | |
| boiled, drained, ½ cup | 79 |
| canned, see "Black-eyed peas" | |
| frozen, boiled, drained, ½ cup | 112 |
| young pods, w/seeds, raw, ½ cup | 21 |
| young pods, w/seeds, boiled, drained, ½ cup | 16 |
| **Cowpeas, leafy-tips:** | |
| raw, chopped, ½ cup | 5 |
| boiled, drained, 4 oz. | 25 |
| **Cowpeas, mature,** dried: | |
| raw, ½ cup | 283 |
| boiled, ½ cup | 100 |
| canned, w/liquid, ½ cup | 92 |
| canned, w/pork, ½ cup | 99 |
| **Crab, imitation:** | |
| from surimi, 4 oz. | 116 |
| (*Icicle Brand*), 3.5 oz. | 99 |
| **Crab,** meat only: | |
| fresh: | |
| Alaska king, raw, 4 lb. | 95 |
| Alaska king, boiled, poached, or steamed, 4 oz. | 110 |

| FOOD AND MEASURE | CALORIES |
|---|---|
| blue, raw, 4 oz. | 99 |
| blue, boiled, poached, or steamed, 4 oz. | 116 |
| Dungeness, raw, 4 oz. | 97 |
| queen, raw, 4 oz. | 103 |
| canned, blue, 4 oz. | 112 |
| canned, blue, 1 cup | 133 |
| canned, Dungeness (*S&W*), 3.25 oz. | 81 |
| frozen, snow (*Wakefield*), 3 oz. | 60 |
| **Crab cake, deviled,** breaded, frozen: | |
| (*Mrs. Paul's*), 1 cake | 180 |
| miniature (*Mrs. Paul's*), 3.5 oz. | 240 |
| **Crab and shrimp,** frozen: | |
| (*Wakefield*), 3 oz. | 60 |
| **Crabapple:** | |
| fresh, w/skin, sliced, ½ cup | 42 |
| canned, spiced (*Lucky Leaf/Musselman's*), 4 oz. | 110 |
| **Cracker:** | |
| all varieties (*Keebler Munch'ems*), ½ oz. | 70 |
| all varieties (*Keebler* Toasteds), 4 pieces | 60 |
| all varieties, except rye and sesame (*Hain*), 1 oz. | 130 |
| bacon flavor (*Nabisco Bacon Flavor Thins*), 7 pieces | 70 |
| w/bacon and cheese (*Handi-Snacks*), 1 pkg. | 130 |
| bran (*FiberRich*), 1 piece | 18 |
| bran, toasted (*Nabisco Bran Thins*), 7 pieces | 60 |
| butter flavor: | |
| (*Escort*), 3 pieces | 70 |
| (*Keebler Club* Low Salt), 4 pieces | 60 |
| (*Keebler Town House* Regular/Low Salt), 4 pieces | 70 |
| (*Ritz* Regular/Low Salt), 4 pieces | 70 |
| (*Ritz Bits* Regular/Low Salt), 22 pieces | 70 |
| dairy (*Nabisco American Classic*), 4 pieces | 70 |
| original (*Pepperidge Farm Flutters*), ¾ oz. | 100 |
| thins (*Pepperidge Farm* Distinctive), 4 pieces | 70 |
| cheese or cheese flavor: | |
| (*Cheese Nips*), 13 pieces | 70 |
| (*Combos*), 1.8 oz. | 240 |
| (*Pepperidge Farm* Goldfish Thins), 4 pieces | 50 |
| (*Ritz Bits*), 22 pieces | 70 |

| FOOD AND MEASURE | CALORIES |
|---|---|
| *Cracker, cheese or cheese flavor, continued* | |
| (*Tid Bits*), 16 pieces | 70 |
| cheddar (*Better Cheddars* Regular/Low Salt), 10 pieces | 70 |
| cheddar (*Guppies*), ¼ oz. | 40 |
| cheddar (*Keebler Town House Jrs.*), 8 pieces | 80 |
| cheddar (*Nabisco Cheddar Wedges*), ½ oz. | 70 |
| cheddar (*Pepperidge Farm* Tiny Goldfish), 1 oz. | 120 |
| cheddar or Parmesan (*Pepperidge Farm* Goldfish), 1 oz. | 120 |
| Swiss (*Nabisco Swiss Cheese*), 7 pieces | 70 |
| (*Pepperidge Farm* Snack Sticks), 8 pieces | 130 |
| cheese sandwich: | |
| (*Ritz Bits*), 6 pieces | 80 |
| cheddar (*Keebler Town House* & Cheddar), 1 piece | 70 |
| and peanut butter (*Keebler*), 2 pieces | 70 |
| wheat and American cheese (*Keebler*), 1 piece | 70 |
| and cheese (*Handi-Snacks*), 1 pkg. | 120 |
| chicken-flavored (*Chicken In A Biskit*), 7 pieces | 80 |
| crackerbread (*Crisp & Light* Regular/Salt Free), 1 slice | 17 |
| crispbread (see also specific grains): | |
| (*Dar-Vida*), 1 piece | 20 |
| (*Kavli* Norwegian), 1 thick piece | 35 |
| (*Kavli* Norwegian), 2 thin pieces | 40 |
| (*Wasa* Breakfast), 1 piece | 50 |
| (*Wasa* Extra Crisp), 1 piece | 25 |
| (*Wasa* Fiber Plus), 1 piece | 35 |
| dark, regular or w/caraway (*Finn Crisp*), 2 pieces | 38 |
| garlic flavor (*Weight Watchers*), 2 pieces | 30 |
| high fiber (*Ryvita* Crisp Bread), 1 piece | 23 |
| high fiber (*Ryvita* Snackbread), 1 piece | 14 |
| croissant (*Carr's*), 1 piece | 25 |
| (*Estee* Unsalted), 4 pieces | 60 |
| (*FFV* Schooners), 33 pieces, approx. ½ oz. | 60 |
| garlic (*Manischewitz Garlic Tams*), 10 pieces | 153 |
| graham, see "cookie" | |
| grain, mixed (*Harvest Crisps* 5 Grain), 6 pieces | 60 |
| herb, garden (*Pepperidge Farm Flutters*), ¾ oz. | 100 |
| (*Manischewitz Tam Tams*), 10 pieces | 147 |
| (*Manischewitz Tam Tams* No Salt), 10 pieces | 138 |
| matzo, 1 board, except as noted: | |
| (*Manischewitz* Daily Unsalted) | 110 |
| (*Manischewitz* Passover) | 129 |

| FOOD AND MEASURE | CALORIES |
|---|---|
| American (*Manischewitz*) | 115 |
| diatetic, thin (*Manischewitz*) | 91 |
| egg (*Manischewitz* Passover) | 132 |
| egg, miniature (*Manischewitz* Passover), 10 pieces | 108 |
| egg n' onion (*Manischewitz*) | 112 |
| miniature (*Manischewitz*), 10 pieces | 90 |
| tea, thin (*Manischewitz* Daily) | 103 |
| thin (*Manischewitz*) | 100 |
| whole wheat, w/bran (*Manischewitz*) | 110 |
| melba toast, ½ oz., except as noted: | |
| (*Devonsheer* Regular/Unsalted), 1 piece | 16 |
| (*Devonsheer* Rounds) | 53 |
| (*Devonsheer* Unsalted Rounds) | 52 |
| bacon (*Old London* rounds) | 53 |
| garlic (*Devonsheer/Old London* rounds) | 56 |
| honey bran (*Devonsheer*), 1 piece | 16 |
| honey bran (*Devonsheer* Rounds) | 52 |
| oat (*Harvest Crisps*), 6 pieces or ½ oz. | 60 |
| onion (*Devonsheer* Rounds) | 51 |
| onion (*Old London* Rounds) | 52 |
| pumpernickel (*Old London*) | 54 |
| rye (*Devonsheer* Regular/Unsalted), 1 piece | 16 |
| rye (*Devonsheer* rounds) | 53 |
| rye (*Old London/Old London* Rounds) | 52 |
| sesame (*Devonsheer*), 1 piece | 16 |
| sesame (*Devonsheer* Rounds) | 57 |
| sesame (*Old London* Regular/Unsalted) | 55 |
| sesame (*Old London* Rounds) | 56 |
| vegetable (*Devonsheer*), 1 piece | 16 |
| wheat (*Estee* 6 calorie), 1 piece | 6 |
| wheat (*Estee* Snax) | 50 |
| wheat (*Old London*) | 51 |
| wheat, whole (*Devonsheer* Regular/Unsalted), 1 piece | 16 |
| white (*Old London* Regular/Unsalted) | 51 |
| white (*Old London* Rounds) | 48 |
| whole grain (*Old London*) | 52 |
| whole grain (*Old London* Rounds) | 54 |
| whole grain (*Old London* Unsalted) | 53 |
| oat (*Oat Thins*), 8 pieces or ½ oz. | 70 |
| oat bran (*Oat Bran Krisp*), 2 triple pieces or ½ oz. | 60 |
| onion (*Manischewitz Onion Tams*), 10 pieces | 150 |

| FOOD AND MEASURE | CALORIES |
|---|---|
| *Cracker, continued* | |
| onion, minced (*Nabisco American Classic*), 4 pieces | 70 |
| oyster, see "soup and oyster," below | |
| peanut butter (*Combos*), 1.8 oz. | 240 |
| peanut butter sandwich (*Handi-Snacks*), 1 pkg. | 190 |
| peanut butter sandwich (*Ritz Bits*), 6 pieces or ½ oz. | 80 |
| peanut butter, toast and (*Keebler*), 2 pieces | 70 |
| (*Pepperidge Farm* Original Tiny Goldfish), 1 oz. | 130 |
| pizza flavor (*Pepperidge Farm* Tiny Goldfish), 1 oz. | 130 |
| poppy, toasted (*Nabisco American Classic*), 4 pieces | 70 |
| pretzel (*Pepperidge Farm* Snack Sticks), 8 pieces | 120 |
| pretzel (*Pepperidge Farm* Tiny Goldfish), 1 oz. | 110 |
| pumpernickel (*Pepperidge Farm* Snack Sticks), 8 pieces | 140 |
| rice, harvest (*Weight Watchers* Crispbread), 2 pieces | 30 |
| rice bran (*Health Valley*), 7 pieces | 130 |
| rye: | |
| (*Hain* Regular/No Salt Added), 1 oz. | 120 |
| (*Rykrisp*), ½ oz. | 40 |
| dark (*Ryvita* Crisp Bread), 1 piece | 26 |
| golden (*Wasa* Crispbread), 1 piece | 35 |
| hearty (*Wasa* Crispbread), 1 piece | 45 |
| light (*Finn Crisp* Hi-Fiber), 1 piece | 35 |
| light (*Ryvita* Crisp Bread), 1 piece | 26 |
| light (*Wasa* Crispbread Lite), 1 piece | 25 |
| original (*Finn Crisp* Hi-Fiber), 1 piece | 40 |
| seasoned (*Rykrisp*/*Rykrisp* Twindividuals), ½ oz. | 45 |
| sesame (*Rykrisp*), ½ oz. | 50 |
| sesame, toasted (*Ryvita* Crisp Bread), 1 piece | 31 |
| saltine: | |
| (*Premium* Regular/Low Salt/Unsalted Tops/Wheat), 5 pieces. | 60 |
| (*Premium* Fat Free), 5 pieces | 50 |
| (*Premium Bits*), 16 pieces | 70 |
| (*Rokeach*), 10 pieces | 120 |
| (*Zesta* Regular/Low Salt/Unsalted Tops/Wheat), 5 pieces | 60 |
| wheat, whole (*Premium Plus*), 5 pieces | 60 |
| sesame: | |
| (*Dar-Vida* Crispbread), 1 piece | 22 |
| (*FFV* Crisp), 1 piece | 60 |
| (*Hain* Regular/No Salt Added), 1 oz. | 140 |
| (*Pepperidge Farm* Distinctive), 4 pieces | 80 |
| (*Pepperidge Farm* Snack Sticks), 8 pieces | 140 |

| FOOD AND MEASURE | CALORIES |
|---|---|
| bread wafer (*Meal mates*), 3 pieces | 70 |
| golden (*Nabisco American Classic*), 4 pieces | 70 |
| golden (*Pepperidge Farm Flutters*), ¾ oz. | 110 |
| savory (*Wasa* Crispbread), 1 piece | 30 |
| wafer (*FFV* Crisp), 4 pieces | 60 |
| sesame and cheese (*Twigs* Snack Sticks), 5 pieces | 70 |
| sesame wheat (*Wasa* Crispbread), 1 piece | 50 |
| snack (*Rokeach*), 9 pieces | 130 |
| soda or water: | |
| (*Carr's* Table Water, Bite Size), 2 pieces | 25 |
| (*Crown Pilot*), ½-oz. piece | 70 |
| (*FFV* Ocean Crisps), 1 piece | 60 |
| (*North Castles* English), 1 piece | 10 |
| (*Pepperidge Farm* English Water Biscuits), 4 pieces | 70 |
| (*Royal Lunch*), ½-oz. piece | 60 |
| (*Sailor Boy* Pilot), 1 piece | 100 |
| soup and oyster (*Dandy*), 20 pieces or ½ oz. | 60 |
| soup and oyster (*OTC*), 1 piece | 25 |
| soup and oyster (*Oysterettes*), 18 pieces or ½ oz. | 60 |
| toast (*Uneeda* Biscuits Unsalted Tops), 3 pieces | 60 |
| vegetable (*Vegetable Thins*), 7 pieces | 70 |
| water, see "soda or water," above | |
| (*Waverly* Regular/Low Salt), 4 pieces | 70 |
| wheat: | |
| (*FFV* Crispy Wafer), 6 pieces | 70 |
| (*FFV* Stoned Wheat Wafer), 4 pieces | 60 |
| (*Manischewitz Wheat Tams*), 10 pieces | 150 |
| (*Ryvita* Original Snackbread), 1 piece | 20 |
| (*Sociables*), 6 pieces | 70 |
| (*Triscuit* Regular/Low Salt), 3 pieces | 60 |
| (*Triscuit Bits*), 8 pieces | 60 |
| (*Wheat Thins* Regular/Low Salt), 8 pieces | 70 |
| (*Wheatsworth* Stone Ground), 4 pieces | 70 |
| all varieties, except sesame (*Health Valley* Stoned Wheat), 13 pieces | 120 |
| cracked (*Nabisco American Classic*), 4 pieces | 70 |
| cracked (*Pepperidge Farm* Distinctive), 3 pieces | 100 |
| hearty (*Pepperidge Farm* Distinctive), 4 pieces | 100 |
| nutty (*Wheat Thins*), 7 pieces | 70 |
| sesame (*Health Valley* Stoned Wheat), 13 pieces | 130 |
| toasted (*Pepperidge Farm* Distinctive), 4 pieces | 80 |

| FOOD AND MEASURE | CALORIES |
|---|---|
| *Cracker, wheat, continued* | |
| toasted (*Pepperidge Farm Flutters*), ¾ oz. | 110 |
| whole (*Carr's*), 2 pieces | 70 |
| whole (*Keebler Wheatables*), 12 pieces | 70 |
| whole grain (*Keebler Harvest Wheats*), 4 pieces | 60 |
| whole grain (*Wasa* Crispbread), 1 piece | 30 |
| wheat'n bran (*Triscuit*), 3 pieces | 60 |
| zwieback toast (*Nabisco*), 2 pieces | 60 |

## Cracker crumbs and meal:

| | |
|---|---|
| (*Golden Dipt*), 1 oz. | 100 |
| matzo (*Manischewitz Farfel*), 1 cup | 180 |
| matzo meal (*Manischewitz* Daily), 1 cup | 514 |

## Cranberry:

| | |
|---|---|
| whole, ½ cup | 23 |
| chopped, ½ cup | 27 |
| (*Ocean Spray*), 2 oz. or ½ cup | 25 |

## Cranberry fruit concentrate:

| | |
|---|---|
| (*Hain*), 1 oz. or 2 tbsp. | 40 |

## Cranberry juice:

| | |
|---|---|
| (*Lucky Leaf*), 6 fl. oz. | 110 |
| (*Smucker's* Naturally 100%), 8 fl. oz. | 130 |

## Cranberry juice cocktail, 6 fl. oz., except as noted:

| | |
|---|---|
| (*Ocean Spray*) | 110 |
| (*Ocean Spray* Low Calorie) | 40 |
| (*Sunkist*) | 110 |
| (*Veryfine*), 8 fl. oz. | 160 |
| frozen, diluted (*Sunkist*) | 110 |
| frozen, diluted (*Welch's*) | 100 |
| frozen, diluted (*Welch's* No Sugar Added) | 40 |

## Cranberry juice drink:

| | |
|---|---|
| (*Tropicana* Sparkler Cranberry Orchard), 8 fl. oz. | 120 |
| blend (*Ocean Spray Cran•Tastic*), 6 fl. oz. | 110 |

## Cranberry-apple juice cocktail:

| | |
|---|---|
| frozen, diluted (*Welch's*), 6 fl. oz. | 120 |

| FOOD AND MEASURE | CALORIES |
|---|---|
| **Cranberry-apple juice drink,** 6 fl. oz.: | |
| (*Ocean Spray Cran•Apple*) | 130 |
| (*Ocean Spray Cran•Apple* Low Calorie) | 40 |
| **Cranberry-apricot juice drink:** | |
| (*Ocean Spray Cranicot*), 6 fl. oz. | 110 |
| **Cranberry-blueberry drink:** | |
| (*Ocean Spray Cran•Blueberry*), 6 fl. oz. | 120 |
| **Cranberry-blueberry juice cocktail:** | |
| frozen, diluted (*Welch's*), 6 fl. oz. | 110 |
| **Cranberry-grape juice cocktail:** | |
| frozen, diluted (*Welch's*), 6 fl. oz. | 110 |
| **Cranberry-grape juice drink:** | |
| (*Ocean Spray Cran•Grape*), 6 fl. oz. | 130 |
| **Cranberry-orange relish,** canned: | |
| ¼ cup | 123 |
| **Cranberry-raspberry drink:** | |
| (*Ocean Spray Cran•Raspberry*), 6 fl. oz. | 110 |
| (*Ocean Spray Cran•Raspberry* Low Calorie), 6 fl. oz. | 40 |
| **Cranberry-raspberry juice cocktail:** | |
| frozen, diluted (*Welch's*), 6 fl. oz. | 110 |
| **Cranberry sauce,** canned: | |
| whole or jellied (*Ocean Spray*), 2 oz. | 90 |
| whole or jellied (*S&W* Old Fashioned), ½ cup | 90 |
| blends, all varieties (*Ocean Spray Cran•Fruit*), 2 oz. | 100 |
| **Crawfish entree,** frozen: | |
| etouffee (*Cajun Cookin'*), 12 oz. | 390 |
| **Crayfish,** meat only: | |
| raw, 1 oz. or 8 medium | 25 |
| boiled or steamed, 4 oz. | 129 |
| **Cream,** fluid: | |
| half and half, 1 cup | 315 |
| half and half, 1 tbsp. | 20 |

| FOOD AND MEASURE | CALORIES |
|---|---|
| *Cream, continued* | |
| half and half (*Crowley*), 1 fl. oz. | 35 |
| half and half (*Knudsen*), 4 fl. oz. | 150 |
| light, coffee or table, 1 cup | 469 |
| light, coffee or table, 1 tbsp. | 29 |
| light, whipping, 1 cup (2 cups whipped) | 699 |
| light, whipping, 1 tbsp. (2 tbsp. whipped) | 44 |
| heavy, whipping, 1 cup (2 cups whipped) | 821 |
| heavy, whipping, 1 tbsp. (2 tbsp. whipped) | 52 |
| heavy, whipping (*Crowley*), 1 fl. oz. | 110 |
| medium, 25% fat, 1 cup | 583 |
| medium, 25% fat, 1 tbsp. | 37 |
| sour, see "Cream, sour" | |
| whipped topping (see also "Cream topping"): | |
| (*La Creme*), 1 tbsp. | 16 |
| frozen (*Kraft* Real Cream), ¼ cup | 30 |
| pressurized, 1 cup | 154 |
| pressurized, 1 tbsp. | 8 |

## Cream, sour:

| | |
|---|---|
| (*Bison*), 1 oz. | 50 |
| (*Crowley*), 1 oz. | 50 |
| (*Friendship*), 1 oz. or 2 tbsp. | 55 |
| French onion (*Crowley*), 1 oz. | 50 |
| half and half (*Breakstone's Light Choice*), 1 tbsp. | 25 |
| imitation (*Pet*), 1 tbsp. | 25 |
| light (*Crowley*), 1 oz. | 30 |
| light (*Weight Watchers*), 1 oz. or 2 tbsp. | 35 |
| lowfat (*Friendship Lite Delight*), 1 oz. or 2 tbsp. | 35 |
| nondairy, 1 cup | 479 |
| nondairy, dressing (*Crowley*), 1 oz. | 40 |

## Cream gravy, canned:

| | |
|---|---|
| (*Franco-American*), 2 oz. | 35 |

## Cream puff, frozen:

| | |
|---|---|
| Bavarian (*Rich's*), 1 piece | 150 |

## Cream of tartar:

| | |
|---|---|
| (*Tone's*), 1 tsp. | 2 |

| FOOD AND MEASURE | CALORIES |
|---|---|
| **Cream topping,** nondairy: | |
| (*Pet Whip*), 1 tbsp. | 14 |
| frozen: | |
| (*Bird's Eye Cool Whip*), 1 tbsp. | 12 |
| (*Bird's Eye Cool Whip* Lite), 1 tbsp. | 8 |
| (*Kraft* Whipped Topping), ¼ cup | 35 |
| extra creamy (*Birds Eye Cool Whip* Dairy Recipe), 1 tbsp. | 14 |
| mix, prepared (*D-Zerta*), 1 tbsp. | 8 |
| mix, prepared (*Dream Whip*), 1 tbsp. | 10 |
| mix, prepared (*Featherweight*), 1 tbsp. | 4 |
| pressurized, 1 tbsp. | 11 |
| pressurized (*Rich's Richwhip*), ¼ oz. | 20 |
| prewhipped (*Estee*), 1 tbsp. | 4 |
| prewhipped (*Rich's Richwhip*), 1 tbsp. | 12 |
| unwhipped (*Rich's Richwhip*), ¼ oz. | 20 |
| **Creamer, nondairy:** | |
| (*Crowley*), ½ oz. | 16 |
| liquid (*Coffee-mate*), 1 tbsp. | 16 |
| liquid, frozen (*Rich's Coffee/Farm/Poly Rich*), ½ oz. | 20 |
| powdered (*Coffee-mate*), 1 tsp. | 10 |
| powdered (*Coffee-mate* Lite), 1 tsp. | 8 |
| powdered (*Cremora*), 1 tsp. | 10 |
| **Creme de menthe:** | |
| 72 proof, 1 fl. oz. | 125 |
| **Creole sauce:** | |
| Cajun (*Enrico's* Light), 4 oz. | 76 |
| **Cress, garden:** | |
| raw, ½ cup | 8 |
| boiled, drained, ½ cup | 16 |
| **Croaker,** Atlantic, meat only: | |
| raw, 4 oz. | 117 |
| **Croissant,** 1 piece: | |
| (*Pepperidge Farm* Sandwich Quartet) | 170 |
| butter (*Awrey's*), 3 oz. | 300 |
| butter (*Awrey's*), 2 oz. | 200 |
| margarine (*Awrey's*), 2.5 oz. | 250 |

| FOOD AND MEASURE | CALORIES |
|---|---|
| *Croissant, continued* | |
| margarine (*Awrey's*), 1.25 oz. | 120 |
| wheat (*Awrey's*), 2.5 oz. | 240 |
| frozen, butter (*Sara Lee*), 1.5 oz. | 170 |
| frozen, butter, petite (*Sara Lee*), 1 oz. | 120 |
| **Crookneck squash,** see "Squash" | |
| **Crouton,** ½ oz.: | |
| all varieties, except cheddar and Romano (*Pepperidge Farm*) | 70 |
| Casear salad (*Brownberry*) | 62 |
| cheddar cheese (*Brownberry*) | 63 |
| cheddar and Romano cheese (*Pepperidge Farm*) | 60 |
| onion and garlic (*Brownberry*) | 60 |
| seasoned (*Brownberry*) | 59 |
| toasted (*Brownberry*) | 56 |
| **Cucumber,** unpeeled: | |
| 1 medium, 8¼" long × 2⅛" diam. | 39 |
| sliced, ½ cup | 7 |
| **Cucumber dip:** | |
| creamy (*Kraft* Premium), 2 tbsp. | 50 |
| **Cumin seed:** | |
| 1 tsp. | 7 |
| **Cupcake,** see "Cake, snack" | |
| **Currant:** | |
| black, European, trimmed, ½ cup | 36 |
| red or white, trimmed, ½ cup | 31 |
| zante, dried, ½ cup | 204 |
| **Curry powder:** | |
| 1 tsp. | 6 |
| **Cusk,** meat only, raw: | |
| raw, 4 oz. | 100 |
| **Custard,** see "Pudding mix" | |

| FOOD AND MEASURE | CALORIES |
| --- | --- |
| **Custard apple:** | |
| trimmed, 1 oz. | 29 |
| **Cuttlefish,** meat only: | |
| raw, 4 oz. | 89 |

# D

| FOOD AND MEASURE | CALORIES |
|---|---|

**Daikon,** see "Radish, Oriental"

**Daiquiri mix:**

| | |
|---|---|
| bottled (*Holland House*), 1 fl. oz. | 36 |
| bottled, raspberry (*Holland House*), 1 fl. oz. | 30 |
| bottled, strawberry (*Holland House*), 1 fl. oz. | 31 |
| instant (*Holland House*), .56 oz. dry | 65 |
| instant, prepared w/liquor (*Bar-Tender's*), 3.5 fl. oz. | 177 |

***Dairy Queen/Brazier,*** 1 serving:

| | |
|---|---|
| sandwiches: | |
| BBQ beef, 4.5 oz. | 225 |
| chicken fillet, breaded, 6.7 oz. | 430 |
| chicken fillet, breaded, w/cheese, 7.2 oz. | 480 |
| chicken fillet, grilled, 6.5 oz. | 300 |
| fish fillet, 6 oz. | 370 |
| fish fillet, w/cheese, 6.5 oz. | 420 |
| hamburger, single, 5 oz. | 310 |
| hamburger, single, w/cheese, 5.5 oz. | 365 |
| hamburger, double, 7 oz. | 460 |
| hamburger, double, w/cheese, 8 oz. | 570 |
| hamburger, *DQ Homestyle*, Ultimate, 9.7 oz. | 700 |
| hot dog, 3.5 oz. | 280 |
| hot dog, w/cheese, 4 oz. | 330 |
| hot dog, w/chili, 4.5 oz. | 320 |
| hot dog, 1/4 lb. *Super Dog*, 7 oz. | 590 |
| side dishes and dressings: | |
| dressing, french, reduced calorie, 2 oz. | 90 |
| dressing, Thousand Island, 2 oz. | 225 |
| french fries, regular, 3.5 oz. | 300 |
| onion rings, 3 oz. | 240 |
| salad, garden, w/out dressing, 10 oz. | 200 |
| desserts and shakes: | |
| banana split, 13 oz. | 510 |
| *Blizzard, Heath*, small, 10.3 oz. | 560 |

| FOOD AND MEASURE | CALORIES |
|---|---|
| *Blizzard, Heath*, regular, 14.3 oz. | 820 |
| *Blizzard*, strawberry, small, 9.4 oz. | 500 |
| *Blizzard*, strawberry, regular, 13.5 oz. | 740 |
| *Breeze, Heath*, small, 9.6 oz. | 450 |
| *Breeze, Heath*, regular, 13.4 oz. | 680 |
| *Breeze*, strawberry, small, 8.7 oz. | 400 |
| *Breeze*, strawberry, regular, 12.5 oz. | 590 |
| *Buster Bar*, 5.3 oz. | 450 |
| *Brownie Delight*, hot fudge, 10.8 oz. | 710 |
| cone, chocolate, regular, 5 oz. | 230 |
| cone, chocolate dipped, regular, 5.5. oz. | 330 |
| cone, vanilla, regular, 5 oz. | 230 |
| *Dilly* Bar, 3 oz. | 210 |
| *DQ* frozen cake slice, undecorated, 5.8 oz. | 380 |
| *DQ* Sandwich, 2.2 oz. | 140 |
| malt, vanilla, regular, 14.7 oz. | 610 |
| *Mr. Misty*, regular, 11.6 oz. | 250 |
| *Nutty Double Fudge*, 9.7 oz. | 580 |
| *Peanut Buster* parfait, 10.8 oz. | 710 |
| *QC Big Scoop*, chocolate, 4.5 oz. | 310 |
| *QC Big Scoop*, vanilla, 4.5 oz. | 300 |
| shake, chocolate, regular, 14 oz. | 540 |
| shake, vanilla, regular, 14 oz. | 520 |
| sundae, chocolate, regular, 6.2 oz. | 300 |
| *Waffle Cone Sundae*, strawberry, 6.1 oz. | 350 |
| yogurt cone, regular, 5 oz. | 180 |
| yogurt cup, regular, 5 oz. | 170 |
| yogurt sundae, strawberry, regular, 12.5 oz. | 200 |

## Dandelion greens:

| | |
|---|---|
| raw, 1 oz. or ½ cup chopped | 13 |
| boiled, drained, chopped, ½ cup | 17 |

## Danish pastry, see specific listings

## Date:

| | |
|---|---|
| (*Bordo*), 2 oz. | 204 |
| (*Dole*), ½ cup | 280 |
| (*Dromedary*), 1 oz. or 5 dates | 100 |
| chopped (*Dromedary*), ¼ cup | 130 |

| FOOD AND MEASURE | CALORIES |
|---|---|
| *Date, continued* | |
| diced (*Bordo*), 2 oz. | 203 |
| domestic, natural and dry, chopped, ½ cup | 245 |
| **Date bar mix,** prepared: | |
| (*Betty Crocker* Classic), 1 bar | 60 |
| **Diable sauce:** | |
| (*Escoffier*), 1 tbsp. | 20 |
| **Dill** seasoning, dried: | |
| (*McCormick/Schilling Parsley Patch* It's a Dilly), 1 tsp. | 9 |
| seed, 1 tsp. | 6 |
| weed, 1 tsp. | 3 |
| **Dips,** see specific listings | |
| **Dock:** | |
| raw, trimmed, chopped, ½ cup | 15 |
| boiled, drained, 4 oz. | 23 |
| **Dolphinfish,** meat only: | |
| raw, 4 oz. | 96 |
| ***Domino's Pizza,*** 2 slices: | |
| cheese | 376 |
| deluxe | 498 |
| double cheese/pepperoni | 545 |
| ham | 417 |
| pepperoni | 460 |
| sausage/mushroom | 430 |
| veggie | 498 |
| **Donut,** 1 piece: | |
| plain: | |
| (*Awrey's*) | 490 |
| (*Hostess Breakfast Bake Shop Donette Gems*) | 60 |
| (*Hostess* Family Pack) | 120 |
| (*Hostess* Pantry) | 190 |
| (*Tastykake* Assorted), 1.6 oz. | 185 |

| FOOD AND MEASURE | CALORIES |
|---|---|
| cinnamon: | |
| (*Hostess Breakfast Bake Shop Donette Gems*) | 60 |
| (*Hostess Breakfast Bake Shop* Family Pack) | 120 |
| (*Hostess Breakfast Bake Shop* Pantry) | 190 |
| (*Tastykake* Assorted), 1.6 oz. | 179 |
| apple-filled (*Hostess Breakfast Bake Shop Donette Gems*) | 70 |
| mini (*Tastykake*), .4 oz. | 48 |
| crumb (*Hostess Breakfast Bake Shop*) | 160 |
| crumb (*Hostess Breakfast Bake Shop Donette Gems*) | 80 |
| crunch (*Awrey's*) | 600 |
| frosted (*Hostess Breakfast Bake Shop*), 1.5 oz. | 190 |
| frosted (*Hostess Breakfast Bake Shop Donette Gems*) | 80 |
| frosted (*Hostess O's*) | 260 |
| frosted, rich (*Tastykake*), 2 oz. | 258 |
| frosted, rich, mini (*Tastykake*), .5 oz. | 61 |
| frosted, strawberry-filled (*Hostess Breakfast Bake Shop Donette Gems*) | 80 |
| glazed (*Hostess Breakfast Bake Shop* Old Fashioned) | 250 |
| glazed, whirl (*Hostess Breakfast Bake Shop*) | 190 |
| honey wheat (*Hostess Breakfast Bake Shop*) | 250 |
| honey wheat (*Tastykake*), 2 oz. | 209 |
| honey wheat, mini (*Tastykake*), .4 oz. | 40 |
| (*Hostess O's*) | 230 |
| (*Hostess Breakfast Bake Shop* Old Fashioned) | 170 |
| orange-glazed (*Tastykake*), 2 oz. | 219 |
| powdered sugar: | |
| (*Hostess Breakfast Bake Shop Donette Gems*) | 60 |
| (*Hostess Breakfast Bake Shop* Family Pack) | 120 |
| (*Hostess Breakfast Bake Shop* Pantry) | 190 |
| (*Tastykake* Assorted), 1.6 oz. | 188 |
| mini (*Tastykake*), .4 oz. | 42 |
| strawberry-filled (*Hostess Breakfast Bake Shop Donette Gems*) | 70 |
| stick (*Little Debbie*), 1.67 oz. | 230 |
| sugared (*Awrey's*) | 610 |
| frozen, glazed (*Rich's Ever Fresh*), 1.2-oz. piece | 141 |
| frozen, jelly (*Rich's Ever Fresh*), 2.17-oz. piece | 213 |

**Drum,** freshwater, meat only:

| | |
|---|---|
| raw, 4 oz. | 135 |

| FOOD AND MEASURE | CALORIES |
|---|---|
| ***Druther's*[1], 1 serving:** | |
| breakfast: | |
| bacon and egg biscuit, 3.1 oz. | 258 |
| bacon and egg plate, fried egg, 10 oz. | 721 |
| bacon and egg plate, scrambled egg, 11.1 oz. | 742 |
| ham and egg biscuit, 3.5 oz. | 217 |
| ham and egg plate, fried egg, 10.9 oz. | 681 |
| ham and egg plate, scrambled egg, 12.1 oz. | 762 |
| sausage and egg biscuit, 3.3 oz. | 246 |
| sausage and egg plate, fried egg, 10.6 oz. | 741 |
| sausage and egg plate, scrambled egg, 10 oz. | 762 |
| 1 sausage, 1 biscuit, 1.7 oz. | 179 |
| 2 sausages, 2 biscuits, 3.4 oz. | 358 |
| biscuits and gravy, 8.1 oz. | 331 |
| cheeseburger: | |
| 4.7 oz. | 380 |
| deluxe quarter, 8.7 oz. | 660 |
| double, 6.4 oz. | 500 |
| chicken: | |
| 8 pieces, 2.6 lbs. | 3,664 |
| 12 pieces, 3.9 lbs. | 5,496 |
| breast and wing, snack, 14 oz. | 970 |
| breast and wing, snack, 7.5 oz. | 595 |
| thigh and leg, snack, 13.4 oz. | 925 |
| thigh and leg, snack, 7 oz. | 549 |
| chicken dinner: | |
| 2-piece, breast and wing, 14 oz. | 970 |
| 2-piece, leg and thigh, 13.4 oz. | 925 |
| 3-piece, breast, thigh, and leg, 1.1 lb. | 1,281 |
| 3-piece, breast, thigh, and wing, 1.1 lb. | 1,309 |
| fish and chips, 11.2 oz. | 729 |
| fish dinner, 13.3 oz. | 770 |
| fish sandwich, 4.8 oz. | 349 |
| hamburger, 4.4 oz. | 327 |
| **Duck,** domesticated: | |
| roasted, meat w/skin, 4 oz. | 382 |
| roasted, meat only, 4 oz. | 228 |

[1]Values for dinners are complete as served, including accompanying biscuits, potatoes, hushpuppies.

| FOOD AND MEASURE | CALORIES |
|---|---|
| **Duck fat:** | |
| 1 tbsp. | 115 |
| **Duck sauce,** see "Sweet and sour sauce" | |
| **Dulcita,** frozen: | |
| apple (*Hormel*), 4 oz. | 290 |
| cherry (*Hormel*), 4 oz. | 300 |
| ***Dunkin' Donuts,*** 1 piece: | |
| apple-filled, w/cinnamon sugar, 2.8 oz. | 250 |
| Bavarian cream-filled, w/chocolate frosting, 2.8 oz. | 240 |
| blueberry-filled, 2.4 oz. | 210 |
| buttermilk ring, glazed, 2.6 oz. | 290 |
| cake ring, plain, 2.2 oz. | 270 |
| cake ring, chocolate, w/glaze, 2.5 oz. | 324 |
| chocolate chunk cookie, 1.5 oz. | 200 |
| chocolate chunk cookie, w/nuts, 1.5 oz. | 210 |
| coffee roll, glazed, 2.9 oz. | 280 |
| croissant, plain, 2.5 oz. | 310 |
| croissant, almond, 3.7 oz. | 420 |
| croissant, chocolate, 3.3 oz. | 440 |
| cruller, French, w/glaze, 1.3 oz. | 140 |
| jelly-filled, 2.4 oz. | 220 |
| lemon-filled, 2.8 oz. | 260 |
| muffin: | |
| apple spice, 3.5 oz. | 300 |
| banana nut, 3.6 oz. | 310 |
| blueberry, 3.6 oz. | 280 |
| bran, w/raisins, 3.7 oz. | 310 |
| corn, 3.4 oz. | 340 |
| cranberry nut, 3.5 oz. | 290 |
| oat bran, 3.4 oz. | 330 |
| oatmeal pecan raisin cookie, 1.6 oz. | 200 |
| whole wheat ring, glazed, 2.9 oz. | 330 |
| yeast ring, chocolate frosted or glazed, 1.9 oz. | 200 |
| **Dutch brand loaf:** | |
| (*Eckrich/Eckrich Smorgas Pac*), 1-oz. slice | 70 |
| (*Eckrich* Lean Supreme), 1-oz. slice | 60 |
| (*Kahn's*), 1 slice | 80 |

# E

| FOOD AND MEASURE | CALORIES |
|---|---|
| **Eclair,** frozen: | |
| chocolate (*Rich's*), 2-oz. piece | 210 |
| **Eel,** meat only: | |
| raw, 4 oz. | 208 |
| baked, broiled, or microwaved, 4 oz. | 268 |
| **Egg, chicken:** | |
| fresh or frozen, raw, 1 whole large egg | 75 |
| fresh or frozen, raw, white from 1 large egg | 17 |
| fresh, raw, yolk from 1 large egg[1] | 59 |
| fresh, hard-boiled, 1 large egg | 77 |
| fresh, poached, 1 large egg | 74 |
| dried, whole, 1 oz. | 168 |
| dried, whole, 1 tbsp. | 30 |
| **Egg, pickled:** | |
| (*Penrose*), 1 egg | 80 |
| **Egg, quail,** fresh: | |
| whole, raw, 1 egg | 14 |
| **Egg, substitute:** | |
| (*Fleischmann's Egg Beaters*), ¼ cup | 25 |
| (*Morningstar Farms Scramblers*), ¼ cup | 60 |
| (*Tofutti Egg Watchers*), 2 oz. | 50 |
| w/cheese (*Fleischmann's Egg Beaters* Cheez), ½ cup | 130 |
| mix, prepared w/tofu (*Tofu Scrambler*), ½ cup | 98 |
| mix, prepared w/tofu and butter (*Tofu Scrambler*), ½ cup | 158 |
| mix, vegetable omelet (*Egg Beaters*), ½ cont. | 50 |
| **Egg breakfast,** frozen, 1 pkg. or serving: | |
| omelet, w/cheese sauce and ham (*Swanson Great Starts*) | 390 |
| reduced cholesterol, w/mini oat bran muffins (*Swanson Great Starts*) | 250 |

[1]Includes small portion of egg white.

| FOOD AND MEASURE | CALORIES |
|---|---|
| scrambled: | |
| and bacon, w/home fries (*Swanson Great Starts*) | 340 |
| cheddar cheese and fried potatoes (*Aunt Jemima*) | 250 |
| w/cheese, and cinnamon pancakes (*Swanson Great Starts*) | 290 |
| w/ham and hash browns (*Downyflake*) | 360 |
| w/ham and pecan twirl (*Downyflake*) | 470 |
| w/hash browns and sausages (*Downyflake*) | 420 |
| and home fries (*Swanson Great Starts*) | 260 |
| and sausage, w/hash browns (*Aunt Jemima*) | 290 |
| and sausages, w/hash browns (*Swanson Great Starts*) | 430 |
| w/sausage and pecan twirl (*Downyflake*) | 510 |

**"Egg" breakfast, vegetarian,** frozen:

| | |
|---|---|
| *Scramblers,* hash browns, and links (*Morningstar Farms* Country Breakfast), 7 oz. | 360 |
| *Scramblers,* pancakes, and links (*Morningstar Farms* Country Breakfast), 6.8 oz. | 380 |

**Egg breakfast sandwich,** frozen:

| | |
|---|---|
| biscuit, Canadian bacon and cheese (*Swanson Great Starts*), 5.2 oz. | 420 |
| biscuit, sausage and cheese (*Swanson Great Starts*), 5.5 oz. | 460 |
| English muffin (*Weight Watchers* Microwave), 4 oz. | 230 |
| muffin, beefsteak and cheese (*Swanson Great Starts*), 4.9 oz. | 360 |
| muffin, Canadian bacon and cheese (*Swanson Great Starts*), 4.1 oz. | 290 |

**Egg foo young mix,** prepared:

| | |
|---|---|
| (*La Choy*), 8.8 oz. | 164 |

**Egg roll,** frozen:

| | |
|---|---|
| chicken (*Chun King*), 3.6 oz. | 220 |
| chicken (*Jeno's* Snacks), 3 oz. or 6 rolls | 190 |
| meat and shrimp (*Chun King*), 3.6 oz. | 220 |
| meat and shrimp (*Jeno's* Snacks), 3 oz. or 6 rolls | 200 |
| pork (*Chun King* Restaurant Style), 3 oz. | 180 |
| shrimp (*Chun King*), 3.6 oz. | 200 |
| shrimp and cheese (*Jeno's* Snacks), 3 oz. or 6 rolls | 190 |
| vegetarian (*Worthington*), 3-oz. roll | 160 |

**Egg roll wrapper:**

| | |
|---|---|
| (*Nasoya*), 1 piece | 23 |

| FOOD AND MEASURE | CALORIES |
|---|---|
| **Eggnog,** nonalcoholic: | |
| canned (*Borden*), 4 fl. oz. | 160 |
| chilled (*Crowley*), 6 fl. oz. | 270 |
| **Eggplant:** | |
| raw, 1 medium, 8½″ × 1⅜″ | 27 |
| raw, 1″ pieces, ½ cup | 11 |
| boiled, drained, 1″ cubes, ½ cup | 13 |
| **Eggplant appetizer:** | |
| (*Progresso* Caponata), ½ can | 70 |
| **Eggplant entree,** frozen: | |
| parmigiana (*Celentano*), 6.25 oz. | 260 |
| parmigiana (*Celentano*), 8 oz. | 280 |
| parmigiana (*Celentano*), 10 oz. | 350 |
| parmigiana (*Mrs. Paul's*), 5 oz. | 240 |
| rollettes (*Celentano*), 11 oz. | 320 |
| **Elderberry:** | |
| ½ cup | 53 |
| **Enchilada dinner,** frozen: | |
| beef (*Banquet*), 12 oz. | 500 |
| beef (*Old El Paso* Festive Dinners), 11 oz. | 390 |
| beef (*Patio*), 13.25 oz. | 520 |
| beef (*Swanson*), 13.75 oz. | 480 |
| beef (*Van de Kamp's* Mexican Dinner), ½ pkg. | 200 |
| cheese (*Banquet*), 12 oz. | 550 |
| cheese (*Old El Paso* Festive Dinners), 11 oz. | 590 |
| cheese (*Patio*), 12.25 oz. | 380 |
| cheese (*Van de Kamp's* Mexican Dinner), ½ pkg. | 220 |
| chicken (*Old El Paso* Festive Dinners), 11 oz. | 460 |
| **Enchilada entree,** frozen: | |
| beef: | |
| (*Hormel*), 1 piece | 140 |
| (*Old El Paso*), 1 pkg. | 210 |
| (*Van de Kamp's* Mexican Entrees), 1 pkg. | 270 |
| (*Van de Kamp's* Mexican Entrees Family Pack), ¼ pkg. | 150 |
| and bean (*Lean Cuisine* Enchanadas), 9.25 oz. | 280 |
| chili gravy and (*Banquet Family Entrees*), 7 oz. | 270 |

| FOOD AND MEASURE | CALORIES |
|---|---|
| Ranchero (*Weight Watchers*), 9.12 oz. | 230 |
| shredded (*Van de Kamp's* Mexican Entrees), 1 pkg. | 360 |
| sirloin Ranchero (*The Budget Gourmet* Slim Selects), 9 oz. | 290 |
| cheese: | |
| (*Hormel*), 1 piece | 151 |
| (*Old El Paso*), 1 pkg. | 250 |
| (*Stouffer's*), 10⅛ oz. | 590 |
| (*Van de Kamp's* Mexican Entrees), 1 pkg. | 300 |
| (*Van de Kamp's* Mexican Entrees Family Pack), ¼ pkg. | 200 |
| Ranchero (*Van de Kamp's* Mexican Entrees), ½ pkg. | 260 |
| Ranchero (*Weight Watchers*), 8.87 oz. | 360 |
| chicken: | |
| (*Le Menu* LightStyle), 8 oz. | 280 |
| (*Lean Cuisine* Enchanadas), 9⅞ oz. | 270 |
| (*Old El Paso*), 1 pkg. | 220 |
| (*Stouffer's*), 10 oz. | 490 |
| (*Van de Kamp's* Mexican Entrees), 1 pkg. | 260 |
| w/sour cream sauce (*Old El Paso*), 1 pkg. | 280 |
| Suiza (*The Budget Gourmet* Slim Selects), 9 oz. | 270 |
| Suiza (*Van de Kamp's* Mexican Entrees), 1 pkg. | 230 |
| Suiza (*Weight Watchers*), 9 oz. | 280 |
| vegetable, w/tofu and sauce (*Legume* Mexican), 11 oz. | 270 |

**Enchilada sauce:**

| | |
|---|---|
| (*La Victoria*), 1 cup | 80 |
| (*Rosarita*), 3 oz. | 20 |
| green (*Old El Paso*), 2 tbsp. | 11 |
| hot (*El Molino*), 2 tbsp. | 16 |
| hot (*Old El Paso*), ¼ cup | 30 |
| hot or mild (*Del Monte*), ½ cup | 45 |
| hot or mild (*Ortega*), 1 oz. | 12 |
| mild (*Old El Paso*), ¼ cup | 25 |

**Enchilada seasoning mix:**

| | |
|---|---|
| (*Lawry's*), 1 pkg. | 152 |
| (*Old El Paso*), 1/18 pkg. | 6 |

**Endive, Belgian,** see "Chicory, witloof"

**Escarole** (curly endive):

| | |
|---|---|
| trimmed, 1 head, 1.3 lb. | 86 |

# F

| FOOD AND MEASURE | CALORIES |
| --- | --- |
| **Fajita entree,** frozen: | |
| beef (*Weight Watchers*), 6.75 oz. | 250 |
| chicken (*Weight Watchers*), 6.75 oz. | 230 |
| **Fajita entree,** refrigerated: | |
| chicken (*Chicken By George*), 5 oz. | 170 |
| **Fajita marinade:** | |
| (*Old El Paso*), ⅛ jar | 14 |
| **Fajita sauce:** | |
| (*Tio Sancho* Skillet Sauce), 1 oz. | 14 |
| **Fajita seasoning blend:** | |
| (*Lawry's*), 1 pkg. | 63 |
| **Falafel mix:** | |
| (*Casbah*), 1 oz. dry | 103 |
| (*Fantastic Foods Falafel*), 6 balls[1], 3 oz. | 129 |
| **Fast-food restaurants,** see specific listings | |
| **Fat,** see specific listings | |
| **Fat, imitation:** | |
| (*Rokeach Neutral Nyafat*), 1 tbsp. | 99 |
| **Fennel,** fresh: | |
| (*Frieda* of California), 1 oz. | 4 |
| **Fennel seed:** | |
| 1 tsp. | 7 |
| **Fenugreek seed:** | |
| 1 tsp. | 12 |

[1]Prepared according to package directions; does not include value for oil or fat used in frying.

| FOOD AND MEASURE | CALORIES |
| --- | --- |
| **Fettuccine,** see "Pasta" | |
| **Fettuccine entree,** frozen: | |
| Alfredo (*Healthy Choice*), 8 oz. | 240 |
| Alfredo (*Stouffer's*), ½ of 10-oz. pkg. | 270 |
| Alfredo (*Weight Watchers*), 9 oz. | 210 |
| w/broccoli (*Dining Lite*), 9 oz. | 290 |
| w/meat sauce (*The Budget Gourmet*), 10 oz. | 290 |
| primavera (*Green Giant*), 1 pkg. | 230 |
| primavera (*Green Giant* Microwave Garden Gourmet), 1 pkg. | 260 |
| **Fettuccine entree mix:** | |
| Alfredo (*Hain* Pasta & Sauce), ¼ pkg. | 180 |
| **Fig:** | |
| fresh, w/stems, 1 lb. | 333 |
| fresh, 1 large | 47 |
| fresh, 1 medium | 37 |
| canned, in light syrup, ½ cup | 87 |
| canned, in heavy syrup, whole (*Del Monte*), ½ cup | 100 |
| canned, in heavy syrup, whole kadota (*S&W* Fancy), ½ cup | 100 |
| canned, in extra heavy syrup, ½ cup | 140 |
| dried, uncooked, ½ cup | 254 |
| dried, uncooked, 10 figs | 477 |
| dried, Calimyrna (*Blue Ribbon/Sun-Maid*), ½ cup | 250 |
| dried, Mission (*Blue Ribbon/Sun-Maid*), ½ cup | 210 |
| **Filberts,** shelled: | |
| dried, unblanched, 1 oz. | 179 |
| dried, blanched, 1 oz. | 191 |
| dry-roasted, unblanched, 1 oz. | 188 |
| oil-roasted, unblanched, 1 oz. | 187 |
| **Filé powder,** see "Gumbo filé powder" | |
| **Finnan haddie,** see "Haddock" | |
| **Fish,** see specific listings | |
| **Fish cakes,** see "Fish entree" and specific listings | |

| FOOD AND MEASURE | CALORIES |
|---|---|

**Fish dinner,** frozen (see also specific fish listings):

(*Morton*), 9.75 oz. .... 370
'n' chips (*Swanson*), 10 oz. .... 500

**Fish entree,** frozen (see also specific fish listings):

(*Banquet* Platters), 8.75 oz. .... 450
battered fillets:
(*Gorton's* Crispy Batter), 2 pieces .... 290
(*Gorton's* Crispy Batter, Large), 1 piece .... 320
(*Gorton's* Crunchy), 2 pieces .... 230
(*Gorton's* Crunchy Microwave), 2 pieces .... 340
(*Gorton's* Crunchy Microwave, Large), 1 piece .... 320
(*Gorton's* Potato Crisp), 2 pieces .... 300
(*Gorton's* Value Pack), 1 piece .... 180
(*Mrs. Paul's*), 2 pieces .... 330
(*Mrs. Paul's* Crunchy), 2 pieces .... 280
(*Van de Kamp's*), 1 piece .... 170
minced (*Mrs. Paul's* Portions), 2 pieces .... 300
tempura (*Gorton's Light Recipe*), 1 piece .... 200
breaded fillets:
(*Gorton's Light Recipe*), 1 piece .... 180
(*Mrs. Paul's* Crispy Crunchy), 2 pieces .... 220
(*Van de Kamp's*), 2 pieces .... 280
crispy (*Van de Kamp's* Microwave), 1 piece .... 140
crispy (*Van de Kamp's* Microwave, Large), 1 piece .... 290
minced (*Mrs. Paul's* Crispy Crunchy Portions), 2 pieces .... 230
in butter sauce, fillets (*Mrs. Paul's* Light), 1 piece .... 140
cakes (*Mrs. Paul's*), 2 pieces .... 190
coated fillets, ranch (*Gorton's* Specialty Microwave, Large), 1 piece .... 330
Dijon (*Mrs. Paul's* Light), 8.75 oz. .... 200
fillet of:
divan (*Lean Cuisine*), 12⅜ oz. .... 260
Florentine (*Lean Cuisine*), 9 oz. .... 230
in herb butter (*Gorton's*), 1 pkg. .... 190
jardiniere, w/potatoes (*Lean Cuisine*), 11.25 oz. .... 290
Florentine (*Mrs. Paul's* Light), 8 oz. .... 220
'n' fries (*Swanson* Homestyle Recipe), 6.5 oz. .... 340
gems, fancy style (*Wakefield*), 4 oz. .... 80
gems, salad style (*Wakefield*), 3 oz. .... 70
Mornay (*Mrs. Paul's* Light), 9 oz. .... 230

| FOOD AND MEASURE | CALORIES |
|---|---|
| sticks, battered: | |
| (*Gorton's* Crispy Batter), 4 pieces | 260 |
| (*Gorton's* Crunchy), 4 pieces | 210 |
| (*Gorton's* Crunchy Microwave), 6 pieces | 340 |
| (*Gorton's* Potato Crisp), 4 pieces | 260 |
| (*Gorton's* Value Pack), 4 pieces | 190 |
| (*Mrs. Paul's*), 4 pieces | 210 |
| (*Van de Kamp's*), 4 pieces | 160 |
| minced (*Mrs. Paul's*), 4 pieces | 220 |
| sticks, breaded: | |
| (*Frionor Bunch O' Crunch*), 4 pieces or 2.7 oz. | 210 |
| (*Mrs. Paul's* Crispy Crunchy), 4 pieces | 140 |
| (*Van de Kamp's*), 4 pieces | 200 |
| (*Van de Kamp's* Value Pack), 4 pieces | 170 |
| crispy (*Van de Kamp's* Microwave), 3 pieces | 130 |
| minced (*Mrs. Paul's* Crispy Crunchy), 4 pieces | 190 |
| whole wheat (*Booth* Microwave), 2 oz. | 150 |

**"Fish" entree, vegetarian,** frozen:

| | |
|---|---|
| (*Worthington Fillets*), 2 pieces or 3 oz. | 180 |

**Fish seasoning and coating mix:**

| | |
|---|---|
| (*Shake'n Bake*), 1/4 pouch | 70 |
| batter, Cajun (*Tone's*), 1 tsp. | 12 |
| batter, fish & chips (*Golden Dipt*), 1.25 oz. | 120 |
| blackened redfish or broiled (*Golden Dipt*), 1/4 tsp. | 2 |
| Chesapeake Bay (*McCormick/Schilling* Spice Blends), 1/4 tsp. | 2 |
| fish fry, regular or Cajun style (*Golden Dipt*), 2/3 oz. | 60 |
| seafood (*Golden Dipt*), 2/3 oz. | 60 |
| seafood, all purpose (*Golden Dipt*), 1/4 tsp. | 2 |
| seafood, lemon pepper (*Golden Dipt*), 1/4 tsp. | 8 |
| shrimp and crab, Cajun style (*Golden Dipt*), 1/4 tsp. | 2 |

**Fish sticks,** see "Fish entree"

**Flatfish,** meat only:

| | |
|---|---|
| raw, 4 oz. | 104 |
| baked, broiled, or microwaved, 4 oz. | 133 |

**Flounder:**

| | |
|---|---|
| fresh, see "Flatfish" | |
| frozen (*Booth*), 4 oz. | 90 |

| FOOD AND MEASURE | CALORIES |
|---|---|
| *Flounder, continued* | |
| frozen (*Gorton's Fishmarket Fresh*), 5 oz. | 110 |
| frozen (*Van de Kamp's* Natural), 4 oz. | 100 |

**Flounder entree,** frozen:

| | |
|---|---|
| battered (*Mrs. Paul's* Crunchy), 2 pieces | 220 |
| breaded (*Van de Kamp's* Light), 1 piece | 260 |
| stuffed (*Gorton's Microwave Entrees*), 1 pkg. | 350 |

**Flour:**

| | |
|---|---|
| amaranth or barley (*Arrowhead Mills*), 2 oz. | 200 |
| arrowroot, 1 cup | 457 |
| buckwheat, 1 cup | 402 |
| buckwheat, whole-grain (*Arrowhead Mills*), 2 oz. | 190 |
| carob, 1 cup | 185 |
| chickpea (*Arrowhead Mills*), 2 oz. | 200 |
| corn (*Quaker Masa Harina* De Maiz), 1.3 oz. or ⅓ cup | 137 |
| corn (*Quaker Masa Trigo*), 1.3 oz. or ⅓ cup | 149 |
| corn, whole-grain, 1 cup | 422 |
| cottonseed, partially defatted, 1 oz. | 102 |
| millet, whole-grain (*Arrowhead Mills*), 2 oz. | 185 |
| oat, whole-grain (*Arrowhead Mills*), 2 oz. | 200 |
| oak blend (*Gold Medal*), 1 cup | 390 |
| peanut, defatted, 1 cup | 196 |
| peanut, low-fat, 1 cup | 257 |
| pecan, 1 oz. | 93 |
| potato, 1 cup | 628 |
| rice (*Featherweight*), 1 cup | 500 |
| rice, brown, 1 cup | 574 |
| rice, brown (*Arrowhead Mills*), 2 oz. | 200 |
| rice, white, 1 cup | 578 |
| rye: | |
| dark, 1 cup | 415 |
| light, 1 cup | 374 |
| medium, 1 cup | 361 |
| medium (*Pillsbury's Best*), 1 cup | 400 |
| stone ground (*Robin Hood*), 1 cup | 360 |
| whole-grain (*Arrowhead Mills*), 2 oz. | 190 |
| rye and wheat (*Pillsbury's Best* Bohemian Style), 1 cup | 400 |
| sesame, high-fat, 1 oz. | 149 |
| sesame, partially defatted, 1 oz. | 109 |

| FOOD AND MEASURE | CALORIES |
|---|---|
| sesame, low-fat, 1 oz. | 95 |
| soy, full-fat, raw, stirred, 1 cup | 371 |
| soy, full-fat, roasted, stirred, 1 cup | 375 |
| soy, defatted, stirred, 1 cup | 329 |
| soy, low-fat, stirred, 1 cup | 287 |
| sunflower seed, partially defatted, 1 cup | 261 |
| teff, whole-grain (*Arrowhead Mills*), 2 oz. | 200 |
| tortilla mix, 1 cup | 449 |
| triticale, whole-grain, 1 cup | 440 |
| white, 1 cup, except as noted: | |
| (*Drifted Snow*) | 400 |
| (*Softasilk*), 1 oz. or ¼ cup | 100 |
| (*Wondra*) | 400 |
| all purpose (*Ballard/Pillsbury's Best*) | 400 |
| all purpose (*Ceresota/Heckers*), 4 oz. | 390 |
| all purpose (*Gold Medal*) | 400 |
| all purpose (*Red Band*) | 390 |
| all purpose (*Robin Hood*) | 400 |
| unbleached (*Gold Medal*) | 400 |
| unbleached (*Pillsbury's Best*) | 400 |
| unbleached (*Robin Hood*) | 400 |
| bread (*Gold Medal Better for Bread*) | 400 |
| bread (*Pillsbury's Best*) | 400 |
| cake | 395 |
| self-rising (*Ballard/Pillsbury's Best*) | 380 |
| self-rising (*Gold Medal*) | 380 |
| self-rising (*Robin Hood*) | 380 |
| self-rising, enriched (*Aunt Jemima*), 1 oz. or ¼ cup | 109 |
| unbleached (*Arrowhead Mills*), 2 oz. | 200 |
| whole wheat, 1 cup, except as noted: | |
| (*Ceresota/Heckers*) | 400 |
| (*Gold Medal*) | 350 |
| (*Pillsbury's Best*) | 400 |
| blend (*Gold Medal*) | 380 |
| pastry (*Arrowhead Mills*), 2 oz. | 180 |
| stone ground (*Arrowhead Mills*), 2 oz. | 200 |

## Forestiera sauce:

| | |
|---|---|
| refrigerated (*Contadina Fresh*), 7.5 oz. | 270 |

| FOOD AND MEASURE | CALORIES |
|---|---|

**Frankfurter,** 1 link, except as noted:

| | |
|---|---|
| (*Eckrich*, 12 oz.) | 110 |
| (*Eckrich*, 1 lb.) | 160 |
| (*Eckrich* Bunsize/Jumbo) | 190 |
| (*Eckrich* Jumbo Lean Supreme) | 140 |
| (*Eckrich Lite*) | 120 |
| (*Eckrich Lite* Bunsize) | 150 |
| (*Hillshire Farm* Bun Size Wieners), 2 oz. | 180 |
| (*Kahn's* Bun Size, Frank, or Jumbo) | 190 |
| (*Kahn's* Wieners) | 140 |
| (*Oscar Mayer* Light Wieners) | 127 |
| (*Oscar Mayer* Wieners), 1.6-oz. link | 144 |
| (*Oscar Mayer* Wieners), 2-oz. link | 181 |
| (*Oscar Mayer Bun-Length* Wieners) | 184 |
| (*Pilgrim's Pride*, 1 lb.), 2-oz. link | 118 |
| (*Pilgrim's Pride*, 12 oz.), 1.5-oz. link | 88 |
| bacon and cheddar cheese (*Oscar Mayer* Hot Dogs) | 137 |
| batter-wrapped, frozen (*Hormel* Corn Dogs) | 220 |
| batter-wrapped, frozen (*Hormel* Tater Dogs) | 210 |
| beef: | |
| (*Boar's Head*), 1 oz. | 80 |
| (*Eckrich*, 12 oz.) | 110 |
| (*Eckrich*, 1 lb.) | 150 |
| (*Eckrich* Bunsize/Jumbo) | 190 |
| (*Hebrew National*) | 149 |
| (*Hillshire Farm* Bun Size Wieners), 2 oz. | 180 |
| (*Hormel* 12 oz.) | 100 |
| (*Hormel* 1 lb.) | 140 |
| (*Kahn's*) | 140 |
| (*Kahn's* Bun Size Franks/Jumbo) | 190 |
| (*Oscar Mayer* Franks), 1.6-oz. link | 143 |
| (*Oscar Mayer* Franks), 2-oz. link | 181 |
| (*Oscar Mayer* Light Franks), 2-oz. link | 131 |
| (*Oscar Mayer Bun-Length*), 4-oz. link | 364 |
| (*Oscar Mayer Bun-Length* Franks), 2-oz. link | 182 |
| w/cheddar (*Kahn's* Beef 'n Cheddar) | 180 |
| w/cheddar (*Oscar Mayer* Franks), 1.6-oz. link | 136 |
| cheese (*Eckrich*) | 180 |
| cheese (*Hillshire Farm* Bun Size Wieners), 2 oz. | 180 |
| cheese (*Kahn's* Cheese Wiener) | 150 |

| FOOD AND MEASURE | CALORIES |
|---|---|
| cheese (*Oscar Mayer* Hot Dogs), 1.6-oz. link | 143 |
| chicken, see "Chicken frankfurter" | |
| chili (*Hormel* Frank 'n Stuff) | 165 |
| cocktail, canned (*Oscar Mayer* Little Wieners), .3-oz. link | 28 |
| hot, regular or beef (*Hillshire Farm* Hot Links), 2 oz. | 190 |
| meat (*Hormel*, 12 oz.) | 110 |
| meat (*Hormel*, 1 lb.) | 140 |
| Mexacali (*Hormel* Mexacali Dogs), 5 oz. | 400 |
| natural casing (*Hillshire Farm* Wieners), 2 oz. | 180 |
| pork and beef (*Boar's Head*), 1 oz. | 80 |
| smoked: | |
| (*Hormel Range Brand Wranglers*) | 170 |
| (*Kahn's* Big Red Smokey) | 170 |
| (*Kahn's* Bun Size Smokey) | 180 |
| beef (*Hormel Wranglers*) | 170 |
| beef (*Kahn's* Bun Size Beef Smokey) | 190 |
| w/cheese (*Hormel Wranglers*) | 180 |
| turkey, see "Turkey frankfurter" | |

**"Frankfurter," vegetarian:**

| | |
|---|---|
| canned (*Worthington Super-Links*), 1.7-oz. link | 100 |
| canned (*Worthington Veja-Links*), 2 links | 140 |
| frozen (*Worthington Leanies*), 1.4-oz. link | 100 |
| frozen, on a stick (*Worthington* Dixie Dogs), 2.5-oz. piece | 200 |

**Frankfurter wrap:**

| | |
|---|---|
| refrigerated (*Weiner Wrap*), 1 piece | 60 |

**French toast,** frozen:

| | |
|---|---|
| (*Aunt Jemima* Original), 3 oz. | 166 |
| (*Downyflake*), 2 slices | 270 |
| (*Downyflake* Extra Thick), 1 slice | 150 |
| w/cinnamon (*Weight Watchers* Microwave), 3 oz. | 160 |
| cinnamon swirl (*Aunt Jemima*), 3 oz. | 171 |
| sticks (*Farm Rich* Original), 3 oz. | 300 |
| sticks, apple cinnamon or blueberry (*Farm Rich*), 3 oz. | 310 |

**French toast breakfast,** frozen:

| | |
|---|---|
| w/sausages (*Swanson Great Starts*), 5.5 oz. | 380 |
| w/sausages, mini (*Swanson Great Starts*), 2.5 oz. | 190 |
| cinnamon swirl, w/sausages (*Swanson Great Starts*), 5.5 oz. | 390 |
| w/links (*Weight Watchers* Microwave), 4.5 oz. | 270 |

| FOOD AND MEASURE | CALORIES |
|---|---|
| *French toast breakfast, continued* | |
| oatmeal, w/lite links (*Swanson Great Starts*), 4.65 oz. | 310 |
| Texas style, w/sausages (*Downyflake*), 4.25 oz. | 400 |
| vegetarian, cinnamon swirl, w/patties (*Morningstar Farms* Country Breakfast), 6.5 oz. | 380 |
| **Frog's legs,** meat only: | |
| raw, 4 oz. | 84 |
| **Frosting, ready-to-spread,** 1/12 can, except as noted: | |
| Amaretto almond (*Betty Crocker Creamy Deluxe*) | 160 |
| butter pecan (*Betty Crocker Creamy Deluxe*) | 170 |
| caramel or coconut pecan (*Pillsbury Frosting Supreme*) | 160 |
| cherry (*Betty Crocker Creamy Deluxe*) | 160 |
| chocolate: | |
| all varieties (*Betty Crocker Creamy Deluxe*) | 160 |
| all varieties (*Betty Crocker Creamy Deluxe* Light) | 130 |
| all varieties (*Duncan Hines*) | 160 |
| all varieties, except double Dutch (*Pillsbury Frosting Supreme*) | 150 |
| double Dutch (*Pillsbury Frosting Supreme*) | 140 |
| fudge (*Pillsbury*), 1/8 cake | 110 |
| fudge (*Pillsbury* Funfetti) | 140 |
| fudge (*Pillsbury Lovin' Lites*) | 120 |
| chocolate chip (*Betty Crocker Creamy Deluxe*) | 170 |
| chocolate chip (*Pillsbury Frosting Supreme*) | 150 |
| chocolate chip, chocolate, candy coated (*Betty Crocker Creamy Deluxe* Party) | 160 |
| chocolate coconut-almond (*Betty Crocker Creamy Deluxe*) | 160 |
| chocolate or white (*Pillsbury* Frost It Hot), 1/8 cake | 50 |
| coconut-almond (*Pillsbury*) | 160 |
| coconut-almond (*Pillsbury Frosting Supreme*) | 150 |
| coconut-pecan (*Betty Crocker Creamy Deluxe*) | 160 |
| coconut-pecan (*Pillsbury*) | 150 |
| cream cheese (*Betty Crocker Creamy Deluxe*) | 160 |
| cream cheese (*Pillsbury Frosting Supreme*) | 160 |
| decorator, all flavors except chocolate (*Pillsbury*), 1 tbsp. | 70 |
| decorator, chocolate (*Pillsbury*), 1 tbsp. | 60 |
| lemon (*Betty Crocker Creamy Deluxe*) | 170 |
| lemon or strawberry (*Pillsbury Frosting Supreme*) | 160 |
| rainbow chip (*Betty Crocker Creamy Deluxe*) | 170 |
| rocky road (*Betty Crocker Creamy Deluxe*) | 150 |

| FOOD AND MEASURE | CALORIES |
|---|---|
| sour cream, all varieties (*Betty Crocker Creamy Deluxe*) | 160 |
| sour cream, vanilla (*Pillsbury Frosting Supreme*) | 160 |
| vanilla: | |
| (*Betty Crocker Creamy Deluxe*) | 160 |
| (*Betty Crocker Creamy Deluxe* Light) | 140 |
| (*Duncan Hines*) | 160 |
| (*Pillsbury*), 1/8 cake | 120 |
| (*Pillsbury Frosting Supreme*) | 160 |
| (*Pillsbury* Funfetti, pink and white) | 150 |
| (*Pillsbury Lovin' Lites*) | 130 |
| white, fluffy (*Pillsbury*) | 60 |

## **Fructose:**

| | |
|---|---|
| (*Estee*), 1 tsp. | 12 |
| (*Featherweight*), 1 pkt. or 1 tsp. | 12 |

## **Fruit,** see specific listings

## **Fruit, mixed** (see also "Fruit salad"):

| | |
|---|---|
| canned, 1/2 cup, except as noted: | |
| (*Del Monte* Fruit Cup), 5 oz. | 100 |
| (*Del Monte* Fruit for Salad) | 90 |
| chunky (*Del Monte*) | 80 |
| chunky (*Del Monte Lite*) | 50 |
| chunky (*S&W/Nutradiet*) | 40 |
| in juice, chunky (*Libby Lite*) | 50 |
| in sweetened clarified juice (*S&W*) | 90 |
| in heavy syrup | 92 |
| fruit cocktail (*Del Monte*) | 80 |
| fruit cocktail (*Del Monte Lite*) | 50 |
| fruit cocktail (*S&W/Nutradiet* Regular/Unsweetened) | 40 |
| fruit cocktail, in juice (*Featherweight*) | 50 |
| fruit cocktail, in juice (*Libby Lite*) | 50 |
| fruit cocktail, in light syrup | 72 |
| fruit cocktail, in heavy syrup (*S&W*) | 90 |
| dried (*Del Monte*), 2 oz. | 130 |
| dried (*Sun-Maid/Sunsweet*), 2 oz. | 150 |
| dried, morsels, w/raisins (*Sunsweet*), 2 oz. | 160 |
| frozen, in syrup (*Birds Eye* Quick Thaw Pouch), 5 oz. | 120 |
| frozen, sweetened, 1/2 cup | 123 |

| FOOD AND MEASURE | CALORIES |
|---|---|
| **Fruit bar,** frozen, 1 bar: | |
| all varieties (*Dole Fresh Lites*) | 25 |
| all varieties (*Dole SunTops*) | 40 |
| berry, wild (*Sunkist* Fruit & Juice Bar) | 103 |
| coconut (*Sunkist*) | 137 |
| lemonade (*Sunkist*) | 68 |
| orange (*Sunkist* Juice Bar) | 72 |
| piña colada (*Dole Fruit'n Juice*) | 90 |
| pineapple, raspberry, or strawberry (*Dole Fruit'n Juice*) | 70 |
| and cream: | |
| blueberry (*Dole* Fruit & Cream) | 90 |
| chocolate/banana (*Dole* Fruit & Cream) | 175 |
| chocolate/strawberry (*Dole* Fruit & Cream) | 140 |
| orange (*Sunkist*) | 84 |
| peach, raspberry, or strawberry (*Dole* Fruit & Cream) | 90 |
| and yogurt, cherry (*Dole* Fruit & Yogurt) | 80 |
| and yogurt, raspberry or strawberry (*Dole* Fruit & Yogurt) | 70 |
| **Fruit drink** (see also specific fruits): | |
| (*Hi-C* Double Fruit Cooler), 6 fl. oz. | 93 |
| (*Hi-C* Ecto Cooler), 6 fl. oz. | 95 |
| (*Hi-C* Hula Cooler), 6 fl. oz. | 97 |
| mix, all flavors, prepared (*Kool-Aid*), 8 fl. oz. | 100 |
| mix, all flavors, prepared (*Kool-Aid* Sugar Free), 8 fl. oz. | 4 |
| mix, all flavors, prepared (*Kool-Aid* Presweetened), 8 fl. oz. | 80 |
| **Fruit juice** (see also specific fruits): | |
| tropical (*Libby's Juicy Juice*), 6 fl. oz. | 100 |
| **Fruit juice cocktail:** | |
| (*Welch's Orchard* Harvest Blend), 6 fl. oz. | 110 |
| **Fruit juice drink:** | |
| mixed (*Tang* Fruit Box), 8.45 fl. oz. | 140 |
| **Fruit and nut mix:** | |
| (*Planters* Fruit'n Nut), 1 oz. | 150 |
| **Fruit punch:** | |
| (*Minute Maid*), 8.45 fl. oz. | 128 |
| (*Minute Maid* Juices to Go), 9.6 fl. oz. | 145 |
| (*Minute Maid On The Go*), 10 fl. oz. | 152 |

| FOOD AND MEASURE | CALORIES |
|---|---|
| (*Veryfine* 100% Juice Punch), 8 fl. oz. | 122 |
| blend (*Libby's Juicy Juice*), 6 fl. oz. | 100 |
| Concord (*Minute Maid*), 8.45 fl. oz. | 131 |
| Concord (*Minute Maid* Juices to Go), 9.6 fl. oz. | 148 |
| Concord (*Minute Maid On The Go*), 10 fl. oz. | 155 |
| tropical (*Minute Maid*), 8.45 fl. oz. | 130 |
| tropical (*Minute Maid* Juices to Go), 9.6 fl. oz. | 147 |
| chilled or frozen, diluted (*Minute Maid*), 6 fl. oz. | 91 |

**Fruit punch cocktail:**

| | |
|---|---|
| (*Welch's Orchard* Fruit Harvest), 10 fl. oz. | 180 |
| island fruit (*Hawaiian Punch*), 6 fl. oz. | 90 |

**Fruit punch drink:**

| | |
|---|---|
| (*Bama*), 8.45 fl. oz. | 130 |
| (*Hi-C*), 6 fl. oz. | 96 |
| (*Hi-C* Hula Punch), 6 fl. oz. | 87 |
| (*Mott's*), 9.5-fl.-oz. can | 161 |
| (*Wylers*), 6 fl. oz. | 84 |
| mountain berry (*Kool-Aid Koolers*), 8.45 fl. oz. | 140 |
| rainbow or tropical (*Kool-Aid Koolers*), 8.45 fl. oz. | 130 |
| red (*Hawaiian Punch* Fruit Juicy), 6 fl. oz. | 90 |
| red (*Hawaiian Punch* Fruit Juicy Lite), 6 fl. oz. | 60 |
| tropical or wild fruit (*Hawaiian Punch*), 6 fl. oz. | 90 |
| tropical (*Wylers*), 6 fl. oz. | 157 |
| chilled (*Crowley*), 8 fl. oz. | 130 |
| chilled (*Minute Maid* Light'N Juicy), 6 fl. oz. | 14 |
| mix, prepared (*Crystal Light* Sugar Free), 8 fl. oz. | 4 |
| mix, prepared, tropical (*Wylers* Crystals), 8 fl. oz. | 85 |

**Fruit salad,** canned or chilled:

| | |
|---|---|
| in juice, ½ cup | 62 |
| in light syrup, ½ cup | 73 |
| in heavy syrup, ½ cup | 94 |
| (*Kraft* Pure), ½ cup | 80 |
| tropical (*Del Monte*), ½ cup | 90 |
| tropical, in heavy syrup, ½ cup | 110 |

**Fruit snack** (see also specific fruits):

| | |
|---|---|
| all varieties (*Grist Mill*), 1 pouch | 100 |
| (*Fruit Corners/Fruit Roll-Ups* Peel-Outs), 1 roll | 50 |

| FOOD AND MEASURE | CALORIES |
|---|---|
| *Fruit snack, continued* | |
| (*Fruit Wrinkles*), 1 pouch | 100 |
| (*Squeezit*), 6.75 oz. | 110 |
| (*Weight Watchers*), 1 pouch | 50 |
| punch, roll (*Flavor Tree*), 1 piece | 74 |

**Fruit spread,** see "Jam and preserves"

**Fruit syrup:**

| | |
|---|---|
| all flavors (*Smucker's*), 2 tbsp. | 100 |

# G

| FOOD AND MEASURE | CALORIES |
|---|---|
| **Garbanzos,** see "Chick-peas" | |
| **Garden salad,** canned: | |
| (*Joan of Arc/Read*), ½ cup | 70 |
| marinated (*S&W*), ½ cup | 60 |
| **Garlic:** | |
| peeled, 1 oz. | 42 |
| 1 clove, 1¼" × ⅝" × ⅜" | 4 |
| **Garlic dip:** | |
| w/tofu (*Life* All Natural Dressing and Dip), 1 tbsp. | 70 |
| and herb (*Nasoya Vegi-Dip*), 1 oz. | 50 |
| **Garlic powder:** | |
| (*Spice Islands*), 1 tsp. | 5 |
| w/parsley (*Lawry's*), 1 tsp. | 12 |
| **Garlic salt:** | |
| (*Lawry's*), 1 tsp. | 4 |
| (*Morton*), 1 tsp. | 3 |
| **Garlic seasoning:** | |
| (*McCormick/Schilling* Season All), ¼ tsp. | 2 |
| (*McCormick/Schilling Parsley Patch*), 1 tsp. | 13 |
| **Garlic spread:** | |
| (*Lawry's* Bread Spread), ½ tbsp. | 47 |
| concentrate (*Lawry's*), 1 tbsp. | 15 |
| **Gefilte fish,** 1 piece: | |
| (*Manischewitz*, 12⁄24 oz.) | 53 |
| (*Manischewitz* Homestyle, 12⁄24 oz.) | 55 |
| (*Manischewitz* Unsalted) | 45 |
| sweet (*Manischewitz*, 12⁄24 oz.) | 65 |
| whitefish and pike (*Manischewitz*, 12⁄24 oz.) | 49 |
| whitefish and pike, sweet (*Manischewitz* 12⁄24 oz.) | 64 |

| FOOD AND MEASURE | CALORIES |
|---|---|
| *Gefilte fish, continued* | |
| in jelled broth: | |
| (*Mother's* Old Fashioned, 12 oz.) | 54 |
| (*Mother's* Old Fashioned, 24 oz.) | 70 |
| (*Mother's* Old World) | 70 |
| (*Rokeach* Old Vienna, 12 oz.), 2 oz. | 54 |
| (*Rokeach* Old Vienna, 24 oz.), 2.6 oz. | 70 |
| (*Rokeach* Old Vienna, 31 oz.), 3 oz. | 81 |
| (*Rokeach Redi-Jelled*), 2 oz. | 46 |
| (*Rokeach Redi-Jelled*), 3 oz. | 65 |
| whitefish (*Mother's*, 24⁄31 oz.) | 60 |
| whitefish or whitefish and pike (*Mother's*, 12 oz.) | 46 |
| whitefish and pike (*Mother's* Old World, 12 oz.) | 54 |
| whitefish and pike (*Mother's* Old World, 24 oz.) | 70 |
| whitefish and pike (*Rokeach*, 24⁄31 oz.), 2.6 oz. | 60 |
| whitefish and pike (*Rokeach*, 12 oz.), 2 oz. | 46 |
| in liquid: | |
| (*Mother's* Old Fashioned, 12 oz.) | 54 |
| (*Mother's* Old Fashioned, 24⁄31 oz.) | 70 |
| natural broth (*Rokeach*), 4 oz. | 60 |
| natural broth (*Rokeach*), 2.6 oz. | 50 |
| sweet (*Mother's* Old World) | 54 |
| whitefish (*Mother's*, 12 oz.) | 54 |
| whitefish (*Mother's*, 24⁄31 oz.) | 70 |

## **Gelatin,** unflavored:

| | |
|---|---|
| (*Knox*), 1 pkt. | 25 |

## **Gelatin bar,** frozen:

| | |
|---|---|
| all flavors (*Jell-O Gelatin Pops*), 1 bar | 35 |

## **Gelatin dessert mix,** prepared:

| | |
|---|---|
| all flavors (*D-Zerta*), ½ cup | 8 |
| all flavors (*Estee*), ½ cup | 8 |
| all flavors (*Featherweight*), ½ cup | 10 |
| all flavors (*Jell-O*), ½ cup | 80 |
| all flavors (*Royal*), ½ cup | 80 |
| all flavors (*Royal* Sugar Free), ½ cup | 6 |

## **Gelatin drink mix:**

| | |
|---|---|
| orange flavor (*Knox*), 1 envelope | 39 |

| FOOD AND MEASURE | CALORIES |
|---|---|

**Gin,** see "Liquor"

**Ginger, ground:**

1 tsp. . . . . . 6

**Ginger, root:**

peeled, 1 oz. . . . . . 20
peeled, sliced, ¼ cup . . . . . 17

**Gingerbread,** see "Bread, sweet, mix"

**Ginkgo nut:**

raw, shelled, 1 oz. . . . . . 52
canned, drained, 1 oz., 22 small, 14 medium, or 9 large . . . . . 32
dried, shelled, 1 oz. . . . . . 99

**Goatfish,** meat only:

raw, 4 oz. . . . . . 108

***Godfather's Pizza:***

original:
cheese, mini, ¼ pie, 2.8 oz. . . . . . 190
cheese, small, ⅙ pie, 3.6 oz. . . . . . 240
cheese, medium, ⅛ pie, 4 oz. . . . . . 270
cheese, large, ⅒ pie, 4.4 oz. . . . . . 297
cheese, large, hot slice, ⅛ pie, 5.5 oz. . . . . . 370
combo, mini, ¼ pie, 3.8 oz. . . . . . 240
combo, small, ⅙ pie, 5.6 oz. . . . . . 360
combo, medium, ⅛ pie, 6.2 oz. . . . . . 400
combo, large, ⅒ pie, 6.8 oz. . . . . . 437
combo, large, hot slice, ⅛ pie, 8.5 oz. . . . . . 550
thin crust:
cheese, small, ⅙ pie, 2.6 oz. . . . . . 180
cheese, medium, ⅛ pie, 3 oz. . . . . . 210
cheese, large, ⅒ pie, 3.4 oz. . . . . . 228
combo, small, ⅙ pie, 4.3 oz. . . . . . 270
combo, medium, ⅛ pie, 4.9 oz. . . . . . 310
combo, large, ⅒ pie, 5.4 oz. . . . . . 336
stuffed pie:
cheese, small, ⅙ pie, 4.4 oz. . . . . . 310
cheese, medium, ⅛ pie, 4.8 oz. . . . . . 350
cheese, large, ⅒ pie, 5.2 oz. . . . . . 381

| FOOD AND MEASURE | CALORIES |
|---|---|
| *Godfather's Pizza, stuffed pie, continued* | |
| combo, small, 1/6 pie, 6.3 oz. | 430 |
| combo, medium, 1/8 pie, 7 oz. | 480 |
| combo, large, 1/10 pie, 7.6 oz. | 521 |

**Goose,** domesticated:

| | |
|---|---|
| roasted, meat w/skin, 4 oz. | 346 |
| roasted, meat only, 4 oz. | 270 |

**Goose fat:**

| | |
|---|---|
| 1 tbsp. | 115 |

**Goose liver,** see "Liver" and "Pâté"

**Gooseberries:**

| | |
|---|---|
| fresh, ½ cup | 34 |
| canned, in light syrup, ½ cup | 93 |

**Gourd:**

| | |
|---|---|
| dishcloth, boiled, drained, 1″ slices, ½ cup | 50 |
| white-flowered, boiled, drained, 1″ cubes, ½ cup | 11 |

**Gourmet loaf:**

| | |
|---|---|
| (*Eckrich*), 1-oz. slice | 30 |

**Granadilla,** see "Passion fruit"

**Granola,** see "Cereal, ready-to-eat"

**Granola and cereal bar,** 1 bar:

| | |
|---|---|
| all varieties (*Kellogg's Nutri•Grain*) | 150 |
| w/almonds, chewy (*Sunbelt*), 1 oz. | 120 |
| apple, date, or raisin (*Health Valley Bakes*) | 100 |
| caramel nut (*Quaker Granola Dipps*), 1 oz. | 148 |
| chocolate chip: | |
| (*Quaker Chewy*), 1 oz. | 128 |
| (*Quaker Granola Dipps*), 1 oz. | 139 |
| chewy (*Sunbelt*), 1.25 oz. | 150 |
| chocolate-coated (*Hershey's*), 1.2 oz. | 170 |
| fudge-dipped, chewy (*Sunbelt*), 1.63 oz. | 220 |
| w/chocolate chips, chewy (*Sunbelt*), 1.75 oz. | 220 |
| chocolate fudge (*Quaker Granola Dipps*), 1 oz. | 160 |
| cinnamon, oats and honey, or peanut butter (*Nature Valley*), .8 oz. | 120 |

| FOOD AND MEASURE | CALORIES |
|---|---|
| cocoa creme, chocolate-coated (*Hershey's*), 1.2 oz. | 180 |
| *Common Sense,* raspberry (*Kellogg's Smart Start*), 1.5 oz. | 170 |
| cookies and creme, chocolate-coated (*Hershey's*), 1.2 oz. | 170 |
| corn flakes, mixed berry (*Kellogg's Smart Start*), 1.5 oz. | 170 |
| fruit (*Health Valley Fruit & Fitness*) | 100 |
| honey and oats (*Quaker Chewy*), 1 oz. | 125 |
| nut and raisin, chunky (*Quaker Chewy*), 1 oz. | 131 |
| *Nutri•Grain,* blueberry or strawberry (*Kellogg's Smart Start*), 1.5 oz. | 180 |
| oat bran: | |
| almond and date (*Health Valley Oat Bran Jumbo Fruit Bars*) | 170 |
| apricot (*Health Valley Oat Bran Apricot Bakes*) | 100 |
| fig and nut (*Health Valley Fig & Nut Bakes*) | 110 |
| fruit and nut (*Health Valley Oat Bran Jumbo Fruit Bars*) | 150 |
| raisin and cinnamon (*Health Valley Oat Bran Jumbo Fruit Bars*) | 140 |
| oat bran-honey graham (*Nature Valley*), .8 oz. | 110 |
| oats and honey, chewy (*Sunbelt*), 1 oz. | 130 |
| oats and honey, fudged-dipped, chewy (*Sunbelt*), 1.38 oz. | 190 |
| peanut butter: | |
| (*Quaker Chewy*), 1 oz. | 128 |
| (*Quaker Granola Dipps*), 1 oz. | 170 |
| and chocolate chip (*Quaker Chewy*), 1 oz. | 131 |
| chocolate chip (*Quaker Granola Dipps*), 1 oz. | 174 |
| chocolate-coated (*Hershey's*), 1.2 oz. | 180 |
| w/peanuts, fudge-dipped, chewy (*Sunbelt*), 1.38 oz. | 190 |
| w/peanuts, fudge-dipped, chewy (*Sunbelt*), 2.25 oz. | 300 |
| raisin bran (*Kellogg's Smart Start*), 1.5 oz. | 160 |
| w/raisins, chewy (*Sunbelt*), 1.25 oz. | 150 |
| w/raisins, fudged-dipped, chewy (*Sunbelt*), 1.5 oz. | 200 |
| raisin and cinnamon (*Quaker Chewy*), 1 oz. | 128 |
| rice bran, almond and date (*Health Valley Rice Bran Jumbo Fruit Bars*) | 190 |
| *Rice Krispies,* w/almonds (*Kellogg's Smart Start*), 1 oz. | 130 |

## Grape:

| | |
|---|---|
| fresh, slipskin (Concord, Delaware Niagara): | |
| untrimmed, 1 lb. | 165 |
| 10 medium | 15 |
| peeled and seeded, ½ cup | 29 |
| fresh, adherent skin (Thompson seedless, Muscat): | |
| seedless, untrimmed, 1 lb. | 309 |

| FOOD AND MEASURE | CALORIES |
|---|---|
| *Grape, fresh, continued* | |
| seedless, 10 medium, 5/8" diam. | 36 |
| seedless or seeded, ½ cup | 57 |
| canned, in heavy syrup (*S&W* Premium Thompson), ½ cup | 100 |

## Grape drink:

| | |
|---|---|
| (*Bama*), 8.45 fl. oz. | 120 |
| (*Crowley*), 8 fl. oz. | 130 |
| (*Minute Maid* Light'N Juicy), 6 fl. oz. | 13 |
| (*Veryfine*), 8 fl. oz. | 130 |

## Grape fruit roll:

| | |
|---|---|
| (*Flavor Tree*), 1 piece | 76 |

## Grape juice:

| | |
|---|---|
| (*Kraft* Pure 100% Unsweetened), 6 fl. oz. | 104 |
| (*Minute Maid*), 8.45 fl. oz. | 150 |
| (*Veryfine* 100%), 8 fl. oz. | 153 |
| blend (*Libby's Juicy Juice*), 6 fl. oz. | 100 |
| Concord (*S&W* Unsweetened), 6 fl. oz. | 100 |
| purple, red, or white (*Welch's*), 6 fl. oz. | 120 |
| red (*Welch's*), 8.45 fl. oz. | 170 |
| sparkling, red (*Welch's*), 6 fl. oz. | 128 |
| sparkling, white (*Welch's*), 6 fl. oz. | 120 |
| white (*Welch's*), 8.45 fl. oz. | 160 |
| chilled or frozen, diluted (*Minute Maid*), 6 fl. oz. | 100 |
| frozen, diluted (*Sunkist*), 6 fl. oz. | 69 |
| frozen, diluted, purple or white (*Welch's*), 6 fl. oz. | 100 |

## Grape juice cocktail:

| | |
|---|---|
| (*Welch's Orchard*), 10 fl. oz. | 170 |
| (*Welch's Orchard*), 6 fl. oz. | 110 |
| (*Welch's Orchard* Cocktails-In-A-Box), 8.45 fl. oz. | 150 |
| frozen, diluted (*Welch's* No Sugar Added), 6 fl. oz. | 40 |

## Grape juice drink:

| | |
|---|---|
| (*Hi-C*), 8.45 fl. oz. | 136 |
| (*Hi-C*), 6 fl. oz. | 96 |
| (*Kool-Aid Koolers*), 8.45 fl. oz. | 140 |
| (*Tang* Fruit Box), 8.45 fl. oz. | 130 |
| frozen, diluted (*Sunkist*), 6 fl. oz. | 69 |

| FOOD AND MEASURE | CALORIES |
|---|---|
| **Grape-apple drink:** | |
| (*Mott's*), 9.5-fl.-oz. can | 158 |
| **Grapeade:** | |
| chilled or frozen, diluted (*Minute Maid*), 6 fl. oz. | 94 |
| **Grapefruit:** | |
| fresh, pink or red: | |
| California or Arizona, ½ fruit, 3¾" diam. | 46 |
| California or Arizona, sections, w/juice, ½ cup | 43 |
| Florida, ½ fruit, 3¾" diam. | 37 |
| Florida, sections, w/juice, ½ cup | 34 |
| fresh, white: | |
| California, ½ fruit, 3¾" diam. | 43 |
| California, sections, w/juice, ½ cup | 42 |
| Florida, ½ fruit, 3¾" diam. | 38 |
| Florida, sections, w/juice, ½ cup | 38 |
| canned or chilled, ½ cup: | |
| (*Kraft* Pure) | 50 |
| (*S&W* Unsweetened/*S&W Nutradiet*) | 40 |
| in juice (*Featherweight*) | 40 |
| in light syrup (*S&W*) | 80 |
| in light syrup (*Stokely*) | 90 |
| **Grapefruit juice:** | |
| fresh, 6 fl. oz. | 72 |
| canned, bottled, boxed, or chilled: | |
| (*Del Monte*), 6 fl. oz. | 70 |
| (*Minute Maid*), 6 fl. oz. | 78 |
| (*Kraft* Pure 100%), 6 fl. oz. | 70 |
| (*Minute Maid On The Go*), 10 fl. oz. | 130 |
| (*Mott's*) 9.5-fl.-oz. can | 118 |
| (*Ocean Spray*), 6 fl. oz. | 70 |
| (*S&W*), 6 fl. oz. | 80 |
| (*Stokely*), 6 fl. oz. | 76 |
| (*Sunkist* Fresh Squeezed), 8 fl. oz. | 96 |
| (*Tree Top*), 6 fl. oz. | 80 |
| (*Veryfine* 100%), 8 fl. oz. | 101 |
| pink (*Ocean Spray Pink Premium*), 6 fl. oz. | 60 |
| regular or pink (*TreeSweet*), 6 fl. oz. | 72 |
| regular or ruby red (*Tropicana* 100% Pure), 8 fl. oz. | 101 |

| FOOD AND MEASURE | CALORIES |
|---|---|
| *Grapefruit juice, canned, bottled, boxed, or chilled, continued* | |
| chilled or frozen, diluted, pink (*Minute Maid*), 6 fl. oz. | 78 |
| frozen, diluted (*Minute Maid*), 6 fl. oz. | 83 |
| frozen, diluted (*Sunkist*), 6 fl. oz. | 56 |
| frozen, diluted (*TreeSweet*), 6 fl. oz. | 78 |
| **Grapefruit juice cocktail,** pink: | |
| (*Minute Maid* Juices to Go), 9.6 fl. oz. | 136 |
| (*Ocean Spray*), 6 fl. oz. | 80 |
| (*TreeSweet* Lite), 6 fl. oz. | 40 |
| (*Tropicana* Twister), 8 fl. oz. | 110 |
| (*Veryfine*), 8 fl. oz. | 120 |
| chilled or frozen, diluted (*Minute Maid*), 6 fl. oz. | 85 |
| **Grapefruit juice drink:** | |
| (*Citrus Hill* Plus Calcium), 6 fl. oz. | 70 |
| (*Tropicana* Sparkler), 8 fl. oz. | 110 |
| **Gravy,** see specific listings | |
| **Grenadine:** | |
| (*Rose's*), 1 fl. oz. | 65 |
| **Grits,** see "Corn grits" | |
| **Ground cherry:** | |
| trimmed, ½ cup | 37 |
| **Grouper,** mixed species, meat only: | |
| raw, 4 oz. | 104 |
| baked, broiled, or microwaved, 4 oz. | 134 |
| **Guacamole,** see "Avocado dip" | |
| **Guacamole seasoning:** | |
| blend (*Lawry's*), 1 pkg. | 60 |
| mix (*Old El Paso*), 1/7 pkg. | 7 |
| **Guava,** common: | |
| 1 medium, 4 oz. | 45 |
| trimmed, ½ cup | 42 |

| FOOD AND MEASURE | CALORIES |
|---|---|
| **Guava, strawberry:** | |
| untrimmed, 1 lb. | 268 |
| 1 medium, .2 oz. | 4 |
| trimmed, ½ cup | 85 |
| **Guava fruit drink,** Hawaiian: | |
| (*Ocean Spray Mauna La'I*), 6 fl. oz. | 100 |
| **Guava juice:** | |
| (*Welch's Orchard Tropicals*), 6 fl. oz. | 100 |
| **Guava nectar:** | |
| (*Libby's*), 6 fl. oz. | 110 |
| **Guava sauce:** | |
| cooked, ½ cup | 43 |
| **Guava-passion fruit drink,** Hawaiian: | |
| (*Ocean Spray Mauna La'I*), 6 fl. oz. | 100 |
| **Guava-strawberry tropical refresher:** | |
| (*Veryfine*), 8 fl. oz. | 120 |
| **Guinea hen,** fresh, raw: | |
| meat w/skin, 1 oz. | 45 |
| meat only, 1 oz. | 31 |
| **Gumbo filé powder:** | |
| (*Tone's*), 1 tsp. | 8 |

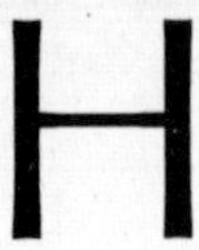

| FOOD AND MEASURE | CALORIES |
|---|---|

**Haddock,** meat only:

| | |
|---|---|
| fresh, raw, 4 oz. | 100 |
| fresh, baked, broiled, or microwaved, 4 oz. | 127 |
| fresh, smoked (finnan haddie), 4 oz. | 132 |
| frozen (*Booth* Individually Wrapped), 4 oz. | 90 |
| frozen (*Gorton's Fishmarket Fresh*), 5 oz. | 110 |
| frozen (*SeaPak*), 4 oz. | 90 |
| frozen (*Van de Kamp's* Natural), 4 oz. | 90 |

**Haddock entree,** frozen:

| | |
|---|---|
| battered (*Mrs. Paul's* Crunchy), 2 pieces | 190 |
| battered (*Van de Kamp's*), 2 pieces | 250 |
| breaded (*Van de Kamp's*), 2 pieces | 270 |
| breaded (*Van de Kamp's* Light), 1 piece | 240 |
| in lemon butter (*Gorton's Microwave Entrees*), 1 pkg. | 360 |

**Hake,** see "Whiting"

**Halibut,** meat only:

| | |
|---|---|
| Atlantic or Pacific, raw, 4 oz. | 124 |
| Atlantic or Pacific, baked, broiled, or microwaved, 4 oz. | 159 |
| Greenland, raw, 4 oz. | 211 |

**Halibut entree,** frozen:

| | |
|---|---|
| battered fillets (*Van de Kamp's*), 2 pieces | 150 |

**Ham,** boneless:

| | |
|---|---|
| fresh, whole leg, roasted, lean and fat, 4 oz. | 333 |
| fresh, whole leg, roasted, lean only, 4 oz. | 249 |
| fresh, rump half, roasted, lean and fat, 4 oz. | 311 |
| fresh, rump half, roasted, lean only, 4 oz. | 251 |
| fresh, shank half, roasted, lean and fat, 4 oz. | 344 |
| fresh, shank half, roasted, lean only, 4 oz. | 244 |
| cured, whole leg, roasted: | |
| lean and fat, 4 oz. | 276 |

| FOOD AND MEASURE | CALORIES |
|---|---|
| lean and fat, chopped or diced, 1 cup not packed | 341 |
| lean only, 4 oz. | 178 |
| lean only, chopped or diced, 1 cup not packed | 219 |
| cured, regular and extra lean, roasted, 4 oz. | 187 |
| cured, regular (11% fat), roasted, 4 oz. | 202 |
| cured, extra lean (5% fat), roasted, 4 oz. | 164 |
| cured, center slice, lean and fat, unheated, 1 oz. | 57 |
| cured, country style, lean only, raw, 1 oz. | 55 |
| cured, steak (*Oscar Mayer* Jubilee), 2-oz. steak | 57 |

**Ham,** canned:

| | |
|---|---|
| (*Black Label,* 5 lb./3 lb.), 4 oz. | 140 |
| (*Black Label* 1½ lb.), 4 oz. | 150 |
| (*EXL*), 4 oz. | 120 |
| (*EXL* Deli Ham, 10 lb.), 4 oz. | 130 |
| (*Holiday Glaze,* 3 lb.), 4 oz. | 130 |
| (*Hormel* Bone-In), 4 oz. | 210 |
| (*Hormel Cure 81*), 4 oz. | 160 |
| (*Hormel Curemaster*), 4 oz. | 140 |
| (*Light & Lean* Boneless), 2 oz. | 60 |
| (*Oscar Mayer* Jubilee), 1 oz. | 29 |
| chopped (*Hormel,* 8 lb.), 3 oz. | 240 |
| chopped (*Hormel,* 12 oz.), 2 oz. | 120 |
| chunk (*Hormel*), 6-¾ oz. | 310 |
| hickory-smoked (*Rath Black Hawk*), 2 oz. | 60 |
| roll (*Hormel*), 4 oz. | 170 |
| spiced (*Hormel*), 3 oz. | 240 |

**"Ham," vegetarian,** frozen:

| | |
|---|---|
| roll or slices (*Worthington Wham*), 3 slices or 2.4 oz. | 120 |

**Ham bologna:**

| | |
|---|---|
| (*Boar's Head*), 1 oz. | 40 |
| (*Kahn's*), 1 slice | 90 |

**Ham breakfast taco:**

| | |
|---|---|
| refrigerated (*Owens Border Breakfasts*), 2.17 oz. | 90 |

**Ham dinner,** frozen:

| | |
|---|---|
| (*Morton*), 10 oz. | 290 |
| steak (*Armour Classics*), 10.75 oz. | 270 |

| FOOD AND MEASURE | CALORIES |
|---|---|
| *Ham dinner, continued* | |
| steak (*Le Menu*), 10 oz. | 300 |
| steak, glazed (*Stouffer's Dinner Supreme*), 10.5 oz. | 380 |

**Ham entree,** frozen:

| | |
|---|---|
| (*Banquet* Platters), 10 oz. | 400 |
| and asparagus bake (*Stouffer's*), 9.5 oz. | 510 |
| scalloped potatoes and (*Swanson* Homestyle Recipe), 9 oz. | 300 |

**Ham luncheon meat:**

| | |
|---|---|
| (*Boar's Head* Lower Salt), 1 oz. | 28 |
| (*Healthy Deli* Deluxe/Taverne), 1 oz. | 31 |
| (*Healthy Deli* Lessalt), 1 oz. | 32 |
| (*Healthy Deli* Light AM), 1 oz. | 27 |
| (*Jones Dairy Farm*), 1 slice | 50 |
| (*Jones Dairy Farm* Family Ham), 1 oz. | 35 |
| (*Kahn's* Low Salt), 1 slice | 30 |
| (*Oscar Mayer* Breakfast Ham), 1.5-oz. slice | 47 |
| (*Oscar Mayer* Jubilee), 1 oz. | 43 |
| (*Oscar Mayer* Lower Salt), .7-oz. slice | 23 |
| (*Swift Premium* Hostess/Sugar Plum), 1 oz. | 30 |
| baked, cooked (*Oscar Mayer*), .75-oz. slice | 21 |
| baked, Virginia (*Healthy Deli*), 1 oz. | 34 |
| baked, Virginia (*Healthy Deli* Lessalt), 1 oz. | 32 |
| barbecue (*Light & Lean*), 2 slices | 50 |
| Black Forest (*Healthy Deli*), 1 oz. | 32 |
| boiled (*Boar's Head* Deluxe), 1 oz. | 28 |
| boiled (*Oscar Mayer*), .75-oz. slice | 23 |
| boiled (*Oscar Mayer* Thin Sliced), .4-oz. slice | 13 |
| breakfast (*Oscar Mayer*), 1.5 oz. | 47 |
| Cajun (*Hillshire Farm* Deli Select), 1 oz. | 31 |
| chopped: | |
|   (*Eckrich*), 1 oz. | 45 |
|   (*Eckrich* Lean Supreme), 1 oz. | 35 |
|   (*Hormel* Perma-Fresh), 2 slices | 88 |
|   (*Kahn's*), 1 oz. | 50 |
|   (*Light & Lean*), 2 slices | 70 |
|   (*Oscar Mayer*), 1 oz. | 41 |
| cooked (*Eckrich Lite*), 1 oz. | 25 |
| cooked (*Kahn's*), 1 slice | 30 |
| cooked (*Light & Lean*), 2 slices | 50 |

| FOOD AND MEASURE | CALORIES |
|---|---|
| fresh, cooked (*Healthy Deli*), 1 oz. | 33 |
| glazed (*Light & Lean*), 2 slices | 50 |
| honey (*Healthy Deli* Honey Valley), 1 oz. | 31 |
| honey (*Hillshire Farm* Deli Select), 1 oz. | 31 |
| honey (*Oscar Mayer*), .75-oz. slice | 23 |
| honey (*Oscar Mayer* Thin Sliced), .4-oz. slice | 13 |
| jalapeño (*Healthy Deli*), 1 oz. | 25 |
| loaf (*Eckrich*), 1 oz. | 50 |
| minced, 1 oz. | 75 |
| peppered, black or red (*Light & Lean*), 2 slices | 50 |
| peppered, black, cracked (*Oscar Mayer*), .75-oz. slice | 22 |
| peppered, chopped (*Oscar Mayer*), 1 oz. | 55 |
| smoked: | |
| (*Eckrich* Slender Sliced), 1 oz. | 40 |
| (*Hillshire Farm* Deli Select), 1 oz. | 31 |
| (*OHSE* 95% Fat Free), 1 oz. | 30 |
| cooked (*Light & Lean*), 2 slices | 50 |
| cooked (*Oscar Mayer*), .75-oz. slice | 22 |

**Ham patty:**

| | |
|---|---|
| grilled, 1 patty, 2.1 oz. (2.3 oz. unheated) | 203 |
| (*Swift Premium* Brown 'N Serve), 1 patty | 130 |
| canned (*Hormel*), 1 patty | 180 |

**Ham spread, deviled,** canned:

| | |
|---|---|
| (*Hormel*), 1 tbsp. | 35 |
| (*Underwood*), 2⅛ oz. | 220 |
| (*Underwood* Light), 2⅛ oz. | 120 |
| smoked (*Underwood*), 2⅛ oz. | 190 |

**Ham and asparagus au gratin:**

| | |
|---|---|
| frozen (*The Budget Gourmet* Slim Selects), 9 oz. | 280 |

**Ham and cheese breakfast sandwich:**

| | |
|---|---|
| frozen, on bagel (*Swanson Great Starts*), 3 oz. | 240 |
| refrigerated (*Owens Border Breakfasts*), 2 oz. | 150 |

**Ham and cheese casserole,** frozen:

| | |
|---|---|
| (*Pillsbury Microwave Classic*), 1 pkg. | 470 |

| FOOD AND MEASURE | CALORIES |
|---|---|
| **Ham and cheese loaf:** | |
| (*Eckrich*), 1-oz. slice | 50 |
| (*Hormel* Perma-Fresh), 2 slices | 110 |
| (*Kahn's*), 1 slice | 70 |
| (*Light & Lean*), 2 slices | 90 |
| (*OHSE*), 1 oz. | 65 |
| (*Oscar Mayer*), 1-oz. slice | 66 |
| canned (*Hormel,* 8 lb.), 3 oz. | 260 |
| **Ham and cheese patty:** | |
| canned (*Hormel*), 1 patty | 190 |
| **Ham and cheese pocket sandwich,** frozen: | |
| (*Hot Pockets*), 5 oz. | 360 |
| **Hamburger,** frozen: | |
| (*MicroMagic*), 4 oz. | 350 |
| **Hamburger entree mix,** prepared: | |
| beef noodle (*Hamburger Helper*), 1 cup | 320 |
| beef Romanoff (*Hamburger Helper*), 1 cup | 350 |
| cheeseburger macaroni (*Hamburger Helper*), 1 cup | 370 |
| chili, w/beans (*Hamburger Helper*), 1¼ cup | 350 |
| chili tomato (*Hamburger Helper*), 1 cup | 330 |
| hamburger hash (*Hamburger Helper*), 1 cup | 320 |
| hamburger stew (*Hamburger Helper*), 1 cup | 300 |
| Italian, cheesy (*Hamburger Helper*), 1 cup | 360 |
| lasagna or zesty Italian (*Hamburger Helper*), 1 cup | 340 |
| meatloaf (*Hamburger Helper*), 1 cup | 360 |
| pizza (*Hamburger Helper Pizzabake*), 4.5 oz. | 320 |
| pizza dish (*Hamburger Helper*), 1 cup | 360 |
| potato au gratin or Stroganoff (*Hamburger Helper*), 1 cup | 320 |
| rice Oriental (*Hamburger Helper*), 1 cup | 340 |
| sloppy Joe (*Hamburger Helper Sloppy Joe Bake*), 5 oz. | 340 |
| spaghetti (*Hamburger Helper*), 1 cup | 340 |
| Stroganoff, creamy (*Hamburger Helper*), 1 cup | 390 |
| taco (*Hamburger Helper Tacobake*), 5.75 oz. | 320 |
| tamale pie (*Hamburger Helper*), 1 cup | 380 |
| **Hamburger seasoning:** | |
| (*McCormick/Schilling*), ¼ pkg. | 33 |

| FOOD AND MEASURE | CALORIES |
|---|---|
| ***Hardee's,*** 1 serving: | |
| *Big Country Breakfast*, bacon, 7.7 oz. | 660 |
| *Big Country Breakfast*, country ham, 9 oz. | 670 |
| *Big Country Breakfast*, ham, 8.9 oz. | 620 |
| *Big Country Breakfast*, sausage, 9.7 oz. | 850 |
| breakfast biscuit: | |
| bacon, 3.3 oz. | 360 |
| bacon and egg, 4.4 oz. | 410 |
| bacon, egg, and cheese, 4.8 oz. | 460 |
| *Biscuit 'N' Gravy*, 7.8 oz. | 440 |
| *Canadian Rise 'N' Shine*, 5.7 oz. | 470 |
| chicken, 5.1 oz. | 430 |
| *Cinnamon 'N' Raisin*, 2.8 oz. | 320 |
| country ham, 3.8 oz. | 350 |
| country ham and egg, 4.9 oz. | 400 |
| ham, 3.7 oz. | 320 |
| ham and egg, 4.9 oz. | 370 |
| ham, egg, and cheese, 5.3 oz. | 420 |
| *Rise 'N' Shine*, 2.9 oz. | 320 |
| sausage, 4.2 oz. | 440 |
| sausage and egg, 5.3 oz. | 490 |
| steak, 5.2 oz. | 500 |
| steak and egg, 6.3 oz. | 550 |
| *Hash Rounds*, 2.8 oz. | 230 |
| pancake syrup, 1.5 oz. | 120 |
| pancakes, 3 pieces, 4.8 oz. | 280 |
| pancakes, 3 pieces, w/2 bacon strips, 5.3 oz. | 350 |
| pancakes, 3 pieces, w/1 sausage patty, 6.2 oz. | 430 |
| sandwiches and burgers: | |
| *Big Deluxe* burger, 7.6 oz. | 500 |
| *Big Roast Beef*, 4.7 oz. | 300 |
| *Big Twin*, 6.1 oz. | 450 |
| cheeseburger, 4.3 oz. | 320 |
| cheeseburger, bacon, 7.7 oz. | 610 |
| cheeseburger, quarter pound, 6.4 oz. | 500 |
| chicken breast sandwich, grilled, 6.8 oz. | 310 |
| *Chicken Fillet*, 6.1 oz. | 370 |
| *Fisherman's Fillet*, 7.3 oz. | 500 |
| hamburger, 3.9 oz. | 270 |
| hot dog, all beef, 4.2 oz. | 300 |

| FOOD AND MEASURE | CALORIES |
|---|---|
| *Hardee's, sandwiches and burgers, continued* | |
| *Hot Ham 'N' Cheese*, 5.3 oz. | 330 |
| *Mushroom 'N' Swiss* burger, 6.6 oz. | 490 |
| roast beef, regular, 4 oz. | 260 |
| *Turkey Club*, 7.3 oz. | 390 |
| salads, side dishes, and special items: | |
| *Chicken Stix*, 9 pieces, 5.3 oz. | 310 |
| *Chicken Stix*, 6 pieces, 3.5 oz. | 210 |
| *Crispy Curls*, 3 oz. | 300 |
| french fries, big, 5.5 oz. | 500 |
| french fries, large, 4 oz. | 360 |
| french fries, regular, 2.5 oz. | 230 |
| salad, chef, 10.4 oz. | 240 |
| salad, chicken 'N' pasta, 14.6 oz. | 230 |
| salad, garden, 8.5 oz. | 210 |
| salad, side, 4 oz. | 20 |
| dressings, sauces, and condiments: | |
| barbecue dipping sauce, 1 oz. | 30 |
| barbecue sauce, .5-oz. pkt. | 14 |
| *Big Twin* sauce, .5 oz. | 50 |
| blue cheese dressing, 2 oz. | 210 |
| French dressing, reduced calorie, 2 oz. | 130 |
| honey sauce, .5 oz. | 45 |
| horseradish, .25-oz. pkt. | 25 |
| house dressing, 2 oz. | 290 |
| Italian dressing, reduced calorie, 2 oz. | 90 |
| sweet mustard dipping sauce, 1 oz. | 50 |
| sweet 'n' sour dipping sauce, 1 oz. | 40 |
| tartar sauce, .7 oz. | 90 |
| Thousand Island dressing, 2 oz. | 250 |
| desserts and shakes: | |
| apple turnover, 3.2 oz. | 270 |
| *Big Cookie*, 1.7 oz. | 250 |
| *Cool Twist*, chocolate, 4.2 oz. | 200 |
| *Cool Twist*, vanilla, 4.2 oz. | 190 |
| *Cool Twist*, vanilla/chocolate, 4.2 oz. | 190 |
| *Cool Twist* sundae, caramel, 6 oz. | 330 |
| *Cool Twist* sundae, hot fudge, 5.9 oz. | 320 |
| *Cool Twist* sundae, strawberry, 5.9 oz. | 260 |
| shake, chocolate, 12 oz. | 460 |

| FOOD AND MEASURE | CALORIES |
|---|---|
| shake, strawberry, 12 oz. | 440 |
| shake, vanilla, 12 oz. | 400 |

**Hazelnuts,** see "Filberts"

**Head cheese:**

| | |
|---|---|
| (*Oscar Mayer*), 1-oz. slice | 55 |

**Heart:**

| | |
|---|---|
| beef, simmered, 4 oz. | 198 |
| chicken, broiler-fryer, simmered, 4 oz. | 210 |
| lamb, simmered, 4 oz. | 210 |
| pork, simmered, 4 oz. | 168 |
| turkey, simmered, 4 oz. | 201 |
| veal, simmered, 4 oz. | 211 |

**Herb gravy mix,** prepared:

| | |
|---|---|
| (*McCormick/Schilling*), ¼ cup | 20 |

**Herb seasoning and coating mix:**

| | |
|---|---|
| Italian (*McCormick/Schilling* Bag'n Season), 1 pkg. | 94 |
| Italian (*Shake'n Bake*), ¼ pouch | 80 |

**Herb and garlic sauce:**

| | |
|---|---|
| w/lemon juice (*Lawry's*), ¼ cup | 36 |

**Herbs,** see specific listings

**Herbs, mixed:**

| | |
|---|---|
| seasoning (*Lawry's* Pinch of Herbs), 1 tsp. | 9 |

**Herring,** fresh, meat only:

| | |
|---|---|
| Atlantic, raw, 4 oz. | 180 |
| Atlantic, baked, broiled, or microwaved, 4 oz. | 230 |
| Atlantic, kippered, 4 oz. | 246 |
| Atlantic, pickled, 4 oz. | 297 |
| Pacific, raw, 4 oz. | 220 |

**Herring,** canned, see "Sardine, canned"

**Herring, lake,** see "Cisco"

**Hickory nuts,** dried:

| | |
|---|---|
| shelled, 1 oz. | 187 |

| FOOD AND MEASURE | CALORIES |
|---|---|
| **Hollandaise sauce:** | |
| (*Great Impressions*), 2 tbsp. | 192 |
| mix (*McCormick/Schilling*), ¼ pkg. | 51 |
| **Homestyle gravy mix,** prepared: | |
| (*French's*), ¼ cup | 20 |
| (*McCormick/Schilling*), ¼ cup | 24 |
| (*Pillsbury*), ¼ cup | 15 |
| **Hominy,** canned (see also "Corn grits"): | |
| golden or Mexican (*Allens*), ½ cup | 80 |
| white (*Allens*), ½ cup | 70 |
| **Honey:** | |
| 1 tbsp. | 60 |
| **Honey butter:** | |
| regular or cinnamon (*Downey's*), 1 tbsp. | 50 |
| **Honey loaf:** | |
| (*Eckrich/Eckrich Smorgas Pac*), 1-oz. slice | 35 |
| (*Hormel* Perma-Fresh), 2 slices | 90 |
| (*Kahn's*), 1 slice | 40 |
| (*Oscar Mayer*), 1-oz. slice | 34 |
| **Honey roll sausage:** | |
| beef, 1 oz. | 52 |
| **Honeydew:** | |
| 1⁄10 melon, 7″ × 2″ slice | 46 |
| cubed, ½ cup | 30 |
| **Horseradish,** prepared: | |
| (*Crowley*), 1 oz. | 10 |
| (*Kraft*), 1 tbsp. | 10 |
| all varieties (*Gold's*), 1 tsp. | 4 |
| cream style (*Kraft*), 1 tbsp. | 12 |
| **Horseradish sauce:** | |
| (*Great Impressions*), 1 tbsp. | 74 |
| (*Heinz*), 1 tbsp. | 74 |
| (*Sauceworks*), 1 tbsp. | 50 |
| strong (*Life* All Natural), .25 fl. oz. or ½ tbsp. | 7 |

| FOOD AND MEASURE | CALORIES |
|---|---|
| **Horseradish tree:** | |
| leafy tips, raw, chopped, ½ cup | 6 |
| leafy tips, boiled, drained, chopped, ½ cup | 13 |
| pods, raw, sliced, ½ cup | 19 |
| pods, boiled, drained, sliced, ½ cup | 21 |
| **Hot dog,** see "Frankfurter" | |
| **Hot sauce,** see "Pepper sauce" and specific listings | |
| **Hummus:** | |
| dip mix (*Fantastic Foods*), 2 oz. or ¼ cup | 111 |
| mix (*Casbah*), 1 oz. | 110 |
| **Hush puppy:** | |
| frozen (*SeaPak* Regular), 4 oz. | 330 |
| mix, all varieties (*Golden Dipt*), 1.25 oz. | 120 |

# I

| FOOD AND MEASURE | CALORIES |
|---|---|

**Ice:**

cherry, Italian (*Good Humor*), 6 fl. oz. .......... 138

**Ice bar** (see also "Fruit bar"):

all flavors (*Good Humor* Ice Stripes), 1.5-fl.-oz. bar .......... 35
cherry (*Good Humor Calippo*), 4.5-fl.-oz. bar .......... 138
lemon (*Good Humor Calippo*), 4.5-fl.-oz. bar .......... 112
orange (*Good Humor Calippo*), 4.5-fl.-oz. bar .......... 111

**Ice cream,** ½ cup, except as noted:

butter almond (*Sealtest*) .......... 160
butter crunch (*Sealtest*) .......... 150
butter pecan:
  (*Breyers*) .......... 180
  (*Frusen Glädjé*) .......... 280
  (*Häagen-Dazs*) .......... 390
  (*Lady Borden*) .......... 180
  (*Sealtest*) .......... 160
caramel nut sundae (*Häagen-Dazs*) .......... 310
cherry vanilla (*Breyers*) .......... 150
chocolate:
  (*Breyers*) .......... 160
  (*Frusen Glädjé*) .......... 240
  (*Häagen-Dazs*) .......... 270
  (*Sealtest*) .......... 140
  deep (*Häagen-Dazs*) .......... 290
  Dutch (*Borden Olde Fashioned Recipe*) .......... 130
  fudge, deep (*Häagen-Dazs*) .......... 290
  swirl (*Borden*) .......... 130
  triple, stripe (*Sealtest*) .......... 140
chocolate almond, Swiss (*Frusen Glädjé*) .......... 270
chocolate chip:
  (*Sealtest*) .......... 150
  chocolate (*Breyers*) .......... 180
  chocolate (*Frusen Glädjé*) .......... 270

| FOOD AND MEASURE | CALORIES |
|---|---|
| chocolate (*Häagen-Dazs*) | 290 |
| mint (*Breyers*) | 170 |
| vanilla (*Frusen Glädjé*) | 280 |
| chocolate-chocolate mint (*Häagen-Dazs*) | 300 |
| chocolate-marshmallow sundae (*Sealtest*) | 150 |
| chocolate-peanut butter, deep (*Häagen-Dazs*) | 330 |
| coffee (*Breyers*) | 150 |
| coffee (*Frusen Glädjé*) | 260 |
| coffee (*Häagen-Dazs*) | 270 |
| coffee (*Sealtest*) | 140 |
| cookies n' cream (*Breyers*) | 170 |
| fudge, marble (*Dreyer's*) | 150 |
| fudge royale (*Sealtest*) | 140 |
| heavenly hash (*Sealtest*) | 150 |
| macadamia brittle (*Häagen-Dazs*) | 280 |
| maple walnut (*Sealtest*) | 160 |
| mocha chip (*Frusen Glädjé*) | 280 |
| peach (*Breyers*) | 130 |
| praline and cream (*Frusen Glädjé*) | 280 |
| rum raisin (*Häagen-Dazs*) | 250 |
| strawberry: | |
| (*Borden*) | 130 |
| (*Breyers*) | 130 |
| (*Frusen Glädjé*) | 230 |
| (*Häagen-Dazs*) | 250 |
| (*Sealtest*) | 130 |
| cream (*Borden Olde Fashioned Recipe*) | 130 |
| vanilla: | |
| (*Borden Olde Fashioned Recipe*) | 130 |
| (*Breyers* Natural) | 150 |
| (*Frusen Glädjé*) | 230 |
| (*Good Humor* Cup), 3 fl. oz. | 98 |
| (*Häagen-Dazs*) | 260 |
| (*Sealtest*) | 140 |
| French (*Sealtest*) | 140 |
| honey (*Häagen-Dazs*) | 250 |
| vanilla fudge (*Häagen-Dazs*) | 270 |
| vanilla fudge (*Sealtest*) | 140 |
| vanilla fudge twirl (*Breyers*) | 160 |
| vanilla peanut butter swirl (*Häagen-Dazs*) | 280 |
| vanilla Swiss almond (*Frusen Glädjé*) | 270 |

| FOOD AND MEASURE | CALORIES |
|---|---|
| *Ice cream, continued* | |
| vanilla Swiss almond (*Häagen-Dazs*) | 290 |
| vanilla toffee chunk (*Frusen Glädjé*) | 270 |
| vanilla-chocolate (*Breyers*) | 160 |
| vanilla-chocolate-strawberry (*Breyers*) | 150 |
| vanilla-chocolate-strawberry (*Sealtest*) | 140 |
| vanilla-chocolate-strawberry (*Sealtest Cubic Scoops*) | 140 |
| vanilla-orange or vanilla-raspberry (*Sealtest Cubic Scoops*) | 130 |
| vanilla-raspberry swirl (*Frusen Glädjé*) | 230 |

**Ice cream, substitute and imitation,** ½ cup, except as noted:

| | |
|---|---|
| all flavors (*Lite-Lite Tofutti*) | 90 |
| all flavors (*Sealtest Free*) | 100 |
| all flavors, except chocolate swirl (*Weight Watchers Grand Collection* Fat Free) | 80 |
| cappuccino or chocolate (*Tofutti* Love Drops) | 230 |
| chocolate (*Simple Pleasures*), 4 oz. | 140 |
| chocolate chip (*Low, Lite'n Luscious*) | 100 |
| chocolate supreme (*Tofutti*) | 210 |
| chocolate swirl (*Weight Watchers Grand Collection* Fat Free) | 90 |
| coffee (*Simple Pleasures*), 4 oz. | 120 |
| Jamoca Swiss almond (*Low, Lite'n Luscious*) | 90 |
| peach (*Simple Pleasures*), 4 oz. | 135 |
| pineapple coconut (*Low, Lite'n Luscious*) | 90 |
| rum raisin (*Simple Pleasures*), 4 oz. | 130 |
| strawberry (*Low, Lite'n Luscious*) | 80 |
| strawberry (*Simple Pleasures*), 4 oz. | 120 |
| vanilla (*Tofutti*) | 200 |
| vanilla (*Tofutti* Love Drops) | 220 |
| vanilla, chocolate-dipped (*Tofutti O's*), 1 piece | 40 |
| vanilla almond bark (*Tofutti*) | 230 |
| wildberry (*Tofutti*) | 210 |

**Ice cream bar,** 1 piece:

| | |
|---|---|
| (*Good Humor* Fat Frog) | 154 |
| (*Good Humor* Halo Bar) | 230 |
| (*Heath*) | 170 |
| (*Klondike*) | 280 |
| (*Klondike* Krispy) | 290 |
| (*Klondike* Lite) | 140 |
| almond, toasted (*Good Humor*), 3 fl. oz. | 212 |
| assorted (*Good Humor Whammy*), 1.6 fl. oz. | 95 |

| FOOD AND MEASURE | CALORIES |
|---|---|
| caramel almond crunch (*Häagen-Dazs*) | 240 |
| chip candy crunch (*Good Humor*), 3 fl. oz. | 255 |
| chocolate: | |
| (*Klondike*) | 270 |
| w/dark chocolate coating (*Häagen-Dazs*) | 390 |
| fudge cake (*Good Humor*), 6.3 fl. oz. | 214 |
| fudge sundae (*Bakers Fudgetastic*) | 220 |
| fudge sundae, crunchy (*Bakers Fudgetastic*) | 230 |
| milk, w/almonds, milk chocolate-coated (*Nestlé* Premium) | 350 |
| w/milk chocolate coating (*Nestlé Quik*) | 210 |
| chocolate eclair (*Good Humor*), 3 fl. oz. | 188 |
| peanut butter crunch (*Häagen-Dazs*) | 270 |
| strawberry shortcake (*Good Humor*), 3 fl. oz. | 176 |
| vanilla: | |
| caramel peanut center, milk chocolate-coated (*Oh! Henry*) | 320 |
| chocolate flavor-coated (*Good Humor*), 3 fl. oz. | 198 |
| crunch (*Häagen-Dazs*) | 220 |
| w/dark chocolate coating (*Häagen-Dazs*) | 390 |
| w/milk chocolate coating (*Häagen-Dazs*) | 360 |
| w/milk chocolate coating and almonds (*Häagen-Dazs*) | 370 |
| w/milk chocolate coating and crisps (*Nestlé Crunch*) | 180 |
| w/white chocolate coating (*Nestlé Alpine* Premium) | 350 |

## **Ice cream bar, substitute and imitation,** 1 piece:

| | |
|---|---|
| (*Good Humor* Cool Shark), 3 fl. oz. | 68 |
| (*Good Humor* Jumbo Jet Star), 4.5 fl. oz. | 85 |
| (*Good Humor* Milky Pop), 1.5 fl. oz. | 47 |
| amaretto-chocolate swirl (*Crystal Light Cool N'Creamy*) | 60 |
| chocolate: | |
| (*Weight Watchers* Treat Bars), 2.75 oz. | 100 |
| dip (*Weight Watchers*), 1.7 oz. | 110 |
| fudge (*Good Humor*), 2.5 fl. oz. | 127 |
| fudge, double (*Crystal Light Cool N'Creamy*) | 50 |
| fudge, double (*Weight Watchers*), 1.75 oz. | 60 |
| fudge swirl (*Sealtest Free*) | 90 |
| mousse (*Weight Watchers*), 1.75 oz. | 35 |
| chocolate/vanilla (*Crystal Light Cool N'Creamy*) | 50 |
| English toffee crunch (*Weight Watchers*), 1.7 oz. | 120 |
| orange-vanilla (*Crystal Light Cool N'Creamy*) | 30 |
| orange-vanilla (*Weight Watchers* Sugar Free Treat), 1.75 oz. | 30 |
| strawberry finger (*Good Humor*), 2.5 fl. oz. | 49 |

| FOOD AND MEASURE | CALORIES |
|---|---|
| *Ice cream bar, substitute and imitation, continued* | |
| vanilla fudge or vanilla raspberry swirl (*Sealtest Free*) | 80 |
| vanilla sandwich (*Weight Watchers*) | 150 |
| **Ice cream cone and cup:** | |
| plain (*Keebler*), 1 cone | 15 |
| plain (*Little Debbie* Ice Cream Cup), 1 cup | 15 |
| filled (*Good Humor* King Cone), 5.5 fl. oz. | 290 |
| filled, boysenberry (*Good Humor* King Cone), 5 fl. oz. | 340 |
| filled, vanilla-chocolate (*Good Humor* Combo), 6 fl. oz. | 201 |
| **Ice cream mix,** prepared: | |
| all flavors (*Salada*), 1 cup | 310 |
| **Ice cream sandwich,** 1 piece: | |
| chocolate chip cookie (*Good Humor*), 2.7 fl. oz. | 204 |
| chocolate chip cookie (*Good Humor*), 4 fl. oz. | 246 |
| vanilla (*Good Humor*), 3 fl. oz. | 191 |
| vanilla (*Good Humor*), 2.5 fl. oz. | 165 |
| vanilla (*Klondike*), 5 fl. oz. | 230 |
| **Ice cream and sorbet,** see "Sorbet" | |
| **Ice milk,** ½ cup: | |
| caramel nut (*Light n' Lively*) | 120 |
| chocolate (*Borden*) | 100 |
| chocolate (*Breyers* Light) | 120 |
| chocolate (*Weight Watchers Grand Collection*) | 110 |
| chocolate chip (*Light n' Lively*) | 120 |
| chocolate chip or swirl (*Weight Watchers Grand Collection*) | 120 |
| chocolate fudge twirl (*Breyers* Light) | 130 |
| coffee (*Light n' Lively*) | 100 |
| cookies n' cream (*Light n' Lively*) | 110 |
| heavenly hash (*Breyers* Light) | 150 |
| heavenly hash (*Light n' Lively*) | 120 |
| Neapolitan (*Weight Watchers Grand Collection*) | 110 |
| pecan pralines'N creme (*Weight Watchers Grand Collection*) | 120 |
| praline almond (*Breyers* Light) | 130 |
| strawberry (*Borden*) | 90 |
| strawberry (*Breyers* Light) | 110 |
| toffee fudge parfait (*Breyers* Light) | 140 |
| vanilla (*Borden*) | 90 |

| FOOD AND MEASURE | CALORIES |
|---|---|
| vanilla (*Breyers* Light) | 120 |
| vanilla (*Light n' Lively*) | 100 |
| vanilla (*Weight Watchers Grand Collection*) | 100 |
| vanilla chocolate almond (*Light n' Lively*) | 120 |
| vanilla-chocolate-strawberry (*Breyers* Light) | 120 |
| vanilla-chocolate-strawberry (*Light n' Lively*) | 100 |
| vanilla fudge or raspberry swirl (*Light n' Lively*) | 110 |
| vanilla raspberry parfait (*Breyers* Light) | 130 |

**Icing, cake,** see "Frosting"

**Iowa Brand loaf:**

| | |
|---|---|
| (*Hormel* Perma-Fresh), 2 slices | 90 |

**Italian sausage:**

| | |
|---|---|
| hot (*Hillshire Farm* Links), 2 oz. | 180 |
| mild (*Hillshire Farm* Links), 2 oz. | 190 |
| smoked (*Hillshire Farm* Flavorseal), 2 oz. | 200 |

# J

| FOOD AND MEASURE | CALORIES |
|---|---|
| **Jack,** see "Mackerel" | |
| ***Jack-in-the-Box,*** 1 serving: | |
| breakfast: | |
| *Breakfast Jack,* 4.4 oz. | 307 |
| crescent, Canadian, 4.7 oz. | 452 |
| crescent, sausage, 5.5 oz. | 584 |
| crescent, supreme, 5.1 oz. | 547 |
| hash browns, 2.2 oz. | 116 |
| jelly, grape, .5 oz. | 38 |
| pancake platter, 8.1 oz. | 612 |
| scrambled egg platter, 8.8 oz. | 662 |
| sandwiches: | |
| bacon cheeseburger, 8.1 oz. | 705 |
| beef fajita pita, 6.2 oz. | 333 |
| cheeseburger, 4 oz. | 315 |
| cheeseburger, double, 5.3 oz. | 467 |
| cheeseburger, ultimate, 10 oz. | 942 |
| chicken fajita pita, 6.7 oz. | 292 |
| chicken fillet, grilled, 7.2 oz. | 408 |
| chicken supreme, 8.1 oz. | 575 |
| fish supreme, 8 oz. | 554 |
| hamburger, 3.4 oz. | 267 |
| *Jumbo Jack,* 7.8 oz. | 584 |
| *Jumbo Jack,* w/cheese, 8.5 oz. | 677 |
| Swiss and bacon burger, 6.6 oz. | 678 |
| Mexican food: | |
| guacamole, 1 oz. | 55 |
| salsa, 1 oz. | 8 |
| taco, 2.9 oz. | 191 |
| taco, super, 4.8 oz. | 288 |
| salads: | |
| chef, 14 oz. | 295 |
| Mexican chicken, 14.6 oz. | 442 |

| FOOD AND MEASURE | CALORIES |
|---|---|
| side, 4 oz. | 51 |
| taco, 14.2 oz. | 503 |
| finger foods: | |
| chicken strips, 4 pieces, 4.4 oz. | 349 |
| chicken strips, 6 pieces, 6.6 oz. | 523 |
| egg rolls, 3 pieces, 6 oz. | 405 |
| egg rolls, 5 pieces, 10 oz. | 675 |
| shrimp, 10 pieces, 3 oz. | 270 |
| shrimp, 15 pieces, 4.4 oz. | 404 |
| taquitos, 5 pieces, 5 oz. | 363 |
| taquitos, 7 pieces, 7 oz. | 508 |
| french fries, small, 2.4 oz. | 221 |
| french fries, regular, 3.9 oz. | 353 |
| french fries, jumbo, 4.8 oz. | 442 |
| onion rings, 3.8 oz. | 382 |
| dressings and sauces: | |
| BBQ sauce, 1 oz. | 44 |
| blue cheese dressing, 2.5 oz. | 262 |
| buttermilk dressing, 2.5 oz. | 362 |
| mayo-mustard sauce, .7 oz. | 124 |
| mayo-onion sauce, .7 oz. | 143 |
| reduced calorie French dressing, 2.5 oz. | 176 |
| seafood cocktail sauce, 1 oz. | 32 |
| sweet and sour sauce, 1 oz. | 40 |
| Thousand Island dressing, 2.5 oz. | 312 |
| desserts: | |
| apple turnover, 4.2 oz. | 410 |
| cheesecake, 3.5 oz. | 309 |
| shake, chocolate | 330 |
| shake, strawberry or vanilla | 320 |

## Jackfruit:

| | |
|---|---|
| trimmed, 1 oz. | 27 |

## Jalapeño dip:

| | |
|---|---|
| bean (*Wise*), 2 tbsp. | 25 |
| bean, medium (*Hain*), 4 tbsp. | 70 |
| pepper (*Kraft*), 2 tbsp. | 50 |

## Jalapeño loaf:

| | |
|---|---|
| (*Kahn's*), 1 slice | 70 |

| FOOD AND MEASURE | CALORIES |
|---|---|

**Jalapeño pepper,** see "Pepper, jalapeño"

**Jalapeño relish,** see "Relish"

**Jam and preserves** (see also "Marmalade"):

all flavors:
(*Bama*), 2 tsp. . . . . . 30
(*Estee*), 1 tsp. . . . . . 2
(*Featherweight*), 1 tsp. . . . . . 4
(*Kraft*), 1 tsp. . . . . . 17
(*Polaner*), 2 tsp. . . . . . 35
(*S&W/Nutradiet*), 1 tsp. . . . . . 4
(*Smucker's*), 1 tsp. . . . . . 18
(*Smucker's Slenderella*), 1 tsp. . . . . . 8
(*Welch's*), 2 tsp. . . . . . 35
fruit spreads, all flavors:
(*Polaner All Fruit* Spreadable Fruit), 1 tsp. . . . . . 14
(*Smucker's* Simply Fruit), 1 tsp. . . . . . 16
(*Weight Watchers*), 2 tsp. . . . . . 16
low sugar (*Smucker's*), 1 tsp. . . . . . 8
strawberry (*Kraft* Reduced Calorie), 1 tsp. . . . . . 6
strawberry (*Smucker's* Imitation), 1 tsp. . . . . . 2

**Java plum:**

3 medium, .4 oz. . . . . . 5
seeded, ½ cup . . . . . . 41

**Jelly:**

all flavors:
(*Bama*), 2 tsp. . . . . . 30
(*Estee*), 1 tsp. . . . . . 2
(*Featherweight*), 1 tsp. . . . . . 4
(*Kraft*), 1 tsp. . . . . . 17
(*Musselman's*), 1 oz. . . . . . 80
(*Polaner*), 2 tsp. . . . . . 35
(*Smucker's*), 1 tsp. . . . . . 18
(*Smucker's Slenderella*), 1 tsp. . . . . . 8
grape (*Kraft* Reduced Calorie), 1 tsp. . . . . . 6
grape (*Smucker's* Imitation), 1 tsp. . . . . . 2
jalapeño (*Great Impressions*), 1 tbsp. . . . . . 58
pepper, green or red (*Great Impressions*), 1 tbsp. . . . . . 50

| FOOD AND MEASURE | CALORIES |
|---|---|
| **Jelly and peanut butter:** | |
| (*Bama*), 2 tbsp. | 150 |
| **Jerusalem artichoke:** | |
| raw, untrimmed, 1 lb. | 238 |
| raw, sliced, ½ cup | 57 |
| **Jicama,** see "Yam bean tuber" | |
| **Jujube:** | |
| raw, seeded, 1 oz. | 22 |
| dried, 1 oz. | 81 |
| **Jute,** potherb: | |
| raw, trimmed, ½ cup | 5 |
| boiled, drained, ½ cup | 16 |

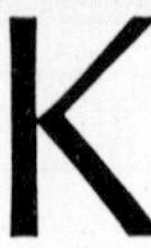

| FOOD AND MEASURE | CALORIES |
|---|---|

**Kale:**

| | |
|---|---|
| fresh, raw, untrimmed, 1 lb. | 137 |
| fresh, raw, chopped, ½ cup | 17 |
| fresh, boiled, drained, chopped, ½ cup | 21 |
| canned, chopped (*Allens*), ½ cup | 25 |
| frozen, chopped (*Southern*), 3.5 oz. | 30 |

**Kale, Scotch:**

| | |
|---|---|
| raw, chopped, ½ cup | 14 |
| boiled, drained, chopped, ½ cup | 18 |

**Kanpyo:**

| | |
|---|---|
| 3 strips, 40¾″ long × ½″ diam. | 49 |

**Kasha,** see "Buckwheat, groats"

***Kentucky Fried Chicken:***

| | |
|---|---|
| chicken, *Original Recipe:* | |
| breast, center, 4.1 oz. | 283 |
| breast, side, 3.2 oz. | 267 |
| drumstick, 2 oz. | 146 |
| thigh, 3.7 oz. | 294 |
| wing, 1.9 oz. | 178 |
| chicken, *Extra Tasty Crispy:* | |
| breast, center, 4.8 oz. | 342 |
| breast, side, 3.9 oz. | 343 |
| drumstick, 2.4 oz. | 204 |
| thigh, 4.2 oz. | 406 |
| wing, 2.3 oz. | 254 |
| chicken, *Kentucky Nuggets,* .6 oz. piece | 46 |
| chicken, *Light N' Crispy:* | |
| breast, center, 3 oz. | 220 |
| breast, side, 2.7 oz. | 204 |
| drumstick, 1.7 oz. | 121 |
| thigh, 2.8 oz. | 246 |

| FOOD AND MEASURE | CALORIES |
|---|---|
| *Chicken Littles* sandwich, 1.7 oz. | 169 |
| *Colonel's* chicken sandwich, 5.9 oz. | 482 |
| Hot Wings, 6 pieces | 376 |
| *Kentucky Nuggets* sauces: | |
| barbecue, 1 oz. | 35 |
| honey, .5 oz. | 49 |
| mustard, 1 oz. | 36 |
| sweet and sour, 1 oz. | 58 |
| side dishes: | |
| buttermilk biscuits, 2.3 oz. | 235 |
| coleslaw, 3.2 oz. | 119 |
| corn-on-the-cob, 5 oz. | 176 |
| french fries, regular, 2.7 oz. | 244 |
| mashed potatoes and gravy, 3.5 oz. | 71 |

**Ketchup,** see "Catsup"

**Kidney beans,** see "Beans, kidney"

**Kidneys:**

| | |
|---|---|
| beef, braised, 4 oz. | 163 |
| lamb, braised, 4 oz. | 155 |
| pork, braised, 4 oz. | 171 |
| veal, braised, 4 oz. | 185 |

**Kielbasa** (see also "Polish sausage"):

| | |
|---|---|
| (*Eckrich Lean Supreme* Polska), 1 oz. | 72 |
| (*Eckrich Lite* Polska), 1 oz. | 70 |
| (*Hillshire Farm* Bun Size), 2 oz. | 180 |
| (*Hillshire Farm* Polska Flavorseal/Links), 2 oz. | 190 |
| (*Hillshire Farm* Polska Flavorseal Lite), 2 oz. | 160 |
| (*Hormel* Kolbase), 3 oz. | 220 |
| skinless (*Eckrich Polska*), 1 link | 180 |
| skinless (*Hormel*), ½ link | 180 |
| turkey, see "Turkey kielbasa" | |

**Kiwifruit:**

| | |
|---|---|
| 1 large | 55 |
| 1 medium | 46 |

**Knockwurst:**

| | |
|---|---|
| (*Hillshire Farm* Links), 2 oz. | 180 |
| beef (*Hebrew National*), 3-oz. link | 263 |

| FOOD AND MEASURE | CALORIES |
|---|---|
| **Kohlrabi:** | |
| raw, untrimmed, 1 lb. | 57 |
| raw, sliced, ½ cup | 19 |
| boiled, drained, sliced, ½ cup | 24 |
| **Kumquat:** | |
| 1 medium, .7 oz. | 12 |
| seeded, 1 oz. | 18 |

# L

| FOOD AND MEASURE | CALORIES |
|---|---|

**Lamb,** domestic, choice grade, boneless, 4 oz.:

| | |
|---|---|
| cubed (leg and shoulder), braised or stewed | 253 |
| cubed (leg and shoulder), broiled | 211 |
| foreshank, braised, separable lean and fat | 276 |
| foreshank, braised, lean only | 212 |
| ground, broiled | 321 |
| leg, shank half, roasted, separable lean and fat | 255 |
| leg, shank half, roasted, lean only | 204 |
| leg, sirloin half, roasted, separable lean and fat | 331 |
| leg, sirloin half, roasted, lean only | 231 |
| loin, roasted, separable lean and fat | 350 |
| loin, roasted, lean only | 229 |
| rib, roasted, separable lean and fat | 407 |
| rib, roasted, lean only | 263 |
| shoulder, arm, braised, separable lean and fat | 392 |
| shoulder, arm, braised, lean only | 316 |
| shoulder, blade, braised, separable lean and fat | 391 |
| shoulder, blade, braised, lean only | 327 |

**Lamb, variety meats,** see specific listings

**Lamb's-quarters:**

| | |
|---|---|
| raw, trimmed, 1 lb. | 195 |
| boiled, drained, chopped, ½ cup | 29 |

**Lard,** pork:

| | |
|---|---|
| 1 tbsp. | 115 |

**Lasagna dinner,** frozen:

| | |
|---|---|
| (*Banquet Extra Helping*), 16.5 oz. | 645 |

**Lasagna entree,** frozen:

| | |
|---|---|
| (*Celentano*), 6.25 oz. | 230 |
| (*Celentano*), 8 oz. | 370 |
| (*Celentano*), 10 oz. | 460 |

| FOOD AND MEASURE | CALORIES |
|---|---|
| *Lasagna entree, frozen, continued* | |
| (*Green Giant Entrees*), 12 oz. | 490 |
| (*Stouffer's*), 10.5 oz. | 360 |
| (*Tyson Gourmet Selection*), 11.5 oz. | 380 |
| cheese (*Dining Lite*), 9 oz. | 260 |
| cheese, Italian (*Weight Watchers*), 11 oz. | 350 |
| cheese, three (*The Budget Gourmet*), 10 oz. | 400 |
| fiesta (*Stouffer's*), 10.25 oz. | 430 |
| garden (*Weight Watchers*), 11 oz. | 290 |
| garden vegetable (*Le Menu* LightStyle), 10.5 oz. | 260 |
| meat (*Buitoni* Single Serving), 9 oz. | 580 |
| w/meat and sauce (*Lean Cuisine*), 10.25 oz. | 270 |
| w/meat sauce: | |
| (*Banquet Family Entrees*), 7 oz. | 270 |
| (*The Budget Gourmet* Slim Selects), 10 oz. | 290 |
| (*Dining Lite*), 9 oz. | 240 |
| (*Freezer Queen Deluxe Family Suppers*), 7 oz. | 200 |
| (*Healthy Choice*), 9 oz. | 260 |
| (*Le Menu* LightStyle), 10 oz. | 290 |
| (*Swanson* Homestyle Recipe), 10.5 oz. | 400 |
| (*Weight Watchers*), 11 oz. | 320 |
| primavera (*Celentano*), 11 oz. | 330 |
| in sauce (*Buitoni* Family Style), 7.3 oz. | 370 |
| sausage, Italian (*The Budget Gourmet*), 10 oz. | 420 |
| seafood (*Mrs. Paul's* Light), 9.5 oz. | 290 |
| w/tofu and sauce (*Legume* Classic), 8 oz. | 210 |
| tuna, w/noodles and vegetables (*Lean Cuisine*), 9.75 oz. | 270 |
| vegetable (*Stouffer's*), 10.5 oz. | 420 |
| vegetable, garden (*Le Menu* LightStyle), 10.5 oz. | 260 |
| vegetable, w/tofu and sauce (*Legume*), 12 oz. | 240 |
| zucchini (*Lean Cuisine*), 11 oz. | 260 |

### **Lasagna entree,** packaged:

| | |
|---|---|
| Italian style (*Hormel Top Shelf*), 1 serving | 360 |
| vegetable (*Hormel Top Shelf*), 10.6 oz. | 275 |

### **Leek:**

| | |
|---|---|
| fresh, raw, 1 medium, 9.9 oz. | 76 |
| fresh, boiled, drained, chopped, ½ cup | 16 |
| freeze-dried, 1 tbsp. | 1 |

| FOOD AND MEASURE | CALORIES |
|---|---|
| **Lemon:** | |
| whole, 1 medium, 2⅛" diam. | 22 |
| peeled, 1 medium, 2⅛" diam. | 17 |
| 1 wedge, ¼ medium lemon | 5 |
| **Lemon and dill seasoning mix:** | |
| (*McCormick/Schilling* Bag'n Season), 1 pkg. | 161 |
| **Lemon drink** (see also "Lemonade"): | |
| chilled (*Crowley*), 8 fl. oz. | 130 |
| **Lemon extract:** | |
| (*Virginia Dare*), 1 tsp. | 22 |
| **Lemon herb marinade:** | |
| (*Golden Dipt*), 1 fl. oz. | 130 |
| **Lemon juice:** | |
| fresh, 1 tbsp. | 4 |
| canned or bottled (*Minute Maid* 100% Pure), 1 tbsp. | 4 |
| canned or bottled, reconstituted (*ReaLemon*), 1 fl. oz. | 6 |
| frozen (*Sunkist*), 1 fl. oz. | 7 |
| **Lemon pepper seasoning:** | |
| (*Lawry's*), 1 tsp. | 6 |
| (*McCormick/Schilling* Spice Blends), 1 tsp. | 7 |
| (*McCormick/Schilling Parsley Patch*), 1 tsp. | 13 |
| **Lemon-lime drink:** | |
| (*Veryfine*), 8 fl. oz. | 120 |
| **Lemonade:** | |
| (*Hi-C*), 8.45 fl. oz. | 109 |
| (*Minute Maid* Light'N Juicy), 6 fl. oz. | 8 |
| (*Sunkist*), 8 fl. oz. | 141 |
| (*Veryfine*), 8 fl. oz. | 120 |
| (*Wylers*), 6 fl. oz. | 64 |
| chilled, all varieties (*Minute Maid*), 6 fl. oz. | 81 |
| frozen, diluted (*Sunkist*), 8 fl. oz. | 92 |
| frozen, diluted, all varieties (*Minute Maid*), 6 fl. oz. | 77 |

| FOOD AND MEASURE | CALORIES |
|---|---|
| **Lemonade flavor drink mix,** prepared: | |
| (*Crystal Light* Sugar Free), 8 fl. oz. | 4 |
| (*Wyler's* Crystals, 4 servings/pkg.), 8 fl. oz. | 92 |
| (*Wyler's* Crystals, 32 servings/pkg.), 8 fl. oz. | 78 |
| all varieties (*Country Time*), 8 fl. oz. | 80 |
| regular or pink (*Country Time* Sugar Free), 8 fl. oz. | 4 |
| **Lentil:** | |
| raw, ½ cup | 324 |
| raw, green (*Arrowhead Mills*), 2 oz. | 190 |
| raw, red (*Arrowhead Mills*), 2 oz. | 195 |
| boiled, ½ cup | 115 |
| **Lentil, sprouted:** | |
| raw, ½ cup | 40 |
| **Lentil dinner,** canned: | |
| w/garden vegetables (*Health Valley Fast Menu*), 7.5 oz. | 160 |
| **Lentil pilaf mix:** | |
| (*Casbah*), 1 oz. dry or ½ cup cooked | 100 |
| **Lentil rice loaf,** frozen: | |
| (*Harvest Bake*), 4 oz. or 2 slices, ½″ each | 190 |
| **Lettuce:** | |
| bibb, Boston, or butterhead, 5″-diam. head | 21 |
| bibb, Boston, or butterhead, 2 inner leaves | 2 |
| cos or romaine, 1 inner leaf | 2 |
| cos or romaine, shredded, ½ cup | 4 |
| iceberg, 6″-diam. head | 70 |
| iceberg, 1 leaf, .7 oz. | 3 |
| looseleaf, trimmed, 1 oz. or ½ cup shredded | 5 |
| **Lima bean,** see "Beans, lima" | |
| **Lime:** | |
| 1 medium, 2″ diam. | 20 |
| **Lime juice:** | |
| fresh, 1 tbsp. | 4 |
| bottled, reconstituted (*ReaLime*), 1 fl. oz. | 6 |
| bottled, sweetened (*Rose's*), 1 fl. oz. | 48 |

| FOOD AND MEASURE | CALORIES |
|---|---|
| **Limeade:** | |
| frozen, diluted (*Minute Maid*), 6 fl. oz. | 71 |
| **Ling,** meat only: | |
| raw, 4 oz. | 99 |
| **Lingcod,** meat only: | |
| raw, 4 oz. | 96 |
| **Linguine entree,** frozen: | |
| w/clam sauce (*Lean Cuisine*), 9⅝ oz. | 270 |
| w/scallops and clams (*The Budget Gourmet*), 9.5 oz. | 280 |
| w/shrimp (*The Budget Gourmet*), 10 oz. | 330 |
| w/shrimp (*Healthy Choice*), 9.5 oz. | 230 |
| **Linguine entree,** packaged: | |
| w/clam sauce (*Hormel Top Shelf*), 1 serving | 330 |
| **Liquor,** pure distilled[1], 1 fl. oz.: | |
| 80 proof | 65 |
| 90 proof | 74 |
| 100 proof | 83 |
| ***Little Caesars,*** 1 serving: | |
| *Little Caesars Meals*, cheese pizza, salad | 600 |
| *Little Caesars Meals*, pizza w/green peppers, onions, mushrooms, salad | 640 |
| pizza, cheese, 2.2-oz. slice | 170 |
| pizza, pepperoni, peppers, onions, mushrooms, 2.7-oz. slice | 190 |
| sandwiches, 1 serving: | |
| ham and cheese | 520 |
| Italian sub | 590 |
| tuna melt | 700 |
| vegetarian | 620 |
| salads, w/low-calorie dressing: | |
| antipasto, 12 oz. | 170 |
| Greek, 11 oz. | 140 |
| tossed, 11 oz. | 80 |

[1]Includes bourbon, brandy, gin, rum, rye, Scotch, tequila, vodka.

| FOOD AND MEASURE | CALORIES |
|---|---|
| **Liver:** | |
| beef, braised, 4 oz. | 183 |
| beef, pan-fried in vegetable oil, 4 oz. | 246 |
| chicken, simmered, 4 oz. | 178 |
| chicken, simmered, chopped or diced, 1 cup | 219 |
| duck, domesticated, raw, 1 oz. | 39 |
| goose, domesticated, raw, 1 oz. | 38 |
| lamb, braised, 4 oz. | 249 |
| lamb, pan-fried in vegetable oil, 4 oz. | 270 |
| pork, braised, 4 oz. | 187 |
| turkey, simmered, 4 oz. | 192 |
| veal (calves), braised, 4 oz. | 187 |
| veal (calves), pan-fried in vegetable oil, 4 oz. | 278 |
| **Liver cheese:** | |
| (*Oscar Mayer*), 1.34-oz. slice | 116 |
| **Liver loaf:** | |
| (*Hormel* Perma-Fresh), 2 slices | 160 |
| (*Kahn's*), 1 slice | 170 |
| **Liverwurst:** | |
| (*Jones Dairy Farm* Chub), 1 oz. | 80 |
| (*Jones Dairy Farm* Slices), 1 slice | 75 |
| **Liverwurst spread,** canned: | |
| (*Hormel*), ½ oz. | 35 |
| (*Underwood*), 2⅛ oz. | 180 |
| **Lobster,** northern, meat only: | |
| raw, 4 oz. | 103 |
| boiled, poached, or steamed, 4 oz. | 111 |
| boiled, poached, or steamed, 1 cup | 142 |
| **Lobster, spiny,** see "Spiny lobster" | |
| **Lobster entree,** frozen: | |
| Newburg (*Stouffer's*), 6½ oz. | 380 |
| **Lobster sauce,** canned: | |
| rock (*Progresso*), ½ cup | 120 |

| FOOD AND MEASURE | CALORIES |
|---|---|
| **Loganberry:** | |
| fresh, trimmed, 1 cup | 89 |
| frozen, ½ cup | 40 |
| **Longan:** | |
| fresh, shelled and seeded, 1 oz. | 17 |
| dried, 1 oz. | 81 |
| **Loquat:** | |
| 1 medium, .6 oz. | 5 |
| peeled and seeded, 1 oz. | 13 |
| **Lotus root:** | |
| raw, 1 root, 9½" × 1⅞" | 64 |
| boiled, drained, 10 slices, 3.1 oz. | 59 |
| **Lotus seed:** | |
| raw, shelled, 1 oz. | 25 |
| dried, 1 oz., 47 small or 36 large | 94 |
| **Lox,** see "Salmon, Chinook, smoked" | |
| **Luncheon meat** (see also specific listings): | |
| (*Oscar Mayer*), 1-oz. slice | 94 |
| pork and beef, 1-oz. slice | 100 |
| canned: | |
| (*Spam*, 12 oz.), 2 oz. | 170 |
| (*Spam*, 7 oz.), 1.75 oz. | 150 |
| w/cheese chunks (*Spam*), 2 oz. | 170 |
| deviled (*Spam*), 1 tbsp. | 35 |
| smoke-flavored (*Spam*), 2 oz. | 170 |
| spiced (*Hormel*), 3 oz. | 280 |
| spiced (*Hormel* Perma-Fresh), 2 slices | 118 |
| spiced (*Kahn's* Luncheon Loaf), 1 slice | 80 |
| spiced (*Light & Lean*), 2 slices | 120 |
| **Luncheon "meat," vegetarian,** canned: | |
| (*Worthington Numete*), ½" slice, 2.4 oz. | 160 |
| (*Worthington Protose*), ½" slice, 2.7 oz. | 180 |

| FOOD AND MEASURE | CALORIES |
| --- | --- |
| **Lupin:** | |
| raw, ½ cup | 334 |
| boiled, ½ cup | 98 |
| **Lychee:** | |
| raw, shelled and seeded, 1 oz. | 19 |
| dried, 1 oz. | 79 |

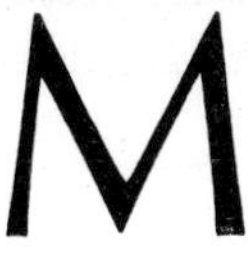

| FOOD AND MEASURE | CALORIES |
|---|---|

**Macadamia nuts:**

dried, shelled, 1 oz. .......... 199
oil-roasted (*Mauna Loa*), 1 oz. .......... 210

**Macaroni** (see also "Pasta"), dry:

uncooked, 2 oz. .......... 210
uncooked, tri-color, 2 oz. .......... 209
uncooked, whole wheat, 2 oz. .......... 198
cooked, elbow, 1 cup .......... 197
cooked, shells, small, 1 cup .......... 162
cooked, tri-color, spirals, 1 cup .......... 171
cooked, whole wheat, elbow, 1 cup .......... 174

**Macaroni and cheese,** see "Macaroni dinner," "Macaroni dishes," and "Macaroni entree"

**Macaroni and cheese loaf:**

(*Eckrich*), 1-oz. slice .......... 75

**Macaroni dinner,** frozen:

and beef (*Swanson*), 12 oz. .......... 370
and cheese (*Banquet*), 10 oz. .......... 420
and cheese (*Swanson*), 12¼ oz. .......... 370

**Macaroni dishes,** mix, prepared:

and cheese:
(*Golden Grain*), 1 serving .......... 310
(*Kraft* Deluxe Dinner), ¾ cup .......... 260
(*Kraft* Regular/Family Size Dinner), ¾ cup .......... 290
cheddar (*Fantastic Foods* Traditional), ½ cup .......... 112
Parmesan and herbs (*Fantastic Foods*), ½ cup .......... 109
shells (*Velveeta* Dinner/*Velveeta* Touch of Mexico Dinner), ½ cup .......... 210
shells, w/bacon (*Velveeta* Bits Of Bacon Dinner), ½ cup .......... 240
spirals (*Kraft* Dinner), ¾ cup .......... 340

| FOOD AND MEASURE | CALORIES |
|---|---|
| *Macaroni dishes, continued* | |
| shells 'n curry, prepared w/tofu (*Tofu Classics*), ½ cup | 103 |
| shells 'n curry, prepared w/tofu and butter (*Tofu Classics*), ½ cup | 143 |
| **Macaroni entree,** canned: | |
| and beef (*Chef Boyardee* Beefaroni Microwave), 7.5 oz. | 220 |
| and beef, in tomato sauce (*Heinz*), 7.25 oz. | 200 |
| and cheese (*Heinz*), 7.5 oz. | 190 |
| and cheese (*Hormel Micro-Cup*), 7.5 oz. | 189 |
| elbows in beef sauce (*Chef Boyardee* Microwave), 7.5 oz. | 210 |
| shells and cheddar (*Lipton Hearty Ones*), 11 oz. | 367 |
| **Macaroni entree,** frozen: | |
| and beef, w/tomatoes (*Stouffer's*), ½ of 11.5-oz. pkg. | 170 |
| and cheese: | |
| (*Banquet* Casserole), 8 oz. | 350 |
| (*Banquet Family Entrees*), 8 oz. | 290 |
| (*The Budget Gourmet* Side Dish), 5.3 oz. | 210 |
| (*Freezer Queen Family Side Dish*), 4 oz. | 110 |
| (*Green Giant* One Serving), 5.7 oz. | 230 |
| (*Stouffer's*), ½ of 12-oz. pkg. | 250 |
| (*Stouffer's*), ¼ of 20-oz. pkg. | 210 |
| (*Swanson* Homestyle Recipe), 10 oz. | 390 |
| pie (*Swanson* Pot Pie), 7 oz. | 200 |
| **Mace,** ground: | |
| 1 tsp. | 8 |
| **Mackerel,** meat only: | |
| fresh: | |
| Atlantic, raw, 4 oz. | 232 |
| Atlantic, baked, broiled, or microwaved, 4 oz. | 297 |
| King, raw, 4 oz. | 119 |
| Pacific or Jack, raw, 4 oz. | 179 |
| Spanish, raw, 4 oz. | 157 |
| Spanish, baked, broiled, or microwaved, 4 oz. | 179 |
| canned, Jack, drained, 1 cup | 296 |
| **Mahi mahi,** see "Dolphinfish" | |
| **Mai tai, mix:** | |
| bottled (*Holland House*), 1 fl. oz. | 32 |
| instant (*Holland House*), .56 oz. | 64 |

| FOOD AND MEASURE | CALORIES |
| --- | --- |
| **Malacca apple:** | |
| seeded, 1 oz. | 9 |
| **Malted milk,** see "Milk, malted" | |
| **Mammy apple:** | |
| peeled and seeded, 1 oz. | 14 |
| 1 medium, 3.1 lb. | 431 |
| **Mandarin orange,** see "Tangerine" | |
| **Mango:** | |
| 1 medium, 10.6 oz. | 135 |
| sliced, ½ cup | 54 |
| **Mango nectar:** | |
| (*Libby's*), 6 fl. oz. | 110 |
| **Manhattan mix:** | |
| bottled (*Holland House*), 1 fl. oz. | 28 |
| **Manicotti entree,** frozen: | |
| (*Buitoni* Single Serving), 9-oz. pkg. | 470 |
| (*Celentano*), 8 oz. | 300 |
| cheese (*Weight Watchers*), 9.25 oz. | 280 |
| cheese, w/meat sauce (*The Budget Gourmet*), 10 oz. | 450 |
| w/sauce (*Celentano*), 7 oz. | 360 |
| w/sauce (*Celentano*), 10 oz. | 380 |
| w/spinach, tofu, and sauce (*Legume* Florentine), 11 oz. | 260 |
| w/three cheeses (*Le Menu*), 11.75 oz. | 390 |
| w/tofu and sauce (*Legume* Classic), 8 oz. | 220 |
| **Maple sugar,** see "Sugar, maple" | |
| **Maple syrup:** | |
| 1 tbsp. | 50 |
| **Margarine,** 1 tbsp., except as noted: | |
| (*Country Morning* Light Stick or Tub), 1 tsp. | 20 |
| (*Country Morning* Stick Regular/Unsalted), 1 tsp. | 35 |
| (*Country Morning* Tub Regular/Unsalted), 1 tsp. | 30 |
| (Diet *Mazola*) | 50 |
| (*Hain* Safflower Regular/Soft/Unsalted) | 100 |

| FOOD AND MEASURE | CALORIES |
|---|---|
| *Margarine, continued* | |
| (*Land O'Lakes* Stick or Tub), 1 tsp. | 35 |
| (*Mazola* Regular/Unsalted) | 100 |
| (*Nucoa*) | 100 |
| (*Nucoa Heart Beat*) | 25 |
| (*Nucoa Heart Beat* Unsalted) | 24 |
| (*Parkay*) | 100 |
| (*Weight Watchers* Regular/Light Spread/Unsalted Tub) | 50 |
| (*Weight Watchers* Stick) | 60 |
| soft: | |
| (*Chiffon* Cup) | 90 |
| (*Chiffon* Stick) | 100 |
| (Diet *Parkay*) | 50 |
| (*Nucoa*) | 90 |
| (*Parkay*) | 100 |
| spread: | |
| (*Kraft Touch of Butter* Bowl) | 50 |
| (*Kraft Touch of Butter* Stick) | 90 |
| (*Land O'Lakes* Tub), 1 tsp. | 25 |
| (*Mazola* Corn Oil Light) | 50 |
| (*Parkay* 50% Vegetable Oil) | 60 |
| (*Parkay* Squeeze Spread) | 90 |
| w/sweet cream (*Land O'Lakes* Stick), 1 tsp. | 30 |
| w/sweet cream (*Land O'Lakes* Tub), 1 tsp. | 25 |
| vegetable (*P&Q* 60% Quarters) | 80 |
| squeeze (*Parkay*) | 100 |
| whipped (*Chiffon*) | 70 |
| whipped (*Miracle* Brand Cup) | 60 |
| whipped (*Miracle* Brand Stick) | 70 |
| whipped (*Parkay* Cup or Stick) | 70 |

**Margarita mix:**

| | |
|---|---|
| bottled (*Holland House*), 1 fl. oz. | 27 |
| instant (*Holland House*), .5 oz. | 57 |
| strawberry, bottled (*Holland House*), 1 fl. oz. | 31 |
| strawberry, instant (*Holland House*), .56 oz. | 66 |

**Marinara sauce,** see "Pasta sauce"

**Marjoram,** dried:

| | |
|---|---|
| 1 tsp. | 2 |

| FOOD AND MEASURE | CALORIES |
|---|---|
| **Marmalade,** orange: | |
| (*Smucker's*), 1 tsp. | 18 |
| **Matzo,** see "Cracker" and "Cracker crumbs and meal" | |
| **Mayonnaise,** 1 tbsp.: | |
| (*Bama*) | 100 |
| (*Bennett's* Real) | 110 |
| (*Hain* Real No Salt Added/Cold Processed) | 110 |
| (*Hellmann's/Best Foods*) | 100 |
| (*Kraft*) | 100 |
| canola (*Hain*) | 100 |
| canola (*Hollywood*) | 100 |
| reduced calorie: | |
| (*Estee*) | 45 |
| (*Featherweight*) | 30 |
| (*Hain* Light Low Sodium) | 60 |
| (*Hellmann's/Best Foods* Light) | 50 |
| (*Kraft* Light) | 50 |
| (*Weight Watchers* Regular/Low Sodium) | 50 |
| canola (*Hain*) | 60 |
| safflower (*Hain*) | 110 |
| soybean (*Featherweight Soyamaise*) | 100 |
| substitute and imitation (see also "Salad dressing") | |
| (*Hain* Eggless No Salt Added) | 110 |
| (*Hellmann's* Cholesterol Free) | 50 |
| (*Kraft Free* Nonfat) | 12 |
| (*Nucoa Heart Beat*) | 40 |
| (*Weight Watchers* Cholesterol Free) | 50 |
| tofu (*Nasoya Nayonaise*) | 40 |
| ***McDonald's,*** 1 serving: | |
| breakfast: | |
| apple bran muffin, 3 oz. | 190 |
| biscuit, w/bacon, egg, and cheese, 5.5 oz. | 440 |
| biscuit, w/biscuit spread, 2.6 oz. | 260 |
| biscuit, w/sausage, 4.3 oz. | 440 |
| biscuit, w/sausage and egg, 6.3 oz. | 520 |
| danish, apple or iced cheese | 390 |
| danish, cinnamon raisin | 440 |
| danish, raspberry | 410 |

| FOOD AND MEASURE | CALORIES |
|---|---|
| *McDonald's, breakfast, continued* | |
| *Egg McMuffin,* 4.9 oz. | 290 |
| eggs, scrambled, 3.5 oz. | 140 |
| English muffin, w/butter, 2.1 oz. | 170 |
| English muffin, w/out butter | 140 |
| hash brown potatoes, 1.9 oz. | 130 |
| hotcakes, w/butter and syrup, 6.2 oz. | 410 |
| sausage, pork, 1.7 oz. | 180 |
| *Sausage McMuffin,* 4.1 oz. | 370 |
| *Sausage McMuffin,* w/egg, 5.9 oz. | 440 |
| sandwiches and chicken: | |
| *Big Mac,* 7.6 oz. | 560 |
| cheeseburger, 4.1 oz. | 310 |
| *Chicken McNuggets,* 4 oz. | 290 |
| *Filet-O-Fish,* 5 oz. | 440 |
| hamburger, 3.6 oz. | 260 |
| *McChicken,* 6.7 oz. | 490 |
| *McD.L.T.,* 8.3 oz. | 580 |
| *McLean* Deluxe, 7.3 oz. | 320 |
| *McLean* Deluxe (patty only), 3 oz. | 130 |
| *McLean* Deluxe, w/cheese, 7.7 oz. | 370 |
| *Quarter Pounder,* 5.9 oz. | 410 |
| *Quarter Pounder,* w/cheese, 6.8 oz. | 520 |
| *Chicken McNuggets* sauces: | |
| barbecue, 1 oz. | 50 |
| honey, 1.5 oz. | 45 |
| hot mustard, 1 oz. | 70 |
| sweet and sour, 1 oz. | 60 |
| french fries, small, 2.4 oz. | 220 |
| french fries, medium, 3.4 oz. | 320 |
| french fries, large, 4.3 oz. | 400 |
| salads: | |
| chef, 10 oz. | 230 |
| chunky chicken, 8.8 oz. | 140 |
| garden, 7.5 oz. | 110 |
| side salad, 4.1 oz. | 60 |
| dressings and condiments: | |
| bacon bits, .1 oz. | 16 |
| bleu cheese dressing, ⅕ pkg. | 70 |
| croutons, .4 oz. | 50 |
| french dressing, red, reduced calorie, ¼ pkg. | 40 |

| FOOD AND MEASURE | CALORIES |
|---|---|
| peppercorn dressing, 1/5 pkg. | 80 |
| Thousand Island dressing, 1/5 pkg. | 78 |
| vinaigrette dressing, lite, 1/4 pkg. | 15 |
| desserts and shakes: | |
| apple pie, 2.9 oz. | 260 |
| cookies, chocolaty chip, 2.3 oz. | 330 |
| cookies, *McDonaldland,* 2.3 oz. | 290 |
| milkshake, lowfat, chocolate or strawberry, 10.3 oz. | 320 |
| milkshake, lowfat, vanilla, 10.3 oz. | 290 |
| yogurt, lowfat, cone, vanilla, 3 oz. | 100 |
| yogurt, lowfat, sundae, hot caramel, 6.1 oz. | 270 |
| yogurt, lowfat, sundae, hot fudge, 6 oz. | 240 |
| yogurt, lowfat, sundae, strawberry, 6 oz. | 210 |

**Meat,** see specific listings

**Meat, potted,** canned:

| | |
|---|---|
| (*Hormel* Food Product), 1 tbsp. | 30 |
| (*Libby's*), 1.83 oz. | 110 |

**Meat loaf dinner,** frozen:

| | |
|---|---|
| (*Armour Classics),* 11.25 oz. | 360 |
| (*Banquet*), 11 oz. | 440 |
| (*Freezer Queen*), 10 oz. | 350 |
| (*Morton*), 10 oz. | 310 |
| (*Swanson*), 10.75 oz. | 360 |
| homestyle (*Stouffer's Dinner Supreme*), 12⅛ oz. | 410 |

**Meat loaf entree,** frozen:

| | |
|---|---|
| (*Banquet Cookin' Bags*), 4 oz. | 200 |
| tomato sauce and (*Freezer Queen Family Suppers*), 7 oz. | 230 |

**Meat loaf entree mix,** prepared:

| | |
|---|---|
| homestyle (*Lipton Microeasy*), 1/4 pkg. | 390 |

**"Meat" loaf entree mix, vegetarian:**

| | |
|---|---|
| (*Natural Touch* Loaf Mix), 4 oz. | 180 |

**Meat loaf seasoning mix:**

| | |
|---|---|
| (*French's*), ⅛ pkg. | 20 |
| (*Lawry's* Seasoning Blends), 1 pkg. | 355 |
| (*McCormick/Schilling*), 1/4 pkg. | 38 |

| FOOD AND MEASURE | CALORIES |
|---|---|
| **Meat marinade mix:** | |
| (*French's*), 1/8 pkg. | 10 |
| (*McCormick/Schilling*), 1/4 pkg. | 28 |
| **Meat tenderizer:** | |
| (*Ac'cent* Flavor Enhancer), 1/2 tsp. | 5 |
| **"Meatball," vegetarian,** canned: | |
| (*Worthington Non-Meat Balls*), 3 pieces or 1.9 oz. | 100 |
| **Meatball dinner,** frozen: | |
| Swedish (*Armour Classics*), 11.25 oz. | 330 |
| **Meatball entree,** frozen: | |
| Italian, w/noodles and peppers (*The Budget Gourmet*), 10 oz. | 310 |
| stew (*Lean Cuisine*), 10 oz. | 250 |
| Swedish: | |
| (*Le Menu* LightStyle), 8.5 oz. | 260 |
| (*Swanson* Homestyle Recipe), 8.5 oz. | 360 |
| in gravy, w/parsley noodles (*Stouffer's*), 11 oz. | 480 |
| w/noodles (*The Budget Gourmet*), 10 oz. | 600 |
| sauce and (*Dining Lite*), 9 oz. | 280 |
| **Meatball seasoning mix:** | |
| (*French's*), 1/4 pkg. | 35 |
| **Meatball stew,** canned: | |
| (*Chef Boyardee*), 8 oz. | 350 |
| (*Dinty Moore*), 8 oz. | 240 |
| **Melon,** see specific listings | |
| **Melon balls** (cantaloupe and honeydew): | |
| frozen, 1/2 cup | 28 |
| **Menudo,** canned: | |
| (*Old El Paso*), 1/2 can | 476 |
| **Mesquite sauce:** | |
| w/lime juice (*Lawry's*), 1/4 cup | 24 |
| **Mexican dinner,** frozen (see also specific listings): | |
| (*Swanson Hungry Man*), 20.25 oz. | 820 |
| fiesta (*Patio*), 12.25 oz. | 470 |

| FOOD AND MEASURE | CALORIES |
|---|---|
| style: | |
| (*Banquet*), 12 oz. | 490 |
| (*Morton*), 10 oz. | 300 |
| (*Patio*), 13.25 oz. | 540 |
| combination (*Banquet*), 12 oz. | 520 |
| combination (*Swanson*), 14.25 oz. | 490 |

**Mexican entree,** frozen (see also specific listings):

| | |
|---|---|
| (*Van de Kamp's*), ½ pkg. | 220 |

**Milk,** cow, fluid, 8 fl. oz.:

| | |
|---|---|
| buttermilk (*Crowley* Regular/Unsalted) | 110 |
| buttermilk, lowfat 2% (*Knudsen*) | 120 |
| buttermilk, lowfat 1.5% (*Borden* Golden Churn) | 120 |
| buttermilk, lowfat 1.5% (*Friendship* Unsalted) | 120 |
| lowfat 2% (*Borden* Hi-Protein) | 140 |
| lowfat 2% (*Crowley*/*Crowley* Tone Acidophilus) | 120 |
| lowfat 2% (*Knudsen*/*Knudsen* Sweet Acidophilus) | 140 |
| lowfat 2% (*Viva*) | 120 |
| lowfat 1% (*Borden*) | 100 |
| lowfat 1% (*Crowley*/*Crowley Lacktaid*) | 100 |
| lowfat 1% (*Knudsen* Nice n' Light) | 130 |
| lowfat 1%, protein fortified (*Crowley*) | 120 |
| skim (*Borden*) | 90 |
| skim (*Borden Skim-Line*) | 100 |
| skim (*Crowley*) | 90 |
| skim (*Knudsen*) | 80 |
| skim (*Weight Watchers*) | 90 |
| whole (*Borden*/*Borden* Hi-Calcium) | 150 |
| whole (*Crowley*) | 150 |
| whole (*Knudsen*) | 160 |

**Milk,** canned:

| | |
|---|---|
| condensed, sweetened (*Borden*), ⅓ cup | 320 |
| condensed, sweetened (*Carnation*), ⅓ cup | 320 |
| condensed, sweetened (*Eagle*), ⅓ cup | 320 |
| evaporated, ½ cup: | |
| (*Carnation*) | 170 |
| (*Pet*) | 170 |
| filled (*Pet*) | 150 |
| lowfat (*Carnation*) | 110 |

| FOOD AND MEASURE | CALORIES |
|---|---|
| *Milk, canned, evaporated, continued* | |
| skim (*Carnation*) | 100 |
| skim (*Pet* Light) | 100 |

**Milk, chocolate,** dairy:

| | |
|---|---|
| (*Hershey's*), 8 fl. oz. | 210 |
| (*Meadow Gold*), 8 fl. oz. | 210 |
| lowfat 2% (*Borden* Dutch Brand), 8 fl. oz. | 180 |
| lowfat 2% (*Hershey's*) 8 fl. oz. | 190 |
| lowfat 1% (*Knudsen*), 8 fl. oz. | 190 |
| mix, see "Milk beverages, flavoring mix" | |

**Milk, dry:**

| | |
|---|---|
| buttermilk, sweet cream, reconstituted, 8 fl. oz. | 464 |
| whole, reconstituted, 8 fl. oz. | 635 |
| nonfat, regular, reconstituted, 8 fl. oz. | 435 |
| nonfat instant (*Carnation*), 5 level tbsp. | 80 |
| nonfat instant (*Sanalac* Dairy Fresh), .8 oz. | 80 |
| nonfat instant (*Weight Watchers* Dairy Creamer), 1 pkt. | 10 |

**Milk, goat's,** fluid:

| | |
|---|---|
| whole, 8 fl. oz. | 168 |

**Milk, imitation:**

| | |
|---|---|
| fluid, 8 fl. oz. | 150 |

**Milk, malted,** powder:

| | |
|---|---|
| natural (*Carnation* Original), 3 heaping tsp. | 90 |
| natural or chocolate (*Kraft* Instant), 3 tsp. | 90 |
| chocolate (*Carnation*), 3 heaping tsp. | 80 |

**Milk, sheep's,** fluid:

| | |
|---|---|
| whole, 8 fl. oz. | 264 |

**Milk, soy,** see "Soy milk"

**Milk beverages, flavored,** canned:

| | |
|---|---|
| all flavors (*Sego*), 10 fl. oz. | 225 |
| all flavors (*Sego* Lite), 10 fl. oz. | 150 |
| chocolate (*Frostee*), 8 fl. oz. | 200 |
| strawberry (*Frostee*), 8 fl. oz. | 180 |

| FOOD AND MEASURE | CALORIES |
|---|---|
| **Milk beverages, flavoring mix,** dry form: | |
| all flavors (*Carnation* Instant Breakfast), 1 pouch | 130 |
| all flavors (*Carnation* Instant Breakfast No Sugar), 1 pouch | 70 |
| all flavors, except vanilla (*Pillsbury* Instant Breakfast), 1 pouch | 130 |
| chocolate (*Hershey's*), .8 oz. or 3 tsp. | 90 |
| chocolate (*Nestlé Quick*), ¾ oz. or 2½ heaping tsp. | 90 |
| chocolate (*Nestlé Quik* Sugar Free), 1 heaping tsp. | 18 |
| eggnog flavor, 1 oz. | 111 |
| strawberry (*Nestlé Quick*), ¾ oz. or 2½ heaping tsp. | 80 |
| vanilla (*Pillsbury* Instant Breakfast), 1 pouch | 140 |
| **Milkfish,** meat only: | |
| raw, 4 oz. | 168 |
| **Milk shake:** | |
| frozen, chocolate (*MicroMagic*), 7 fl. oz. | 200 |
| frozen, chocolate or strawberry (*MicroMagic*), 11.5 fl. oz. | 340 |
| frozen, vanilla (*MicroMagic*), 11.5 fl. oz. | 380 |
| mix, all flavors (*Weight Watchers*), 1 pkt. | 70 |
| **Millet:** | |
| raw, 1 cup | 756 |
| raw, hulled (*Arrowhead Mills*), 1 oz. | 90 |
| cooked, 1 cup | 287 |
| **Mincemeat,** see "Pie filling" | |
| **Miso:** | |
| plain, 1 oz. | 58 |
| w/barley malt (mugi-koji), 1 oz. | 56 |
| w/rice malt, dark yellow (kome-koji), 1 oz. | 53 |
| w/rice malt, sweet (kome-koji), 1 oz. | 62 |
| w/soybean malt (mame-koji), 1 oz. | 62 |
| **Molasses:** | |
| dark or light (*Brer Rabbit*), 1 tbsp. | 60 |
| gold or green (*Grandma's*), 1 tbsp. | 70 |
| **Monkfish,** fillet: | |
| raw, 4 oz. | 88 |
| **Monosodium glutamate:** | |
| (*Tone's*), 1 tsp. | 0 |

| FOOD AND MEASURE | CALORIES |
|---|---|
| **Mortadella:** | |
| beef and pork, 1 oz. | 88 |
| **Mostaccioli entree,** frozen: | |
| and meat sauce (*Banquet Family Entrees*), 7 oz. | 170 |
| **Mothbean:** | |
| boiled, ½ cup | 103 |
| **Mother's loaf luncheon meat:** | |
| pork, 1 oz. | 80 |
| **Mousse,** see specific listings | |
| **Muffin,** 1 piece, except as noted: | |
| apple (*Awrey's*), 2.5 oz. | 220 |
| apple or blueberry (*Awrey's*), 1.5 oz. | 130 |
| apple streusel (*Awrey's* Grande), 4.2 oz. | 340 |
| banana-nut (*Awrey's* Grande), 4.2 oz. | 370 |
| banana-walnut, mini (*Hostess*), 5 pieces or 1 pkg. | 260 |
| blueberry (*Awrey's*), 2.5 oz. | 210 |
| blueberry (*Awrey's* Grande), 4.2 oz. | 360 |
| blueberry, mini (*Hostess*), 5 pieces or 1 pkg. | 240 |
| cinnamon-apple, mini (*Hostess*), 5 pieces or 1 pkg. | 260 |
| corn (*Awrey's*), 2.5 oz. | 220 |
| corn (*Awrey's*), 1.5 oz. | 130 |
| cranberry (*Awrey's*), 1.5 oz. | 120 |
| English: | |
| (*Hi Fiber*) | 110 |
| (*Pepperidge Farm*) | 140 |
| (*Roman Meal* Original) | 146 |
| (*Thomas'*) | 130 |
| (*Wonder*) | 130 |
| cinnamon-apple (*Pepperidge Farm*) | 140 |
| cinnamon-chip (*Pepperidge Farm*) | 160 |
| cinnamon-raisin (*Hi Fiber*) | 110 |
| cinnamon-raisin (*Pepperidge Farm*) | 150 |
| cinnamon and raisin oatmeal (*Oatmeal Goodness*) | 140 |
| honey and oatmeal (*Oatmeal Goodness*) | 140 |
| multigrain (*Hi Fiber*) | 120 |
| oat bran (*Thomas'*) | 116 |

| FOOD AND MEASURE | CALORIES |
|---|---|
| raisin (*Thomas'*) | 153 |
| rye (*Thomas'*) | 120 |
| sourdough (*Pepperidge Farm*) | 135 |
| wheat, honey (*Thomas'*) | 129 |
| oat bran (*Awrey's*), 2.75 oz. | 180 |
| oat bran (*Hostess*) | 160 |
| oat bran, all varieties (*Health Valley Fancy Fruit Muffins*) | 180 |
| oat bran, banana-nut (*Hostess*) | 140 |
| pineapple-raisin oat bran (*Awrey's*), 2.75 oz. | 180 |
| raisin (*Wonder* Raisin Rounds) | 140 |
| raisin bran (*Awrey's*), 2.5 oz. | 190 |
| raisin bran (*Awrey's*), 1.5 oz. | 110 |
| raisin bran (*Awrey's* Grande), 4.2 oz. | 320 |
| rice bran, raisin (*Health Valley Fancy Fruit Muffins*) | 215 |
| sourdough (*Wonder*) | 130 |

**Muffin,** frozen, 1 piece:

| | |
|---|---|
| apple-spice (*Sara Lee*), 2.5 oz. | 220 |
| apple-spice (*Weight Watchers*), 2.5 oz. | 160 |
| banana-nut or blueberry (*Weight Watchers*), 2.5 oz. | 170 |
| blueberry (*Pepperidge Farm*) | 170 |
| blueberry (*Sara Lee*), 2.5 oz. | 200 |
| blueberry (*Sara Lee Free & Light*), 2.25 oz. | 120 |
| cheese streusel or chocolate chunk (*Sara Lee*) | 220 |
| corn (*Pepperidge Farm*) | 180 |
| corn, golden (*Sara Lee*), 2.5 oz. | 240 |
| oat bran (*Sara Lee*) | 210 |
| oat bran-apple (*Pepperidge Farm* Cholesterol Free) | 190 |
| oat bran-apple (*Sara Lee*) | 190 |
| raisin bran (*Pepperidge Farm* Cholesterol Free) | 170 |
| raisin bran (*Sara Lee*), 2.5 oz. | 220 |

**Muffin,** refrigerated:

| | |
|---|---|
| English (*Roman Meal*), ½ piece | 71 |
| English, honey nut and oat bran (*Roman Meal*), ½ piece | 81 |

**Muffin mix,** prepared:

| | |
|---|---|
| apple-cinnamon or banana-nut (*Betty Crocker*), 1/12 pkg. | 120 |
| apple-cinnamon (*Martha White*), 1/6 pkg. | 140 |
| apple streusel, Dutch (*Betty Crocker* Bake Shop), 1/12 pkg. | 200 |
| applesauce (*Robin Hood/Gold Medal* Pouch Mix), 1/6 pkg. | 160 |

| FOOD AND MEASURE | CALORIES |
|---|---|
| *Muffin mix, prepared, continued* | |
| banana (*Robin Hood/Gold Medal* Pouch Mix), 1/6 pkg. | 150 |
| blackberry (*Martha White*), 1/6 pkg. | 140 |
| blueberry: | |
| (*Duncan Hines* Bakery Style), 1 piece | 190 |
| (*Martha White*), 1/6 pkg. | 140 |
| (*Robin Hood/Gold Medal* Pouch Mix), 1/6 pkg. | 170 |
| double, oat bran (*Martha White*), 1 piece | 120 |
| streusel (*Betty Crocker* Bake Shop), 1/12 pkg. | 210 |
| wild (*Betty Crocker*), 1/12 pkg. | 120 |
| wild (*Betty Crocker* Light), 1 piece | 70 |
| wild (*Duncan Hines*), 1 piece | 110 |
| bran (*Martha White*), 1/6 pkg. | 150 |
| bran and honey (*Duncan Hines*), 1 piece | 120 |
| bran and honey (*Duncan Hines* Bakery Style), 1 piece | 200 |
| caramel (*Robin Hood/Gold Medal* Pouch mix), 1/6 pkg. | 150 |
| carrot-nut or chocolate chip (*Betty Crocker*), 1/12 pkg. | 150 |
| cinnamon streusel (*Betty Crocker*), 1/10 pkg. | 200 |
| cinnamon swirl (*Duncan Hines* Bakery Style), 1 piece | 200 |
| corn (*Dromedary*), 1 piece | 120 |
| corn (*Flako*), 1 serving | 116 |
| corn (*Robin Hood/Gold Medal*), 1/6 pkg. | 130 |
| corn, blue (*Arrowhead Mills*), 1 piece | 110 |
| cranberry-orange nut (*Duncan Hines* Bakery Style), 1 piece | 200 |
| honey bran (*Robin Hood/Gold Medal* Pouch Mix), 1/6 pkg. | 170 |
| oat (*Robin Hood/Gold Medal* Pouch Mix), 1/6 pkg. | 150 |
| oat bran (*Betty Crocker*), 1 pkg. | 190 |
| oat bran, all varieties (*Hain*), 1 piece | 140 |
| oat bran, apple spice (*Arrowhead Mills*), 1 piece | 120 |
| oat bran, wheat free (*Arrowhead Mills*), 1 piece | 100 |
| oatmeal raisin (*Betty Crocker*), 1/12 pkg. | 140 |
| orangeberry (*Martha White*), 1/6 pkg. | 140 |
| pecan crunch (*Duncan Hines* Bakery Style), 1 piece | 220 |
| raspberry or strawberry (*Martha White*), 1/6 pkg. | 140 |
| strawberry crown (*Betty Crocker*), 1/10 pkg. | 150 |
| wheat bran (*Arrowhead Mills*), 2 pieces | 270 |
| **Mulberries:** | |
| 1/2 cup | 31 |
| **Mullet,** striped, meat only: | |
| raw, 4 oz. | 132 |
| baked, broiled, or microwaved, 4 oz. | 170 |

| FOOD AND MEASURE | CALORIES |
|---|---|
| **Mung bean,** see "Beans, mung" | |
| **Mung bean long rice,** dehydrated: | |
| ½ cup | 246 |
| **Mushroom:** | |
| fresh, raw, untrimmed, 1 lb. | 111 |
| fresh, raw, pieces, ½ cup | 9 |
| fresh, boiled, drained, pieces, ½ cup | 21 |
| canned (*B in B*), ¼ cup | 12 |
| canned, whole, pieces and stems (*Green Giant*), ¼ cup | 12 |
| canned, pieces and stems (*Allens*), ¼ cup | 20 |
| canned, in butter sauce (*Green Giant*), ½ cup | 30 |
| frozen, whole (*Birds Eye* Deluxe), 2.6 oz. | 20 |
| frozen, battered (*Stilwell Quick Krisp*), 2 oz. | 140 |
| **Mushroom, Japanese honey,** trimmed: | |
| (*Frieda* of California), 1 oz. | 9 |
| **Mushroom, Oriental straw,** canned: | |
| (*Green Giant*), 2 oz. | 12 |
| **Mushroom, oyster:** | |
| (*Frieda* of California), 1 oz. | 7 |
| **Mushroom, shiitake:** | |
| fresh, cooked, 4 medium or ½-cup pieces | 40 |
| dried, 1 oz. | 84 |
| **Mushroom gravy:** | |
| canned (*Franco-American*), 2 oz. | 25 |
| canned (*Heinz*), 2 oz. or ¼ cup | 25 |
| mix, prepared (*French's*), ¼ cup | 20 |
| mix, prepared (*McCormick/Schilling*), ¼ cup | 19 |
| **Mushroom sauce mix:** | |
| prepared w/whole milk, ½ cup | 114 |
| **Mushroom and herb dip:** | |
| (*Breakstone's* Gourmet), 2 tbsp. | 50 |

| FOOD AND MEASURE | CALORIES |
|---|---|
| **Mussel,** blue, meat only: | |
| raw, 4 oz. | 97 |
| boiled or steamed, 4 oz. | 195 |
| **Mustard,** prepared: | |
| (*Hain* Stone Ground Regular/No Salt Added), 1 tbsp. | 14 |
| (*Kraft* Pure), 1 tbsp. | 11 |
| brown, spicy (*Gulden's*), ¼ oz. | 8 |
| Dijon (*French's*), 1 tsp. | 8 |
| Dijon (*Grey Poupon*), 1 tbsp. | 18 |
| English (*Life* All Natural), 1 tbsp. | 22 |
| w/horseradish or Medford (*French's*), 1 tbsp. | 16 |
| horseradish (*Kraft*), 1 tbsp. | 14 |
| hot (*Gulden's* Diablo), ¼ oz. | 8 |
| jalapeño (*Great Impressions*), 2 tsp. | 7 |
| mild, creamy (*Gulden's*), ¼ oz. | 6 |
| w/onion (*French's*), 1 tsp. | 8 |
| spicy (*French's* Bold'n Spicy), 1 tsp. | 6 |
| yellow (*French's*), 1 tbsp. | 10 |
| yellow (*Heinz*), 1 tsp. | 3 |
| **Mustard greens:** | |
| fresh, raw, trimmed, 1 oz. or ½ cup chopped | 7 |
| fresh, boiled, drained, chopped, ½ cup | 11 |
| canned, chopped (*Allens*), ¼ cup | 20 |
| frozen, chopped (*Seabrook*), 3.3 oz. | 20 |
| frozen, chopped (*Southern*), 3.5 oz. | 25 |
| **Mustard powder:** | |
| (*Spice Islands*), 1 tsp. | 9 |
| **Mustard seed,** yellow: | |
| 1 tsp. | 15 |
| **Mustard spinach:** | |
| raw, chopped, ½ cup | 17 |
| boiled, drained, chopped, ½ cup | 14 |

# N

| FOOD AND MEASURE | CALORIES |
|---|---|
| **Nacho seasoning:** | |
| (*Lawry's* Seasoning Blends), 1 pkg. | 141 |
| **Natto:** | |
| ½ cup | 187 |
| **Nectarine:** | |
| 1 medium, 2½″ diam. | 67 |
| sliced, ½ cup | 34 |
| **New England Brand sausage:** | |
| (*Eckrich*), 1 oz. or 1 slice | 35 |
| (*Light & Lean*), 2 slices | 90 |
| (*Oscar Mayer*), .8-oz. slice | 29 |
| **New Zealand spinach:** | |
| raw, trimmed, 1 oz. or ½ cup chopped | 4 |
| boiled, drained, chopped, ½ cup | 11 |
| **Newberg sauce,** canned: | |
| w/sherry (*Snow's*), ⅓ cup | 120 |
| **Noodle,** egg: | |
| plain, dry: | |
| (*Creamette*), 2 oz. | 221 |
| (*Goodman's* Country Style), 2 oz. | 220 |
| (*Mrs. Grass*), 2 oz. | 220 |
| (*Mueller's*), 2 oz. | 220 |
| (*Prince*), 2 oz. | 210 |
| (*San Giorgio*), 2 oz. | 220 |
| plain, cooked, 1 cup | 212 |
| spinach, cooked, 1 cup | 211 |
| **Noodle, Chinese:** | |
| cellophane or long rice, dehydrated, 2 oz. | 199 |
| chow mein, 1 oz. | 149 |

| FOOD AND MEASURE | CALORIES |
|---|---|
| **Noodle, Japanese:** | |
| soba, cooked, 1 cup or 4 oz. | 113 |
| somen, cooked, 1 cup | 230 |
| udon, cooked, 4 oz. | 115 |
| **Noodle and chicken dinner,** frozen: | |
| (*Banquet*), 10 oz. | 350 |
| (*Banquet Family Favorites*), 10 oz. | 340 |
| (*Swanson*), 10.5 oz. | 280 |
| **Noodle dishes,** mix, prepared, ½ cup, except as noted: | |
| Alfredo (*Lipton* Noodles and Sauce) | 220 |
| Alfredo (*Minute* Microwave Family Size) | 170 |
| Alfredo (*Minute* Microwave Single Size) | 160 |
| Alfredo (*Mueller's Chef's Series*) | 190 |
| beef (*Lipton* Noodles and Sauce) | 180 |
| butter (*Lipton* Noodles and Sauce) | 200 |
| butter and herb (*Lipton* Noodles and Sauce) | 190 |
| carbonara Alfredo (*Lipton* Noodles and Sauce) | 210 |
| cheese (*Kraft* Dinner), ¾ cup | 340 |
| cheese (*Lipton* Noodles and Sauce) | 190 |
| chicken or chicken flavor: | |
| (*Kraft* Dinner), ¾ cup | 240 |
| (*Lipton* Noodles and Sauce) | 180 |
| (*Minute* Microwave Family/Single Size) | 160 |
| (*Mueller's Chef's Series*) | 160 |
| broccoli (*Lipton* Noodles and Sauce) | 200 |
| mushroom (*Noodle Roni*), 1 serving | 160 |
| fettuccini (*Noodle Roni*), 1 serving | 300 |
| garlic and butter (*Mueller's Chef's Series*) | 170 |
| garlic butter (*Noodle Roni*), 1 serving | 300 |
| herb butter (*Noodle Roni*), 1 serving | 160 |
| Parmesan (*Lipton* Noodles and Sauce) | 210 |
| Parmesan (*Minute* Microwave Family Size) | 170 |
| Parmesan (*Minute* Microwave Single Size) | 160 |
| Parmesan (*Noodle Roni* Parmesano), 1 serving | 240 |
| pesto (*Noodle Roni*), 1 serving | 220 |
| Romanoff (*Noodle Roni*), 1 serving | 240 |
| sour cream and chives (*Lipton* Noodles and Sauce) | 200 |
| sour cream and chives (*Mueller's Chef's Series*) | 190 |

| FOOD AND MEASURE | CALORIES |
|---|---|
| Stroganoff (*Lipton* Noodles and Sauce) | 200 |
| Stroganoff (*Mueller's Chef's Series*) | 190 |
| Stroganoff (*Noodle Roni*), 1 serving | 350 |
| **Noodle entree,** canned: | |
| and beef, in sauce (*Heinz*), 7.5 oz. | 170 |
| and chicken (*Heinz*), 7.5 oz. | 160 |
| and chicken (*Hormel/Dinty Moore Micro-Cup*), 7.5 oz. | 180 |
| w/franks (*Van Camp's Noodle Weenee*), 1 cup | 245 |
| **Noodle entree,** frozen: | |
| and beef w/gravy (*Banquet Family Entrees*), 8 oz. | 200 |
| and julienne beef w/sauce (*Banquet Family Entrees*), 7 oz. | 170 |
| Romanoff (*Stouffer's*), ⅓ of 12-oz. pkg. | 170 |
| **Nutmeg,** ground: | |
| (*Spice Islands*), 1 tsp. | 11 |
| **Nuts,** see specific listings | |
| **Nuts, mixed:** | |
| dry-roasted (*Planters*), 1 oz. | 160 |
| dry-roasted (*Planters* Unsalted), 1 oz. | 170 |
| oil-roasted (*Flavor House*), 1 oz. | 180 |
| w/peanuts (*Guy's*), 1 oz. | 170 |

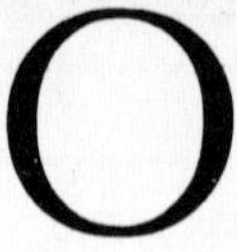

| FOOD AND MEASURE | CALORIES |
|---|---|
| **Oat** (see also "Cereal"): | |
| whole-grain, dry, 1 cup | 607 |
| rolled or oatmeal, dry, 1 cup | 311 |
| rolled or oatmeal, cooked, 1 cup | 145 |
| steel-cut (*Arrowhead Mills*), 2 oz. | 220 |
| **Oat bran** (see also "Cereal"): | |
| raw, 1 cup | 231 |
| cooked, 1 cup | 87 |
| **Oat flakes:** | |
| (*Arrowhead Mills*), 2 oz. | 220 |
| **Oat flour,** see "Flour" | |
| **Oat groats:** | |
| (*Arrowhead Mills*), 2 oz. | 220 |
| **Ocean perch,** meat only: | |
| fresh, Atlantic, raw 4 oz. | 107 |
| fresh, Atlantic, baked, broiled, or microwaved, 4 oz. | 137 |
| frozen (*Booth*), 4 oz. | 100 |
| frozen (*Gorton's Fishmarket Fresh*), 5 oz. | 140 |
| frozen (*Van de Kamp's* Natural), 4 oz. | 130 |
| **Ocean perch entree,** frozen: | |
| breaded (*Van de Kamp's* Light), 1 piece | 280 |
| **Octopus,** meat only: | |
| raw, 4 oz. | 92 |
| **Oheloberry:** | |
| ½ cup | 20 |
| **Oil:** | |
| almond, coconut, corn, cottonseed, palm, safflower, sesame, soybean, sunflower, vegetable, or walnut, 1 tbsp. | 120 |

| FOOD AND MEASURE | CALORIES |
|---|---|
| avocado or canola, 1 tbsp. | 124 |
| olive or peanut, 1 tbsp. | 119 |
| vegetable spray, regular or butter flavor (*Weight Watchers*), 1 second spray | 2 |

**Okra:**

| | |
|---|---|
| fresh, raw, untrimmed, 1 lb. | 148 |
| fresh, raw, sliced, ½ cup | 19 |
| fresh, boiled, drained, sliced, ½ cup | 25 |
| frozen, whole (*Seabrook*), 3.3 oz. | 30 |
| frozen, whole (*Southern*), 3.5 oz. | 35 |
| frozen, cut (*Seabrook*), 3.3 oz. | 25 |
| frozen, cut (*Southern*), 3.5 oz. | 31 |

**Old-fashioned drink mix:**

| | |
|---|---|
| bottled (*Holland House*), 1 fl. oz. | 33 |

**Old-fashioned loaf:**

| | |
|---|---|
| (*Oscar Mayer*), 1-oz. slice | 62 |

**Olive appetizer:**

| | |
|---|---|
| (*Progresso*), ½ cup | 180 |
| salad (*Progresso*), ½ cup | 120 |

**Olive condite:**

| | |
|---|---|
| (*Progresso*), ½ cup | 130 |

**Olive loaf:**

| | |
|---|---|
| (*Boar's Head*), 1 oz. | 60 |
| (*Eckrich*), 1-oz. slice | 80 |
| (*Hormel* Perma-Fresh), 2 slices | 110 |
| (*Oscar Mayer*), 1-oz. slice | 63 |

**Olives,** pickled:

| | |
|---|---|
| all varieties, all sizes (*S&W*), 1 oz. | 46 |
| green, 10 small, select or standard | 33 |
| green, 10 large | 45 |
| green, 10 giant | 76 |
| green, pitted, 1 oz. | 33 |
| ripe: | |
| Manzanillo or Mission (*Lindsay*), 10 small | 37 |
| Manzanillo or Mission (*Lindsay*), 10 medium | 44 |

| FOOD AND MEASURE | CALORIES |
|---|---|
| *Olives, ripe, continued* | |
| Manzanillo or Mission (*Lindsay*), 10 large | 50 |
| Manzanillo or Mission (*Lindsay*), 10 extra large | 63 |
| Manzanillo or Mission, pitted (*Lindsay*), 1 oz. | 32 |
| mixed varieties, pitted (*Vlasic*), 1 oz. | 37 |
| mixed varieties, pitted or chopped (*Lindsay*), 1 oz. | 29 |
| mixed varieties, pitted, sliced (*Lindsay*), ½ cup | 70 |
| salt-cured, oil-coated, Greek style, 10 medium | 65 |
| salt-cured, oil-coated, Greek style, 10 extra large | 89 |
| salt-cured, oil-coated, Greek style, pitted, 1 oz. | 96 |
| Sevillano and Ascolano (*Lindsay*), 10 jumbo | 66 |
| Sevillano and Ascolano (*Lindsay*), 10 colossal | 90 |
| Sevillano and Ascolano (*Lindsay*), 10 super colossal | 122 |
| Sevillano and Ascolano, pitted (*Lindsay*), 1 oz. | 23 |

**Omelet,** see "Egg breakfast"

**Onion, cocktail:**

| | |
|---|---|
| lightly spiced (*Vlasic*), 1 oz. | 4 |

**Onion, dried:**

| | |
|---|---|
| flakes, 1 tbsp. | 16 |
| minced, w/green onion (*Lawry's*), 1 tsp. | 7 |

**Onion, green** (scallion):

| | |
|---|---|
| untrimmed, 1 lb. | 140 |
| trimmed, w/top, chopped, ½ cup | 16 |
| trimmed, w/top, chopped, 1 tbsp. | 2 |

**Onion,** mature:

| | |
|---|---|
| fresh, raw, untrimmed, 1 lb. | 154 |
| fresh, raw, chopped, ½ cup | 30 |
| fresh, raw, chopped, 1 tbsp. | 4 |
| fresh, boiled, drained, chopped, ½ cup | 47 |
| canned, whole, small (*S&W*), ½ cup | 35 |
| canned, whole, sweet (*Heinz*), 1 oz. | 40 |
| frozen, whole, small (*Birds Eye*), 4 oz. | 40 |
| frozen, whole, small (*Seabrook*), 3.3 oz. | 35 |
| frozen, chopped (*Ore-Ida*), 2 oz. | 20 |
| frozen, w/cream sauce (*Birds Eye* Combinations), 5 oz. | 140 |
| frozen, rings, see "Onion ring" | |

| FOOD AND MEASURE | CALORIES |
|---|---|
| **Onion, Welsh:** | |
| trimmed, 1 oz. | 10 |
| **Onion dip:** | |
| creamy or French (*Kraft* Premium), 2 tbsp. | 45 |
| French (*Bison*), 1 oz. | 60 |
| French (*Nasoya Vegi-Dip*), 1 oz. | 50 |
| French or green onion (*Kraft*), 2 tbsp. | 60 |
| **Onion-flavored snack:** | |
| (*Funyuns*), 1 oz. | 140 |
| rings (*Wise*), 1 oz. | 130 |
| **Onion gravy mix,** prepared: | |
| (*French's*), ¼ cup | 25 |
| (*McCormick/Schilling*), ¼ cup | 22 |
| **Onion powder:** | |
| (*Spice Islands*), 1 tsp. | 8 |
| **Onion ring,** frozen: | |
| (*Ore-Ida Onion Ringers*), 2 oz. | 140 |
| battered (*Stilwell*), 3 oz. | 250 |
| battered, precooked (*Farm Rich* Batter Dipt), 4 oz. | 260 |
| crispy (*Farm Rich Onion O's*), 5 rings | 190 |
| crispy (*Mrs. Paul's*), 2.5 oz. | 190 |
| **Onion ring batter mix:** | |
| (*Golden Dipt*), 1 oz. | 100 |
| **Onion salt:** | |
| (*Tone's*), 1 tsp. | 1 |
| **Orange:** | |
| California navel, 1 medium, 2⅞" diam. | 65 |
| California navel, sections, w/out membrane, ½ cup | 38 |
| California Valencia, 1 medium, 2⅝" diam. | 59 |
| California Valencia, sections, w/out membrane, ½ cup | 44 |
| Florida, 1 medium, 2 11/16" diam. | 69 |
| Florida, sections, w/out membrane, ½ cup | 42 |
| Mandarin, see "Tangerine" | |

| FOOD AND MEASURE | CALORIES |
|---|---|
| **Orange danish:** | |
| w/icing, refrigerated (*Pillsbury*) | 150 |
| **Orange drink** (See also "Orange flavor drink"): | |
| (*Crowley*), 8 fl. oz. | 130 |
| (*Hawaiian Punch*), 6 fl. oz. | 100 |
| (*Hi-C*), 6 fl. oz. | 95 |
| (*Veryfine*), 8 fl. oz. | 130 |
| **Orange extract:** | |
| (*Virginia Dare*), 1 tsp. | 22 |
| **Orange flavor drink,** breakfast, 6 fl. oz.: | |
| frozen, diluted, or chilled (*Bright & Early*) | 90 |
| mix, prepared, crystals (*Tang*) | 90 |
| mix, prepared, crystals (*Tang* Sugar Free) | 6 |
| **Orange fruit juice blend:** | |
| (*Mott's*), 9.5-fl.-oz. can | 139 |
| **Orange juice:** | |
| fresh, 6 fl. oz. | 83 |
| canned, bottled or boxed: | |
| (*Del Monte* Unsweetened), 6 fl. oz. | 80 |
| (*Minute Maid*), 8.45 fl. oz. | 129 |
| (*Ocean Spray*), 6 fl. oz. | 90 |
| (*S&W*), 6 fl. oz. | 83 |
| (*Stokely* Unsweetened), 6 fl. oz. | 89 |
| (*Tree Top*), 6 fl. oz. | 90 |
| (*TreeSweet*), 6 fl. oz. | 78 |
| (*Tropicana* 100% Pure), 8 fl. oz. | 109 |
| (*Veryfine* 100%), 8 fl. oz. | 121 |
| blend (*Minute Maid* Juices to Go), 9.6 fl. oz. | 149 |
| blend (*Minute Maid On The Go*), 10 fl. oz. | 155 |
| blend (*Veryfine* 100%), 8 fl. oz. | 120 |
| canned or chilled (*Sunkist*), 6 fl. oz. | 84 |
| chilled: | |
| (*Citrus Hill* Plus Calcium/Select), 6 fl. oz. | 90 |
| (*Crowley*), 8 fl. oz. | 110 |
| (*Kraft* Pure 100% Unsweetened), 6 fl. oz. | 80 |
| (*Sunkist*), 6 fl. oz. | 84 |
| (*Sunkist* Fresh Squeezed), 6 fl. oz. | 77 |

| FOOD AND MEASURE | CALORIES |
|---|---|
| chilled or frozen, diluted (*Minute Maid*), 6 fl. oz. | 91 |
| frozen, diluted (*Sunkist*), 8 fl. oz. | 112 |
| frozen, diluted (*TreeSweet*), 6 fl. oz. | 84 |

**Orange juice cocktail:**

(*Welch's Orchard*), 10 fl. oz. .......... 150

**Orange juice drink:**

(*Citrus Hill* Lite Premium), 6 fl. oz. .......... 60
(*Kool-Aid Koolers*), 8.45 fl. oz. .......... 110
(*Minute Maid* Light'n Juicy), 6 fl. oz. .......... 16
(*Tang* Fruit Box), 8.45 fl. oz. .......... 130
tropical (*Tang* Fruit Box), 8.45 fl. oz. .......... 150
tropical (*Tropicana* Sparkler), 8 fl. oz. .......... 110

**Orange pastry:**

swirl (*Hostess Breakfast Bake Shop*), 1 piece .......... 230

**Orange sauce:**

Mandarin (*La Choy*), 1 tbsp. .......... 24

**Orange-apricot juice cocktail:**

(*Musselman's* Breakfast), 6 fl. oz. .......... 90

**Orange-banana juice:**

(*Smucker's* Naturally 100%), 8 fl. oz. .......... 120

**Orange-grapefruit juice:**

chilled (*Kraft* Pure 100%), 6 fl. oz. .......... 80

**Orange-grapefruit juice cocktail:**

(*Musselman's* Breakfast), 6 fl. oz. .......... 90

**Orange-pineapple juice:**

(*Kraft* Pure 100%), 6 fl. oz. .......... 80
(*Tropicana* 100% Pure), 8 fl. oz. .......... 111

**Orange-pineapple juice cocktail:**

(*Musselman's* Breakfast), 6 fl. oz. .......... 90

**Orange-strawberry-banana juice:**

(*Tropicana* 100% Pure), 8 fl. oz. .......... 141

| FOOD AND MEASURE | CALORIES |
|---|---|
| **Oregano,** dried: | |
| (*Spice Islands*), 1 tsp. | 6 |
| **Oriental spice:** | |
| 5-spice (*Tone*), 1 tsp. | 9 |
| **Oyster:** | |
| fresh, Eastern, meat only: | |
| raw, 4 oz. | 78 |
| raw, 1 cup | 170 |
| raw, 6 medium, 70 per qt. | 58 |
| boiled, poached, or steamed, 4 oz. | 155 |
| boiled, poached, or steamed, 6 medium | 58 |
| fresh, Pacific, meat only, raw, 4 oz. | 92 |
| fresh, Pacific, meat only, raw, 1 medium, 20 per qt. | 41 |
| canned (*Bumble Bee*), 1 cup | 218 |
| canned, Eastern, w/liquid, 1 cup | 170 |
| canned, whole (*S&W Fancy*), 2 oz. | 95 |

**Oyster stew,** see "Soup, canned, condensed"

# P

| FOOD AND MEASURE | CALORIES |
|---|---|

**P&B loaf:**

| | |
|---|---|
| (*Kahn's*), 1 slice | 40 |

**Pancake,** frozen:

| | |
|---|---|
| (*Aunt Jemima* Original Microwave), 3.5 oz. | 211 |
| (*Downyflake*), 3 pieces | 280 |
| (*Pillsbury* Original Microwave), 3 pieces | 240 |
| blueberry (*Aunt Jemima*), 3.5 oz. | 220 |
| blueberry (*Downyflake*), 3 pieces | 290 |
| blueberry (*Pillsbury* Microwave), 3 pieces | 250 |
| buttermilk (*Aunt Jemima* Lite Microwave), 3.5 oz. | 140 |
| buttermilk (*Aunt Jemima* Microwave), 3.5 oz. | 210 |
| buttermilk (*Downyflake*), 3 pieces | 280 |
| buttermilk (*Pillsbury* Microwave), 3 pieces | 260 |
| buttermilk (*Weight Watchers* Microwave), 2.5 oz. | 140 |
| wheat, harvest (*Pillsbury* Microwave), 3 pieces | 240 |

**Pancake batter,** frozen, 3.6 oz.:

| | |
|---|---|
| (*Aunt Jemima* Original) | 183 |
| blueberry (*Aunt Jemima*) | 204 |
| buttermilk (*Aunt Jemima*) | 180 |

**Pancake breakfast,** frozen:

| | |
|---|---|
| w/bacon (*Swanson Great Starts*), 4.5 oz. | 400 |
| w/blueberry topping (*Weight Watchers* Microwave), 4.75 oz. | 200 |
| w/links (*Weight Watchers* Microwave), 4 oz. | 220 |
| lite, and lite syrup (*Aunt Jemima*), 6 oz. | 260 |
| lite, and two lite links (*Aunt Jemima*), 6 oz. | 310 |
| and sausages (*Downyflake*), 5.5 oz. | 430 |
| and sausages (*Swanson Great Starts*), 6 oz. | 460 |
| silver dollar, w/sausages (*Swanson Great Starts*), 3.75 oz. | 310 |
| w/strawberry topping (*Weight Watchers* Microwave), 4.75 oz. | 200 |
| whole wheat, w/lite links (*Swanson Great Starts*), 5.5 oz. | 350 |

| FOOD AND MEASURE | CALORIES |
|---|---|

**Pancake syrup** (see also "Maple syrup"):

| | |
|---|---|
| (*Aunt Jemima* ButterLite), 2 tbsp. | 50 |
| (*Aunt Jemima* Lite), 2 tbsp. | 54 |
| (*Aunt Jemima* Original), 2 tbsp. | 109 |
| (*Estee*), 1 tbsp. | 4 |
| (*Featherweight*), 1 tbsp. | 16 |
| (*Log Cabin* Country Kitchen/Pancake and Waffle), 2 tbsp. | 100 |
| (*Log Cabin* Lite), 2 tbsp. | 50 |
| (*Vermont Maid*), 1 tbsp. | 50 |
| maple flavored (*S&W*), 1 tsp. | 4 |

**Pancake and waffle mix,** prepared:

| | |
|---|---|
| (*Aunt Jemima* Original), 3 pieces, 4″ each | 116 |
| (*Aunt Jemima* Original Complete), 3 pieces, 4″ each | 253 |
| (*Bisquick Shake'N Pour*), 3 pieces, 4″ each | 260 |
| (*Hungry Jack Extra Lights*), 3 pieces, 4″ each | 210 |
| (*Hungry Jack Extra Lights* Complete), 3 pieces, 4″ each | 190 |
| (*Hungry Jack* Panshakes), 3 pieces, 4″ each | 250 |
| (*Martha White FlapStax*), 1 piece | 100 |
| apple cinnamon (*Bisquick Shake'N Pour*), 3 pieces, 4″ each | 270 |
| blueberry (*Bisquick Shake'N Pour*), 3 pieces, 4″ each | 280 |
| blueberry (*Hungry Jack*), 3 pieces, 4″ each | 320 |
| buckwheat (*Aunt Jemima*), 3 pieces, 4″ each | 143 |
| buttermilk, 3 pieces, 4″ each: | |
| (*Aunt Jemima*) | 122 |
| (*Aunt Jemima* Complete) | 231 |
| (*Aunt Jemima* Lite Complete) | 130 |
| (*Betty Crocker*) | 280 |
| (*Bisquick Shake'N Pour*) | 260 |
| (*Hungry Jack*) | 240 |
| (*Hungry Jack* Complete/Complete Packets) | 180 |
| oat bran (*Bisquick Shake'N Pour*), 3 pieces, 4″ each | 240 |
| whole wheat (*Aunt Jemima*), 3 pieces, 4″ each | 161 |

**Pancreas:**

| | |
|---|---|
| beef, braised, 4 oz. | 307 |
| lamb, braised, 4 oz. | 265 |
| pork, braised, 4 oz. | 248 |
| veal, braised, 4 oz. | 290 |

| FOOD AND MEASURE | CALORIES |
|---|---|
| **Papaya:** | |
| cubed, ½ cup | 27 |
| (*Calavo Growers*), ½ medium | 80 |
| (*Del Monte*), ⅓ medium | 60 |
| **Papaya nectar:** | |
| (*Libby's*), 6 fl. oz. | 110 |
| **Papaya punch:** | |
| (*Veryfine*), 8 fl. oz. | 120 |
| **Paprika:** | |
| 1 tsp. | 6 |
| **Parsley:** | |
| fresh, 10 sprigs | 3 |
| fresh, chopped, ½ cup | 10 |
| dried, 1 tbsp. | 4 |
| dried, 1 tsp. | 1 |
| freeze-dried, 1 tbsp. | 1 |
| **Parsley seasoning:** | |
| all purpose (*McCormick/Schilling Parsley Patch*), 1 tsp. | 6 |
| **Parsnip:** | |
| raw, sliced, ½ cup | 50 |
| boiled, drained, 1 medium, 9″ × 2¼″ diam. | 130 |
| boiled, drained, sliced, ½ cup | 63 |
| **Passion fruit,** purple: | |
| 1 medium, 1.2 oz. | 18 |
| **Passion fruit juice,** fresh: | |
| purple, 6 fl. oz. | 95 |
| yellow, 6 fl. oz. | 112 |
| **Passion fruit juice cocktail:** | |
| (*Welch's Orchard Tropicals* Cocktails-In-A-Box), 8.45 fl. oz. | 140 |
| bottled (*Welch's Orchard Tropicals*), 6 fl. oz. | 100 |
| **Passion fruit–orange refresher:** | |
| tropical (*Veryfine*), 8 fl. oz. | 110 |

| FOOD AND MEASURE | CALORIES |
|---|---|

**Pasta** (see also "Macaroni" and "Noodle"):

| | |
|---|---|
| dry, 2 oz.: | |
| (*Creamette*) | 210 |
| (*Ronzoni*) | 210 |
| all varieties (*Antoine's*) | 210 |
| all varieties, except whole wheat (*Al Dente*) | 220 |
| all varieties, except vegetable, tomato and basil, and whole wheat (*De Boles*) | 210 |
| all varieties, except oat bran (*Health Valley*) | 170 |
| w/egg (*Creamette*) | 221 |
| oat bran (*Health Valley* Spaghetti) | 120 |
| spinach, w/egg (*Creamette*) | 220 |
| tomato and basil (*De Boles*) | 200 |
| vegetable, tri-color (*Creamette*) | 210 |
| vegetable, tri-color (*De Boles* Primavera) | 200 |
| whole wheat (*Al Dente* Fettucine) | 210 |
| whole wheat (*De Boles* Natural Gourmet) | 200 |
| whole wheat, w/bran (*Misura*) | 197 |
| cooked: | |
| 1 cup | 197 |
| corn, 1 cup | 176 |
| spinach, 1 cup | 183 |
| whole wheat, 1 cup | 174 |

**Pasta dinner,** frozen (see also specific pasta listings):

| | |
|---|---|
| shells, stuffed, 3-cheese (*Le Menu* LightStyle), 10 oz. | 280 |

**Pasta dishes,** canned (see also specific pasta listings), 7.5 oz., except as noted:

| | |
|---|---|
| in tomato and cheese sauce (*Franco-American* SportyO's) | 170 |
| garden medley (*Lipton Hearty Ones*), 11 oz. | 323 |
| Italiano (*Lipton Hearty Ones*), 11 oz. | 328 |
| w/meatballs, in tomato sauce (*Franco-American* SportyO's) | 210 |
| rings or twists, in sauce (*Buitoni*) | 150 |
| rings or twists and meatballs, in sauce (*Buitoni*) | 210 |
| shells, in meat sauce (*Chef Boyardee* Microwave) | 210 |
| shells, in mushroom sauce (*Chef Boyardee* Microwave) | 170 |

**Pasta dishes,** frozen (see also "Pasta entree"):

| | |
|---|---|
| Alfredo, w/broccoli (*The Budget Gourmet* Side Dish), 5.5 oz. | 200 |
| angel hair (*Weight Watchers*), 10 oz. | 210 |

| FOOD AND MEASURE | CALORIES |
|---|---|
| creamy cheddar (*Green Giant Pasta Accents*), ½ cup | 100 |
| Dijon (*Green Giant* Garden Gourmet), 1 pkg. | 260 |
| Florentine (*Green Giant* Garden Gourmet), 1 pkg. | 230 |
| garden herb (*Green Giant Pasta Accents*), ½ cup | 80 |
| garlic seasoning (*Green Giant Pasta Accents*), ½ cup | 110 |
| marinara (*Green Giant* One Serving), 5.5 oz. | 180 |
| Parmesan, w/sweet peas (*Green Giant* One Serving), 5.5 oz. | 170 |
| primavera (*Green Giant Pasta Accents*), ½ cup | 110 |
| rigati (*Weight Watchers*), 10.63 oz. | 300 |
| and vegetables, in creamy Stroganoff sauce (*Birds Eye Custom Cuisine*), 4.6 oz. w/out added ingredients | 120 |
| and vegetables w/white cheese sauce (*Birds Eye Custom Cuisine*), 4.6 oz. w/out added ingredients | 150 |

**Pasta dishes, mix**[1], ½ cup, except as noted:

| | |
|---|---|
| (*Kraft Light Rancher's Choice* Pasta Salad & Dressing) | 170 |
| (*Kraft Rancher's Choice* Pasta Salad & Dressing) | 250 |
| Alfredo (*Hain* Pasta & Sauce), ¼ pkg. | 180 |
| Alfredo (*McCormick/Schilling Pasta Prima*), 1 cup | 253 |
| bacon vinaigrette (*Country Recipe* Pasta Salad) | 140 |
| broccoli, cheddar, fusilli (*Lipton* Pasta & Sauce) | 200 |
| broccoli, creamy (*Lipton* Pasta Salad)[2] | 200 |
| broccoli and vegetables (*Kraft* Pasta Salad & Dressing) | 210 |
| buttermilk, country (*Mueller's* Salad Bar) | 250 |
| carbonara Alfredo (*Lipton* Pasta and Sauce) | 140 |
| cheese, all varieties, except chicken w/herbs (*Kraft* Pasta & Cheese) | 180 |
| cheese, cheddar (*Minute* Microwave Family/Single) | 160 |
| cheese, cheddar tangy (*Hain* Pasta & Sauce), ¼ pkg. | 180 |
| cheese, chicken w/herbs (*Kraft* Pasta & Cheese) | 170 |
| cheese, Parmesan, creamy (*Hain* Pasta & Sauce), ¼ pkg. | 150 |
| cheese, supreme (*Lipton* Pasta and Sauce) | 139 |
| chicken broccoli (*Lipton* Pasta and Sauce) | 129 |
| cucumber, creamy (*Mueller's* Salad Bar) | 250 |
| Dijon, creamy (*Country Recipe* Pasta Salad) | 190 |
| garlic, creamy (*Lipton* Pasta & Sauce) | 210 |
| garlic, creamy (*McCormick/Schilling Pasta Prima*), 1 pkg. dry | 107 |
| herb, Italian (*Hain* Pasta & Sauce), ⅕ pkg. | 110 |
| herb and garlic (*McCormick/Schilling Pasta Prima*), 1 cup | 326 |

[1]Prepared according to package directions, except as noted.
[2]Prepared with 3 tbsp. milk and 3 tbsp. mayonnaise or salad dressing.

| FOOD AND MEASURE | CALORIES |
|---|---|
| *Pasta dishes, mix, continued* | |
| herb tomato (*Lipton* Pasta & Sauce) | 180 |
| homestyle (*Kraft* Pasta Salad & Dressing) | 240 |
| homestyle (*Mueller's* Salad Bar) | 250 |
| Italian (*Kraft* Pasta Salad & Dressing) | 130 |
| Italian, creamy (*Country Recipe* Pasta Salad) | 160 |
| Italian, creamy (*Mueller's* Salad Bar) | 290 |
| Italian, robust (*Lipton* Pasta Salad) | 190 |
| Italian, zesty (*Mueller's* Salad Bar) | 140 |
| marinara (*McCormick/Schilling Pasta Prima*), 1 cup | 329 |
| mushroom, chicken flavors (*Lipton* Pasta and Sauce) | 124 |
| mushroom, creamy (*Lipton* Pasta & Sauce) | 210 |
| Oriental, w/fusilli (*Lipton* Pasta and Sauce) | 130 |
| pasta salad (*McCormick/Schilling Pasta Prima*), 1 cup | 390 |
| pesto (*McCormick/Schilling Pasta Prima*) | 193 |
| primavera (*Hain* Pasta & Sauce), ¼ pkg. | 140 |
| primavera, garden (*Kraft* Pasta Salad & Dressing) | 170 |
| ranch (*Country Recipe* Pasta Salad) | 140 |
| seafood, creamy (*McCormick/Schilling Pasta Prima*) | 135 |
| Swiss, creamy (*Hain* Pasta & Sauce), ⅕ pkg. | 170 |

**Pasta entree,** frozen (see also "Pasta dishes, frozen" and specific pasta listings):

| FOOD AND MEASURE | CALORIES |
|---|---|
| baked, and cheese (*Celentano*), 6 oz. | 290 |
| carbonara (*Stouffer's*), 9.75-oz. pkg. | 620 |
| casino (*Stouffer's*), 9.25-oz. pkg. | 300 |
| Dijon (*Green Giant* Microwave Garden Gourmet), 1 pkg. | 300 |
| Mexicali (*Stouffer's*), 10-oz. pkg. | 490 |
| Oriental (*Stouffer's*), 9⅞-oz. pkg. | 300 |
| primavera (*Stouffer's*), 10⅝-oz. pkg. | 540 |
| primavera (*Weight Watchers*), 8.5 oz. | 260 |
| rigati (*Weight Watchers*), 10.63 oz. | 300 |
| shells, and beef (*The Budget Gourmet*), 10 oz. | 340 |
| shells, cheese, w/tomato sauce (*Stouffer's*), 9.25 oz. | 330 |
| shells, stuffed: | |
| (*Buitoni* Single Serving), 9 oz. | 460 |
| (*Celentano*), 8 oz. | 330 |
| w/sauce (*Celentano*), 10 oz. | 410 |
| w/sauce (*Celentano*), 6.25 oz. | 340 |
| w/vegetables, tofu, and sauce (*Legume* Provencale), 11 oz. | 240 |
| trio (*Tyson Gourmet Selection*), 11 oz. | 450 |

| FOOD AND MEASURE | CALORIES |
|---|---|
| **Pasta sauce** (see also "Tomato sauce" and specific listings), canned or in jars: | |
| (*Enrico's* All Natural Regular/No Salt Added), 4 oz. | 60 |
| (*Hunt's* Traditional), 4 oz. | 70 |
| (*Pastorelli Italian Chef*), 4 oz. | 81 |
| (*Prego*), 4 oz. | 130 |
| (*Prego* No Salt Added), 4 oz. | 110 |
| (*Progresso* Spaghetti Sauce), ½ cup | 110 |
| (*Ragu*), 4 oz. | 80 |
| (*Ragu* Chunky Garden Style), 4 oz. | 70 |
| (*Ragu* Homestyle), 4 oz. | 50 |
| (*Ragu* Italian), 4 oz. | 90 |
| (*Ragu* Thick & Hearty), 4 oz. | 100 |
| cheese, three (*Prego*), 4 oz. | 100 |
| garden combination (*Prego* Extra Chunky), 4 oz. | 80 |
| marinara (*Buitoni*), ½ cup | 70 |
| marinara (*Prego*), 4 oz. | 100 |
| marinara (*Progresso*), ½ cup | 90 |
| marinara (*Progresso* Authentic Pasta Sauces), ½ cup | 110 |
| marinara (*Rokeach*), 3 oz. | 60 |
| meat (*Hunt's*), 4 oz. | 70 |
| meat (*Prego*), 4 oz. | 140 |
| meat (*Progresso* Spaghetti Sauce), ½ cup | 110 |
| meat (*Weight Watchers*), ⅓ cup | 50 |
| mushroom or mushroom flavor: | |
| (*Enrico's*), 4 oz. | 60 |
| (*Featherweight*), 4 oz. | 60 |
| (*Hunt's*), 4 oz. | 70 |
| (*Prego*), 4 oz. | 130 |
| (*Progresso* Spaghetti Sauce), ½ cup | 110 |
| (*Weight Watchers*), ⅓ cup | 40 |
| w/fresh sliced mushrooms (*Enrico's* Pasta Sauce), 4 oz. | 60 |
| mushroom and green pepper (*Enrico's* All Natural), 4 oz. | 60 |
| mushroom and green pepper, and onion, or w/extra spice (*Prego* Extra Chunky), 4 oz. | 100 |
| mushroom and tomato (*Prego* Extra Chunky), 4 oz. | 110 |
| onion and garlic (*Prego*), 4 oz. | 110 |
| primavera, creamy (*Progresso* Authentic Pasta Sauces), ½ cup | 190 |
| sausage and green pepper (*Prego* Extra Chunky), 4 oz. | 160 |
| Sicilian (*Progresso* Authentic Pasta Sauces), ½ cup | 30 |

| FOOD AND MEASURE | CALORIES |
|---|---|
| *Pasta sauce, canned, continued* | |
| tomato and basil (*Prego*), 4 oz. | 100 |
| tomato and onion (*Prego* Extra Chunky), 4 oz. | 110 |

**Pasta sauce,** refrigerated:

| | |
|---|---|
| marinara or plum, w/basil (*Contadina Fresh*), 7.5 oz. | 100 |

**Pasta sauce mix:**

| | |
|---|---|
| (*Lawry's* Rich & Thick), 1 pkg. | 147 |
| (*McCormick/Schilling*), ¼ pkg. | 32 |
| cheese and garlic or Italian (*French's Pasta Toss*), 2 tsp. | 25 |
| Italian style or w/mushrooms, prepared (*French's*), ⅝ cup. | 100 |
| w/mushrooms, imported (*Lawry's*), 1 pkg. | 143 |
| Romanoff (*French's Pasta Toss*), 2 tsp. | 30 |

**Pastrami:**

| | |
|---|---|
| (*Boar's Head* Round), 1 oz. | 40 |
| (*Healthy Deli* Round), 1 oz. | 34 |
| (*Hillshire Farm* Deli Select), 1 oz. | 31 |
| (*Oscar Mayer*), .6-oz. slice | 16 |
| turkey, see "Turkey pastrami" | |

**Pastry pocket,** refrigerated:

| | |
|---|---|
| (*Pillsbury*), 1 piece | 240 |

**Pastry shells** (see also "Puff pastry"):

| | |
|---|---|
| tart (*Pet-Ritz*, 3″), 1 piece | 150 |

**Pâté,** canned:

| | |
|---|---|
| 1 oz. | 90 |
| 1 tbsp. | 41 |
| chicken liver, 1 oz. | 57 |
| chicken liver, 1 tbsp. | 26 |
| goose liver, smoked, 1 oz. | 131 |
| goose liver, smoked, 1 tbsp. | 60 |
| liver (*Sells*), 2⅛ oz. | 190 |

**Pea pod, Chinese,** see "Peas, edible-podded"

**Peach:**

| | |
|---|---|
| fresh, 1 medium 2½″ diam., 4 per lb. | 37 |
| fresh, peeled, sliced, ½ cup | 37 |

| FOOD AND MEASURE | CALORIES |
|---|---|
| canned, ½ cup, except as noted: | |
| (*Mott's* Peach Fruit Pak), 3.75 oz. | 75 |
| cling, halves or slices (*Del Monte*) | 80 |
| cling, halves or slices (*Del Monte Lite*) | 50 |
| cling, diced (*Del Monte* Fruit Cup), 5 oz. | 110 |
| cling, spiced, w/pits (*Del Monte*), 3.5 oz. | 80 |
| freestone, halves or slices (*Del Monte*) | 90 |
| freestone, halves or slices (*Del Monte Lite*) | 60 |
| freestone or cling (*S&W/Nutradiet*) | 30 |
| in water, cling, halves or slices | 29 |
| in juice, cling, halves or slices (*Featherweight*) | 50 |
| in juice, cling, halves or slices (*Libby Lite*) | 50 |
| in light syrup, cling, halves or slices | 68 |
| in heavy syrup, all varieties (*S&W*) | 100 |
| spiced, whole (*S&W*) | 90 |
| dehydrated, sulfured, uncooked, 2 oz. | 185 |
| dried, uncooked (*Sun-Maid/Sunsweet*), 2 oz. | 140 |
| dried, uncooked (*Del Monte*), 2 oz. | 140 |
| dried, sulfured, uncooked, havles, ½ cup | 192 |
| dried, sulfured, uncooked, 10 halves | 311 |
| frozen, sliced, sweetened, ½ cup | 118 |

**Peach butter:**

| | |
|---|---|
| (*Smucker's*), 1 tsp. | 15 |

**Peach cobbler,** frozen:

| | |
|---|---|
| (*Pet-Ritz*), ⅙ pkg. | 260 |
| (*Stilwell*), 4 oz. | 270 |

**Peach drink:**

| | |
|---|---|
| (*Hi-C*), 6 fl. oz. | 101 |

**Peach juice:**

| | |
|---|---|
| (*Smucker's* Naturally 100%), 8 fl. oz. | 120 |
| orchard blend (*Dole Pure & Light*), 6 fl. oz. | 90 |

**Peach nectar:**

| | |
|---|---|
| (*Libby's*), 6 fl. oz. | 100 |

**Peach parfait,** frozen:

| | |
|---|---|
| (*Pepperidge Farm* Dessert Lights), 4.25 oz. | 150 |

| FOOD AND MEASURE | CALORIES |
|---|---|
| **Peach turnover,** frozen: | |
| (*Pepperidge Farm*), 1 piece | 310 |
| **Peanut,** shelled: | |
| (*Beer Nuts*), 1 oz. | 180 |
| (*Weight Watchers*), 1 pouch | 100 |
| dry-roasted (*Flavor House* Salted/Unsalted), 1 oz. | 180 |
| dry-roasted (*Frito-Lay's*), 1⅛ oz. | 190 |
| dry-roasted (*Planters*), 1 oz. | 160 |
| dry-roasted (*Planters* Unsalted), 1 oz. | 170 |
| honey-roasted (*Eagle Honey Roast*), 1 oz. | 170 |
| honey-roasted (*Flavor House*), 1 oz. | 160 |
| honey-roasted (*Planters*), 1 oz. | 170 |
| honey-roasted, dry-roasted (*Planters*), 1 oz. | 160 |
| oil-roasted (*Flavor House*), 1 oz. | 170 |
| oil-roasted (*Planters/Planters* Cocktail/Redskin), 1 oz. | 170 |
| Spanish, dry-roasted (*Planters*), 1 oz. | 160 |
| Spanish, oil-roasted (*Flavor House*), 1 oz. | 170 |
| **Peanut butter:** | |
| (*Estee*), 1 tbsp. | 100 |
| (*S&W Nutradiet*), 1 tbsp. | 93 |
| chunky or creamy: | |
| (*Arrowhead Mills*), 2 tbsp. | 190 |
| (*Bama*), 2 tbsp. | 200 |
| (*Featherweight*), 1 tbsp. | 90 |
| (*Health Valley* No Salt Added), 2 tbsp. | 180 |
| (*Jif*), 2 tbsp. | 190 |
| (*Peter Pan*), 2 tbsp. | 190 |
| (*Skippy*), 2 tbsp. | 190 |
| (*Smucker's* Natural Regular/No Salt), 2 tbsp. | 200 |
| creamy (*Peter Pan* Creamy Salt Free), 2 tbsp. | 195 |
| **Peanut butter flavor baking chips:** | |
| (*Reese's*), 1.5 oz. or ¼ cup | 230 |
| **Pear:** | |
| untrimmed, 1 lb. | 247 |
| w/skin, sliced, ½ cup | 49 |
| Bartlett, 1 pear, 2½" diam. × 3½" | 98 |

| FOOD AND MEASURE | CALORIES |
|---|---|
| canned, ½ cup: | |
| all varieties, peeled (*S&W/Nutradiet*) | 35 |
| Bartlett, halves or slices (*Del Monte*) | 80 |
| Bartlett, halves or slices (*Del Monte Lite*) | 50 |
| in juice, halves (*Featherweight*) | 60 |
| in juice, halves or slices (*Libby Lite*) | 60 |
| in juice, slices, sweetened (*S&W* Natural Style) | 80 |
| in extra light syrup, halves | 58 |
| in heavy syrup, halves (*S&W*) | 100 |
| dried, sulfured, uncooked, 2 oz. | 149 |
| dried, sulfured, uncooked, halves, ½ cup | 236 |

**Pear nectar,** canned:

| | |
|---|---|
| 6 fl. oz. | 112 |

**Peas, black-eyed,** see "Black-eyed peas" and "Cowpeas"

**Peas, cream,** canned:

| | |
|---|---|
| (*Allens* Fresh), ½ cup | 90 |

**Peas, crowder:**

| | |
|---|---|
| canned (*Allens* Fresh), ½ cup | 80 |
| frozen (*Seabrook*), 3 oz. | 130 |

**Peas, edible-podded:**

| | |
|---|---|
| fresh, raw, untrimmed, 1 lb. | 180 |
| fresh, raw, ½ cup | 30 |
| fresh, boiled, drained, ½ cup | 34 |
| frozen: | |
| Chinese (*Chun King*), 1.5 oz. | 20 |
| Chinese (*Seabrook*), 2 oz. | 20 |
| snow (*Birds Eye* Deluxe), 3 oz. | 35 |
| sugar snap (*Birds Eye* Deluxe), 2.6 oz. | 45 |
| sugar snap (*Green Giant Harvest Fresh*), ½ cup | 30 |
| sugar snap, w/baby carrots and waterchestnuts (*Birds Eye* Farm Fresh), 3.2 oz. | 50 |

**Peas, field,** canned:

| | |
|---|---|
| plain or w/snaps (*Allens* Fresh), ½ cup | 100 |
| tiny, w/snaps (*Allens* Fresh), ½ cup | 70 |

| FOOD AND MEASURE | CALORIES |
|---|---|
| **Peas, green or sweet:** | |
| fresh, raw, in pod, 1 lb. | 140 |
| fresh, raw, shelled, ½ cup | 58 |
| fresh, boiled, drained, ½ cup | 67 |
| canned, ½ cup: | |
| (*S&W* Perfection/Petit Pois) | 70 |
| (*Stokely* No Salt or Sugar Added) | 50 |
| w/liquid (*Del Monte*/*Del Monte* No Salt/Seasoned) | 60 |
| dry early June (*Allens*) | 80 |
| early or sweet (*Stokely*) | 60 |
| early June or sweet (*Green Giant*/*Green Giant* Mini) | 50 |
| small, w/liquid (*Del Monte*) | 50 |
| sweet (*Featherweight*) | 70 |
| sweet (*S&W*/*Nutradiet*) | 40 |
| frozen: | |
| (*Birds Eye*), 3.3 oz. | 80 |
| (*Birds Eye* Portion Pack), 3 oz. | 70 |
| (*Seabrook*), 3.3 oz. | 80 |
| (*Southern*), 3.5 oz. | 79 |
| (*Stokely Singles*), 3 oz. | 65 |
| early June (*Green Giant Harvest Fresh*), ½ cup | 60 |
| petite (*Southern*), 3.5 oz. | 64 |
| sweet (*Green Giant*/*Green Giant Harvest Fresh*), ½ cup | 50 |
| tender tiny (*Birds Eye* Deluxe), 3.3 oz. | 60 |
| tiny (*Seabrook*), 3.3 oz. | 60 |
| in butter sauce, early (*Green Giant* One Serving), 4.5 oz. | 90 |
| in butter sauce, early (*LeSueur*), ½ cup | 80 |
| in butter sauce, sweet (*Green Giant*), ½ cup | 80 |
| in butter sauce, sweet (*Stokely Singles*), 4 oz. | 90 |
| w/cream sauce (*Birds Eye* Combinations), 5 oz. | 180 |
| **Peas, green, combinations,** frozen: | |
| and carrots, see "Peas and carrots" | |
| and cauliflower, in cream sauce (*The Budget Gourmet* Side Dish), 5.75 oz. | 170 |
| *LeSueur* style (*Green Giant Valley Combination*), ½ cup | 70 |
| mini, w/pea pods and waterchestnuts, in butter sauce (*LeSueur*), ½ cup | 80 |
| and onions, see "Peas and onions" | |
| w/onions and carrots, in butter sauce (*LeSueur*), ½ cup | 80 |

| FOOD AND MEASURE | CALORIES |
|---|---|
| and potatoes, w/cream sauce (*Birds Eye* Combinations), 5 oz. | 190 |
| and waterchestnuts Oriental (*The Budget Gourmet*), 5 oz. | 120 |
| **Peas, pigeon,** see "Pigeon peas" | |
| **Peas, purple hull:** | |
| canned (*Allens* Fresh), ½ cup | 100 |
| frozen (*Frosty Acres*), 3.3 oz. | 130 |
| **Peas, snow,** see "Peas, edible-podded" | |
| **Peas, split,** see "Split peas" | |
| **Peas, sprouted,** mature seeds: | |
| raw, ½ cup | 77 |
| boiled, drained, 4 oz. | 134 |
| **Peas, sugar snap,** see "Peas, edible-podded" | |
| **Peas, white acre,** canned: | |
| fresh (*Allens*), ½ cup | 90 |
| **Peas and carrots:** | |
| canned (*Del Monte*), ½ cup | 50 |
| canned (*S&W*), ½ cup | 50 |
| canned (*S&W/Nutradiet*), ½ cup | 35 |
| canned (*Stokely*), ½ cup | 50 |
| canned (*Stokely* No Salt/Sugar), ½ cup | 45 |
| frozen (*Seabrook*), 3.3 oz. | 60 |
| frozen (*Southern*), 3.5 oz. | 64 |
| **Peas and onions:** | |
| canned, w/liquid, ½ cup | 30 |
| canned, sweet (*Green Giant*), ½ cup | 50 |
| canned, sweet, w/tiny pearl onions (*S&W*), ½ cup | 60 |
| frozen (*Birds Eye* Combinations), 3.3 oz. | 70 |
| frozen (*Seabrook*), 3.3 oz. | 70 |
| frozen, w/cheese sauce (*Birds Eye* Combinations), 5 oz. | 140 |
| **Pecan,** shelled: | |
| all varieties (*Planters*), 1 oz. | 190 |
| dried, halves, 1 cup | 721 |
| dry-roasted, 1 oz. | 187 |
| oil-roasted, 1 oz. or 15 halves | 195 |

| FOOD AND MEASURE | CALORIES |
|---|---|
| **Pecan pastry:** | |
| caramel swirl (*Hostess Breakfast Bake Shop*), 1 piece | 240 |
| spinners (*Hostess Breakfast Bake Shop*), 1 piece | 220 |
| **Pepper,** ground: | |
| black, 1 tsp. | 5 |
| red or cayenne, 1 tsp. | 6 |
| white, 1 tsp. | 7 |
| seasoned (*Lawry's*), 1 tsp. | 9 |
| **Pepper, bell,** see "Pepper, sweet" | |
| **Pepper, cherry:** | |
| mild (*Vlasic*), 1 oz. | 8 |
| hot (*Progresso*), ½ cup | 190 |
| hot, pickled (*Progresso*), ½ cup | 130 |
| **Pepper, chili, hot:** | |
| fresh, green and red, raw, 1 medium, 1.6 oz. | 18 |
| fresh, green and red, raw, chopped, ½ cup | 30 |
| canned, green, whole or diced (*Del Monte*), ½ cup | 20 |
| canned, whole (*Old El Paso*), 1 chili | 8 |
| canned, whole, diced, sliced, or strips (*Ortega*), 1 oz. | 10 |
| canned, chopped (*Old El Paso*), 2 tbsp. | 8 |
| **Pepper, green or red,** see "Pepper, sweet" | |
| **Pepper, hot** (see also specific listings): | |
| whole or diced (*Ortega*), 1 oz. | 8 |
| **Pepper, jalapeño,** canned or in jars: | |
| whole or diced (*Oretga*), 1 oz. | 10 |
| whole or sliced, w/liquid (*Del Monte*), ½ cup | 30 |
| hot (*Vlasic*), 1 oz. | 10 |
| marinated (*La Victoria*), 1 tbsp. | 4 |
| nacho (*La Victoria*), 1 tbsp. | 2 |
| **Pepper, pepperoncini:** | |
| (*Progresso* Tuscan), ½ cup | 20 |
| salad (*Vlasic*), 1 oz. | 4 |
| **Pepper, piccalilli:** | |
| (*Progresso*), ½ cup | 190 |

| FOOD AND MEASURE | CALORIES |
|---|---|
| **Pepper, stuffed, entree,** frozen: | |
| green, w/beef, in tomato sauce (*Stouffer's*), 7¾ oz. | 200 |
| sweet red (*Celentano*), 13 oz. | 350 |
| **Pepper, sweet,** green and red: | |
| fresh, raw, 1 medium, 3¾″ × 3″ diam. | 20 |
| fresh, raw, chopped, ½ cup | 13 |
| fresh, boiled, drained, chopped, ½ cup | 19 |
| in jars (*Heinz* Sweet Pepper Mementos), 1 oz. | 6 |
| in jars, roasted (*Progresso*), ½ cup | 20 |
| in jars, sweet, fried (*Progresso*), ½ jar | 37 |
| frozen, boiled, drained, chopped, 4 oz. | 20 |
| frozen, green (*Seabrook*), 1 oz. | 6 |
| frozen, red (*Seabrook*), 1 oz. | 8 |
| **Pepper rings:** | |
| hot (*Vlasic*), 1 oz. | 4 |
| **Pepper sauce, hot:** | |
| (*Gebhardt* Louisiana Style), ½ tsp. | 0 |
| (*Tabasco*), ¼ tsp. | <1 |
| **Pepper steak,** see "Beef dinner" and "Beef entree, frozen" | |
| **Peppered loaf:** | |
| (*Eckrich*), 1-oz. slice | 35 |
| (*Kahn's*), 1 slice | 40 |
| (*Oscar Mayer*), 1-oz. slice | 39 |
| **Pepperoni:** | |
| (*Hormel/Hormel* Chunk), 1 oz. | 140 |
| (*Hormel* Leoni Brand), 1 oz. | 130 |
| (*Hormel* Perma-Fresh), 2 slices | 80 |
| (*Hormel* Rosa/Rosa Grande), 1 oz. | 140 |
| **Pepperoni bits:** | |
| (*Hormel*), 1 tbsp. | 35 |
| **Perch,** meat only: | |
| fresh, raw, 4 oz. | 104 |
| fresh, baked, broiled, or microwaved, 4 oz. | 133 |
| frozen (*Booth*), 4 oz. | 100 |

| FOOD AND MEASURE | CALORIES |
|---|---|
| **Perch, ocean,** see "Ocean perch" | |
| **Perch entree,** frozen: | |
| battered (*Van de Kamp's*), 2 pieces | 310 |
| **Persimmon:** | |
| Japanese, fresh, 1 medium, 2½" × 3½" | 118 |
| Japanese, fresh, trimmed, 1 oz. | 20 |
| Japanese, dried, 1 oz. | 78 |
| native, fresh, 1 medium, 1.1 oz. | 32 |
| native, fresh, trimmed, 1 oz. | 36 |
| **Pesto sauce:** | |
| mix (*French's Pasta Toss*), 2 tsp. dry | 20 |
| refrigerated (*Contadina Fresh*), 2⅓ oz. | 350 |
| **Pheasant,** fresh, raw: | |
| meat w/skin, 4 oz. | 205 |
| meat only, 4 oz. | 151 |
| **Picante sauce** (see also "Salsa"): | |
| (*Estee*), 2 tbsp. | 8 |
| (*Gebhardt*), 1 tbsp. | 4 |
| (*Pace*), 2 tsp. | 3 |
| (*Wise*), 2 tbsp. | 12 |
| all styles (*Old El Paso*), 2 tbsp. | 8 |
| all styles, chunky (*Old El Paso*), 2 tbsp. | 7 |
| mild (*Azteca*), 1 tbsp. | 4 |
| mild (*Rosarita* Chunky), 3.5 oz. | 45 |
| **Pickle loaf:** | |
| (*Eckrich/Eckrich Smorgas Pac*), 1-oz. slice | 80 |
| (*Hormel* Perma-Fresh), 2 slices | 102 |
| (*Kahn's*), 1 slice | 80 |
| (*Kahn's* Family Pack), 1 slice | 70 |
| (*Light & Lean*), 2 slices | 100 |
| beef (*Kahn's* Family Pack), 1 slice | 60 |
| **Pickle relish,** see "Relish" | |
| **Pickle and pimiento loaf:** | |
| (*Oscar Mayer*), 1-oz. slice | 66 |

| FOOD AND MEASURE | CALORIES |
|---|---|
| **Pickles,** 1 oz., except as noted: | |
| bread and butter: | |
| (*Vlasic* Old Fashioned Chunks/Sweet Butter Chips) | 25 |
| slices (*Claussen* Bread 'n Butter) | 20 |
| slices (*Heinz* Cucumber Slices) | 25 |
| slices (*Mrs. Fanning's*), 2 slices or ⅔ oz. | 16 |
| sweet (*Vlasic* Sweet Butter Stix) | 18 |
| dill: | |
| all varieties, except hamburger chips (*Vlasic*) | 4 |
| whole (*Featherweight*), 1 pickle | 4 |
| whole (*Heinz* Genuine) | 2 |
| halves (*Heinz* Genuine) | 4 |
| spears (*Claussen*) | 4 |
| hamburger chips, half salt (*Vlasic*) | 2 |
| hamburger slices (*Heinz*) | 2 |
| kosher, all varieties (*Heinz*) | 4 |
| no garlic (*Claussen*) | 6 |
| Polish style, whole or spears (*Heinz*) | 4 |
| kosher, all varieties (*Heinz* Old Fashioned) | 4 |
| kosher, whole or slices (*Claussen*) | 3 |
| kosher, halves (*Claussen*) | 4 |
| mixed, garden, hot and spicy (*Vlasic*) | 4 |
| salad cubes, sweet (*Heinz*) | 30 |
| sour | 3 |
| sweet: | |
| (*Heinz* Cucumber Stix/Slices) | 25 |
| gherkins, regular or midget (*Heinz*) | 35 |
| half salt (*Vlasic* Sweet Butter Chips) | 30 |
| mixed (*Heinz*) | 40 |
| sliced (*Featherweight*), 3–4 slices | 24 |
| **Pickling spice:** | |
| (*Tone's*), 1 tsp. | 10 |
| **Picnic loaf:** | |
| (*Oscar Mayer*), 1-oz. slice | 61 |
| **Pie,** frozen: | |
| apple: | |
| (*Banquet* Family Size), ⅙ pie | 250 |
| (*Mrs. Smith's "Pie In Minutes"*), ⅛ pie | 210 |

| FOOD AND MEASURE | CALORIES |
|---|---|
| *Pie, frozen, apple, continued* | |
| (*Pet-Ritz*), 1/6 pie | 330 |
| (*Weight Watchers*), 1/2 pkg. | 200 |
| streusel (*Sara Lee Free & Light*), 1/8 pie | 170 |
| banana cream (*Banquet*), 1/6 pie | 180 |
| banana cream (*Pet-Ritz*), 1/6 pie | 170 |
| blackberry or blueberry (*Banquet* Family Size), 1/6 pie | 270 |
| blueberry (*Mrs. Smith's "Pie In Minutes"*), 1/8 pie | 220 |
| blueberry (*Pet-Ritz*), 1/6 pie | 370 |
| Boston cream, see "Cake, frozen" | |
| cherry (*Banquet* Family Size), 1/6 pie | 250 |
| cherry (*Mrs. Smith's "Pie In Minutes"*), 1/8 pie | 220 |
| cherry (*Pet-Ritz*), 1/6 pie | 300 |
| cherry streusel (*Sara Lee Free & Light*), 1/10 pie | 160 |
| chocolate cream or coconut cream (*Banquet*), 1/6 pie | 190 |
| chocolate cream or coconut cream (*Pet-Ritz*), 1/6 pie | 190 |
| egg custard (*Pet-Ritz*), 1/6 pie | 200 |
| lemon cream (*Banquet*), 1/6 pie | 170 |
| lemon cream (*Pet-Ritz*), 1/6 pie | 190 |
| lemon meringue (*Mrs. Smith's*), 1/8 pie | 210 |
| mince (*Pet-Ritz*), 1/6 pie | 280 |
| mincemeat (*Banquet* Family Size), 1/6 pie | 260 |
| Neapolitan cream (*Pet-Ritz*), 1/6 pie | 180 |
| peach (*Banquet* Family Size), 1/6 pie | 245 |
| peach (*Mrs. Smith's "Pie In Minutes"*), 1/8 pie | 210 |
| peach (*Pet-Ritz*), 1/6 pie | 320 |
| pecan (*Mrs. Smith's "Pie In Minutes"*), 1/8 pie | 330 |
| pumpkin (*Banquet* Family Size), 1/6 pie | 200 |
| pumpkin (*Mrs. Smith's "Pie In Minutes"*), 1/8 pie | 190 |
| pumpkin custard (*Pet-Ritz*), 1/6 pie | 250 |
| raspberry (*Sara Lee* Homestyle), 1/10 pie | 280 |
| strawberry cream (*Banquet*), 1/6 pie | 170 |
| strawberry cream (*Pet-Ritz*), 1/6 pie | 170 |
| sweet potato (*Pet-Ritz*), 1/6 pie | 150 |
| **Pie, snack,** 1 piece: | |
| apple: | |
| (*Hostess*) | 430 |
| (*Tastykake*), 4 oz. | 296 |
| Dutch (*Little Debbie*), 2.5 oz. | 270 |

| FOOD AND MEASURE | CALORIES |
|---|---|
| French (*Hostess*) | 430 |
| French (*Tastykake*), 4.2 oz. | 353 |
| apple, blueberry-apple, or lemon (*Drake's*) | 210 |
| banana creme (*Tastykake*), 4.2 oz. | 382 |
| blackberry or blueberry (*Hostess*) | 420 |
| blueberry (*Tastykake*), 4 oz. | 308 |
| cherry (*Hostess*) | 460 |
| cherry (*Tastykake*), 4 oz. | 298 |
| cherry-apple (*Drake's*), approx. 2 oz. | 220 |
| coconut cream (*Tastykake*), 4 oz. | 377 |
| lemon (*Hostess*) | 440 |
| lemon (*Tastykake*), 4 oz. | 319 |
| lemon-lime (*Tastykake*), 4 oz. | 310 |
| marshmallow, banana or chocolate (*Little Debbie*), 1.4 oz. | 170 |
| oatmeal creme (*Little Debbie*), 2.75 oz. | 350 |
| peach (*Hostess*) | 420 |
| peach (*Tastykake*), 4 oz. | 295 |
| pecan (*Little Debbie*), 3 oz. | 280 |
| pineapple cheese (*Tastykake*), 4.2 oz. | 343 |
| pumpkin (*Tastykake*), 4 oz. | 324 |
| raisin creme (*Little Debbie*), 2.5 oz. | 290 |
| strawberry (*Hostess*) | 410 |
| strawberry (*Tastykake*), 3.7 oz. | 342 |
| (*Tastykake* Tasty Klair), 4 oz. | 402 |

**Pie, snack,** frozen, 1 piece:

| | |
|---|---|
| Boston cream, see "Cake, snack, frozen" | |
| Mississippi mud (*Pepperidge Farm*), 2¼ oz. | 310 |

**Pie crust mix:**

| | |
|---|---|
| (*Betty Crocker*), 1⁄16 pkg. | 120 |
| (*Flako*), prepared, 1 serving | 247 |

**Pie crust shell,** frozen or refrigerated:

| | |
|---|---|
| (*Mrs. Smith's*, 8"), ⅛ shell | 80 |
| (*Mrs. Smith's*, 9"), ⅛ shell | 90 |
| (*Mrs. Smith's*, 9⅝"), ⅛ shell | 120 |
| (*Pet-Ritz*), ⅙ shell | 110 |
| (*Pet-Ritz*, 9⅝"), ⅙ shell | 170 |
| (*Pillsbury* All Ready), ⅛ of 2 crust pie | 240 |
| deep dish (*Pet-Ritz*), ⅙ shell | 130 |

| FOOD AND MEASURE | CALORIES |
|---|---|
| *Pie crust shell, continued* | |
| graham cracker or vegetable shortening (*Pet-Ritz*), 1/6 shell | 110 |
| vegetable shortening, deep dish (*Pet-Ritz*), 1/6 shell | 140 |

## Pie crust stick:

| | |
|---|---|
| (*Betty Crocker*), 1/8 stick | 120 |

## Pie filling, canned:

| | |
|---|---|
| apple: | |
| (*Comstock*), 3.5 oz. | 120 |
| (*Comstock* Lite), 3.5 oz. | 80 |
| (*Lucky Leaf/Musselman's*), 4 oz. | 120 |
| (*Lucky Leaf/Musselman's* Plus), 4 oz. | 121 |
| (*White House*), 3.5 oz. | 121 |
| deluxe or diced (*Lucky Leaf/Musselman's*), 4 oz. | 120 |
| apricot (*Comstock*), 3.5 oz. | 110 |
| apricot (*Lucky Leaf/Musselman's*), 4 oz. | 150 |
| banana (*Comstock*), 3.5 oz. | 110 |
| blackberry (*Lucky Leaf/Musselman's*), 4 oz. | 120 |
| blackberry (*Lucky Leaf/Musselman's* Plus), 4 oz. | 121 |
| blueberry: | |
| (*Comstock*), 3.5 oz. | 110 |
| (*Comstock* Lite), 3.5 oz. | 75 |
| (*Lucky Leaf/Musselman's* Plus), 4 oz. | 145 |
| (*White House*), 3.5 oz. | 118 |
| cultivated (*Lucky Leaf/Musselman's*), 4 oz. | 120 |
| boysenberry (*Lucky Leaf/Musselman's*), 4 oz. | 120 |
| cherry: | |
| (*Comstock*), 3.5 oz. | 110 |
| (*Comstock* Lite), 3.5 oz. | 75 |
| (*Lucky Leaf/Musselman's*), 4 oz. | 120 |
| (*Lucky Leaf/Musselman's* Plus), 4 oz. | 108 |
| (*White House*), 3.5 oz. | 141 |
| chocolate (*Comstock*), 3.5 oz. | 130 |
| coconut (*Comstock*), 3.5 oz. | 120 |
| gooseberry (*Lucky Leaf/Musselman's*), 4 oz. | 180 |
| lemon (*Comstock*), 3.5 oz. | 140 |
| lemon (*Lucky Leaf/Musselman's*), 4 oz. | 200 |
| lemon, French (*Lucky Leaf/Musselman's*), 4 oz. | 180 |
| mincemeat: | |
| (*Borden None Such*), 1/3 cup | 200 |

| FOOD AND MEASURE | CALORIES |
|---|---|
| (*Comstock*), 3.5 oz. | 150 |
| (*Lucky Leaf/Musselman's*), 4 oz. | 190 |
| w/brandy (*S&W* Old Fashioned), 4 oz. | 234 |
| w/brandy and rum (*Borden None Such*), ⅓ cup | 220 |
| condensed (*Borden None Such*), ¼ pkg. | 220 |
| peach (*Comstock*), 3.5 oz. | 110 |
| peach (*Lucky Leaf/Musselman's*), 4 oz. | 150 |
| peach (*Lucky Leaf/Musselman's* Plus), 4 oz. | 113 |
| peach (*White House*), 3.5 oz. | 117 |
| pineapple (*Comstock*), 3.5 oz. | 100 |
| pineapple (*Lucky Leaf/Musselman's*), 4 oz. | 110 |
| pumpkin (*Comstock*), 3.5 oz. | 100 |
| pumpkin (*Lucky Leaf/Musselman's*), 4 oz. | 170 |
| pumpkin (*Stokely*), ½ cup | 170 |
| pumpkin pie mix (*Libby's*), 1 cup | 260 |
| raisin (*Comstock*), 3.5 oz. | 120 |
| raisin (*Lucky Leaf/Musselman's*), 4 oz. | 130 |
| raspberry, black or red (*Lucky Leaf/Musselman's*), 4 oz. | 190 |
| strawberry (*Comstock*), 3.5 oz. | 100 |
| strawberry (*Lucky Leaf/Musselman's*), 4 oz. | 120 |
| strawberry (*Lucky Leaf/Musselman's* Plus), 4 oz. | 138 |
| strawberry-rhubarb (*Lucky Leaf/Musselman's*), 4 oz. | 120 |
| vanilla creme (*Lucky Leaf/Musselman's*), 4 oz. | 150 |

**Pie filling mix,** see "Pudding mix"

**Pie mix,** prepared:

| | |
|---|---|
| banana cream (*Jell-O* No Bake), ⅛ pie | 240 |
| cheesecake, see "Cake mix" | |
| chocolate mint (*Royal No-Bake*), ⅛ pie | 260 |
| chocolate mousse (*Jell-O* No Bake), ⅛ pie | 260 |
| chocolate mousse (*Royal No-Bake*), ⅛ pie | 230 |
| coconut cream (*Jell-O* No Bake), ⅛ pie | 260 |
| lemon meringue (*Royal No-Bake*), ⅛ pie | 310 |
| pumpkin (*Jell-O* No Bake), ⅛ pie | 250 |
| pumpkin (*Libby's*), ⅙ pie | 390 |

**Pigeon peas:**

| | |
|---|---|
| fresh, raw, shelled, ½ cup | 105 |
| fresh, boiled, drained, ½ cup | 86 |
| dried, raw, ½ cup | 350 |
| dried, boiled, ½ cup | 102 |

| FOOD AND MEASURE | CALORIES |
|---|---|
| **Pignolias,** see "Pine nuts" | |
| **Pig's ear,** frozen: | |
| simmered, 4 oz. | 188 |
| **Pig's feet:** | |
| simmered, 4 oz. | 220 |
| pickled (*Penrose*), 6-oz. piece | 220 |
| pickled, cured, 1 oz. | 58 |
| **Pig's knuckles,** pickled: | |
| (*Penrose*), 6-oz. piece | 290 |
| **Pike,** meat only: | |
| northern, raw, 4 oz. | 100 |
| northern, baked, broiled, or microwaved, 4 oz. | 128 |
| walleye, raw, 4 oz. | 105 |
| **Pili nut,** dried: | |
| shelled, 1 oz. or 15 kernels | 204 |
| shelled, 1 cup | 863 |
| **Pimiento,** canned or in jars: | |
| 2 oz. | 13 |
| 1 tbsp. | 3 |
| all varieties, drained (*Dromedary*), 1 oz. | 10 |
| **Pimiento spread:** | |
| (*Price's*), 1 oz. | 80 |
| **Piña colada mix:** | |
| bottled (*Holland House*), 1 fl. oz. | 33 |
| instant (*Holland House*), .56 oz. | 82 |
| **Pine nuts,** dried: | |
| pignolia, shelled, 1 oz. | 146 |
| pignolia, shelled, 1 tbsp. | 51 |
| piñon, shelled, 1 oz. | 161 |
| piñon, 10 kernels | 6 |
| **Pineapple:** | |
| fresh, untrimmed, 1 lb. | 117 |
| fresh, sliced, 1 slice, 3½" diam. × ¾" | 42 |

| FOOD AND MEASURE | CALORIES |
|---|---|
| fresh, diced, ½ cup | 39 |
| canned, ½ cup, except as noted: | |
| (*Mott's* Pineapple Fruit Pak), 3.75 oz. | 86 |
| in water, tidbits | 40 |
| in juice, all cuts (*Dole*) | 70 |
| in juice, slices (*Featherweight*) | 70 |
| in juice, slices (*S&W* 100% Hawaiian) | 70 |
| in juice, all cuts, except spears (*Del Monte*) | 70 |
| in juice, spears (*Del Monte*), 2 spears | 50 |
| in juice, crushed (*Empress*) | 70 |
| in syrup, all cuts (*Del Monte*) | 90 |
| in syrup, all cuts (*Dole*) | 95 |
| in light syrup | 66 |
| in heavy syrup, slices (*S&W* 100% Hawaiian), 2 slices | 90 |
| in extra heavy syrup, chunks or crushed | 109 |
| unsweetened, sliced (*S&W/Nutradiet*) | 60 |
| frozen, sweetened, chunks | 104 |

**Pineapple danish:**

| | |
|---|---|
| miniature (*Awrey's*), 1.7 oz. | 157 |

**Pineapple juice,** 6 fl. oz., except as noted:

| | |
|---|---|
| canned, bottled, or boxed: | |
| (*Del Monte* Unsweetened) | 100 |
| (*Dole*) | 103 |
| (*Minute Maid*), 8.45 fl. oz. | 139 |
| (*Minute Maid On The Go*), 10 fl. oz. | 165 |
| (*Mott's*), 9.5-fl.-oz. can | 169 |
| (*S&W* Unsweetened) | 100 |
| (*Veryfine* 100%), 8 fl. oz. | 125 |
| chilled or frozen, diluted (*Dole*) | 100 |
| chilled or frozen, diluted (*Minute Maid*) | 99 |

**Pineapple nectar:**

| | |
|---|---|
| (*Libby's*), 6 fl. oz. | 110 |

**Pineapple-banana juice cocktail:**

| | |
|---|---|
| (*Welch's Orchard Tropicals*), 6 fl. oz. | 100 |
| (*Welch's Orchard Tropicals* Cocktails-In-A-Box), 8.45 fl. oz. | 140 |

| FOOD AND MEASURE | CALORIES |
|---|---|

**Pineapple-grapefruit juice:**

(*Dole*), 6 fl. oz. .......... 90
(*Tropicana* 100% Pure), 8 fl. oz. .......... 120
w/pink grapefruit (*Dole*), 6 fl. oz. .......... 101

**Pineapple-grapefruit juice cocktail:**

(*Ocean Spray*), 6 fl. oz. .......... 110

**Pineapple-grapefruit juice drink:**

(*Tropicana* Twister), 8 fl. oz. .......... 125
regular or pink grapefruit (*Del Monte*), 6 fl. oz. .......... 90

**Pineapple-orange drink:**

(*Veryfine*), 8 fl. oz. .......... 130

**Pineapple-orange juice:**

(*Dole*), 6 fl. oz. .......... 100
chilled or frozen, diluted (*Minute Maid*), 6 fl. oz. .......... 98

**Pineapple-orange juice drink:**

(*Del Monte*), 6 fl. oz. .......... 90

**Pineapple-orange-banana juice:**

(*Dole*), 6 fl. oz. .......... 90

**Piñon,** see "Pine nuts"

**Pinto bean,** see "Beans, pinto"

**Pistachio nuts:**

dried, in shell, 4 oz. .......... 327
dried, shelled, 1 oz. or 47 kernels .......... 164
dry-roasted, in shell, 4 oz. .......... 357
dry-roasted (*Planters*), 1 oz. .......... 170
roasted (*Dole*), 1 oz. .......... 163

**Pitanga:**

1 medium .......... 2
trimmed, ½ cup .......... 29

**Pizza,** frozen:

Canadian bacon (*Jeno's* Crisp'n Tasty), ½ pie .......... 250
Canadian bacon (*Tombstone*), ¼ pie .......... 340

| FOOD AND MEASURE | CALORIES |
|---|---|
| Canadian bacon (*Totino's Party*), ½ pie | 290 |
| (*Celentano* 9-Slice Pizza), 2.7 oz. | 150 |
| (*Celentano* Thick Crust), 4.3 oz. | 290 |
| (*Celeste* Suprema), ¼ pie | 381 |
| (*Celeste* Supreme Pizza For One), 1 pie | 678 |
| cheese: | |
| (*Celeste*), ¼ pie | 317 |
| (*Celeste* Pizza For One), 1 pie | 497 |
| (*Jeno's* Crisp'n Tasty), ½ pie | 270 |
| (*Jeno's* 4-Pack), 1 pie | 160 |
| (*Pillsbury* Microwave), ½ pie | 240 |
| (*Stouffer's*), ½ of 8.5-oz. pkg. | 320 |
| (*Stouffer's* Extra Cheese), ½ of 9.25-oz. pkg. | 370 |
| (*Tombstone*), ¼ pie | 330 |
| (*Totino's* Microwave), 1 pie | 250 |
| (*Totino's Party*), ½ pie | 280 |
| (*Totino's Party* Family Size), ⅓ pie | 310 |
| (*Weight Watchers*), 5.86-oz. pkg. | 300 |
| snack tray (*Jeno's* Snacks), 4 pies or ⅓ pkg. | 130 |
| three cheese (*Tombstone* Double Top), ¼ pie | 490 |
| three cheese (*Tombstone* Microwave), 7.7-oz. pkg. | 520 |
| two cheese (*Tombstone* Thin Crust), ¼ pie | 330 |
| cheese combination: | |
| and hamburger (*Tombstone*), ¼ pie | 360 |
| and hamburger (*Tombstone* Italian Thin Crust), ¼ pie | 320 |
| and pepperoni (*Tombstone*), ¼ pie | 380 |
| and pepperoni (*Tombstone* Microwave), 7.5-oz. pkg. | 530 |
| and pepperoni (*Tombstone* Thin Crust), ¼ pie | 330 |
| and sausage (*Tombstone*), ¼ pie | 350 |
| and sausage, Italian (*Tombstone* Thin Crust), ¼ pie | 330 |
| sausage and mushroom (*Tombstone*), ¼ pie | 360 |
| combination: | |
| (*Jeno's* 4-Pack), 1 pie | 180 |
| (*Pillsbury* Microwave), ½ pie | 310 |
| (*Totino's* Microwave), 1 pie | 290 |
| (*Totino's Party*), ½ pie | 340 |
| (*Totino's Party* Family Size), ⅓ pie | 290 |
| (*Weight Watchers* Deluxe), 7.15-oz. pkg. | 330 |
| deluxe (*Celeste*), ¼ pie | 378 |
| deluxe (*Celeste* Pizza For One), 1 pie | 582 |
| deluxe (*Stouffer's*), ½ of 10-oz. pkg. | 370 |

| FOOD AND MEASURE | CALORIES |
|---|---|
| *Pizza, continued* | |
| hamburger (*Jeno's* Crisp'n Tasty), ½ pie | 290 |
| hamburger (*Jeno's* 4-Pack), 1 pie | 180 |
| hamburger (*Totino's Party*), ½ pie | 320 |
| pepperoni: | |
| (*Celeste*), ¼ pie | 368 |
| (*Celeste* Pizza For One), 1 pie | 546 |
| (*Jeno's* Crisp'n Tasty), ½ pie | 280 |
| (*Jeno's* 4-Pack), 1 pie | 170 |
| (*Pillsbury* Microwave), ½ pie | 300 |
| (*Stouffer's*), ½ of 8.75-oz. pkg. | 350 |
| (*Tombstone* Real Deluxe), ¼ pie | 380 |
| (*Totino's* Microwave), 1 pie | 270 |
| (*Totino's Party*), ½ pie | 330 |
| (*Totino's Party* Family Size), ⅓ pie | 360 |
| (*Weight Watchers*), 6.09-oz. pkg. | 320 |
| double cheese (*Tombstone* Double Top), ¼ pie | 560 |
| double cheese (*Tombstone* Double Top Deluxe), ¼ pie | 550 |
| snack tray (*Jeno's* Snacks), 4 pies or ⅓ pkg. | 140 |
| sausage: | |
| (*Celeste*), ¼ pie | 376 |
| (*Celeste* Pizza For One), 1 pie | 571 |
| (*Jeno's* Crisp'n Tasty), ½ pie | 300 |
| (*Jeno's* 4-Pack), 1 pie | 180 |
| (*Pillsbury* Microwave), ½ pie | 280 |
| (*Stouffer's*), ½ of 9⅜-oz. pkg. | 360 |
| (*Tombstone* Deluxe), ¼ pie | 350 |
| (*Tombstone* Deluxe Microwave), 8.7-oz. pkg. | 520 |
| (*Totino's* Microwave), 1 pie | 280 |
| (*Totino's Party*), ½ pie | 340 |
| (*Totino's Party* Family Size), ⅓ pie | 370 |
| (*Weight Watchers*), 6.26-oz. pkg. | 320 |
| Italian (*Tombstone* Microwave), 8-oz. pkg. | 550 |
| smoked, w/pepperoni seasoning (*Tombstone*), ¼ pie | 350 |
| snack tray (*Jeno's* Snacks), 4 pies or ⅓ pkg. | 140 |
| sausage combination: | |
| (*Tombstone*), ¼ pie | 370 |
| and mushroom (*Celeste* Pizza For One), 1 pie | 592 |
| and pepperoni (*Jeno's* Crisp'n Tasty), ½ pie | 300 |
| and pepperoni (*Stouffer's*), ½ of 9⅜-oz. pkg. | 380 |

| FOOD AND MEASURE | CALORIES |
|---|---|
| and pepperoni (*Tombstone* Double Top), ¼ pie | 540 |
| and pepperoni (*Tombstone* Microwave), 8-oz. pkg. | 560 |
| (*Tombstone* Thin Crust Supreme), ¼ pie | 340 |
| vegetable (*Celeste*), ¼ pie | 310 |
| vegetable (*Celeste* Pizza For One), 1 pie | 490 |

**Pizza, croissant pastry,** frozen, 1 pie:

| FOOD AND MEASURE | CALORIES |
|---|---|
| cheese (*Pepperidge Farm*) | 430 |
| deluxe (*Pepperidge Farm*) | 440 |
| pepperoni (*Pepperidge Farm*) | 420 |

**Pizza, French bread,** frozen:

| FOOD AND MEASURE | CALORIES |
|---|---|
| Canadian style bacon (*Stouffer's*), ½ pkg. | 360 |
| cheese: | |
| (*Banquet Zap*), 4.5 oz. | 310 |
| (*Lean Cuisine*), 5⅛-oz. pkg. | 310 |
| (*Lean Cuisine* Extra Cheese), 5.5-oz. pkg. | 350 |
| (*Pillsbury* Microwave), 1 piece | 370 |
| (*Stouffer's*), ½ pkg. | 340 |
| (*Stouffer's* Double Cheese), ½ pkg. | 410 |
| deluxe (*Banquet Zap*), 4.8 oz. | 330 |
| deluxe (*Lean Cuisine*), 6⅛-oz. pkg. | 350 |
| deluxe (*Stouffer's*), ½ pkg. | 430 |
| deluxe (*Weight Watchers*), 6.12-oz. pkg. | 330 |
| hamburger (*Stouffer's*), ½ pkg. | 410 |
| pepperoni: | |
| (*Banquet Zap*), 4.5 oz. | 350 |
| (*Lean Cuisine*), 5.25-oz. pkg. | 340 |
| (*Pillsbury* Microwave), 1 piece | 430 |
| (*Stouffer's*), ½ pkg. | 410 |
| (*Weight Watchers*), 5.25-oz. pkg. | 320 |
| pepperoni and mushroom (*Stouffer's*), ½ pkg. | 430 |
| sausage (*Lean Cuisine*), 6-oz. pkg. | 350 |
| sausage (*Pillsbury* Microwave), 1 piece | 410 |
| sausage (*Stouffer's*), ½ pkg. | 420 |
| sausage and mushroom (*Stouffer's*), ½ pkg. | 410 |
| sausage and pepperoni (*Pillsbury* Microwave), 1 piece | 450 |
| sausage and pepperoni (*Stouffer's*), ½ pkg. | 450 |
| vegetable deluxe (*Stouffer's*), ½ pkg. | 420 |

| FOOD AND MEASURE | CALORIES |
|---|---|
| **Pizza crust:** | |
| (*Pillsbury* All Ready), 1/8 of crust | 90 |
| mix (*Chef Boyardee* Q & Easy), 1/6 pkg. | 150 |
| mix (*Robin Hood/Gold Medal* Pouch Mix), 1/6 pkg. | 110 |
| ***Pizza Hut:*** | |
| hand-tossed, 2 slices of medium pie: | |
| cheese, 7.8 oz. | 518 |
| pepperoni, 6.9 oz. | 500 |
| supreme, 8.4 oz. | 540 |
| super supreme, 8.6 oz. | 463 |
| pan pizza, 2 slices of medium pie: | |
| cheese, 7.2 oz. | 492 |
| pepperoni, 7.4 oz. | 540 |
| supreme, 9 oz. | 589 |
| super supreme, 9.1 oz. | 563 |
| *Personal Pan Pizza,* 1 whole pie: | |
| pepperoni, 9 oz. | 675 |
| supreme, 9.3 oz. | 647 |
| *Thin 'n Crispy,* 2 slices of medium pie: | |
| cheese, 5.2 oz. | 398 |
| pepperoni, 5.1 oz. | 413 |
| supreme, 7.1 oz. | 459 |
| super supreme, 7.2 oz. | 463 |
| **Pizza pocket sandwich,** frozen: | |
| (*Lean Pockets* Pizza Deluze), 1 pkg. | 280 |
| pepperoni (*Hot Pockets*), 5 oz. | 380 |
| sausage (*Hot Pockets*), 5 oz. | 360 |
| **Pizza roll,** frozen, 3 oz. or 6 rolls: | |
| cheese or hamburger (*Jeno's*) | 240 |
| pepperoni and cheese (*Jeno's*) | 230 |
| pepperoni and cheese (*Jeno's* Microwave) | 240 |
| sausage and cheese (*Jeno's* Microwave) | 250 |
| sausage and pepperoni (*Jeno's*) | 230 |
| **Pizza sauce:** | |
| (*Contadina* Pizza Squeeze), 1/4 cup | 30 |
| (*Contadina* Quick & Easy Original), 1/4 cup | 30 |
| (*Enrico's* Homemade Style), 4 oz. | 60 |

| FOOD AND MEASURE | CALORIES |
|---|---|
| (*Pastorelli Italian-Chef*), 4 oz. | 90 |
| (*Ragu Pizza Quick* Traditional), 3 tbsp. | 35 |
| w/cheese (*Chef Boyardee*), 2.63 oz. | 70 |
| w/cheese (*Chef Boyardee,* Jars), 3.88 oz. | 90 |
| garlic basil (*Ragu Pizza Quick*), 3 tbsp. | 40 |
| w/Italian cheese (*Contadina*), ¼ cup | 30 |
| w/pepperoni (*Contadina*), ¼ cup | 40 |

**Plantain:**

| | |
|---|---|
| raw, 1 medium, 9.7 oz. | 218 |
| raw, sliced, ½ cup | 91 |
| cooked, sliced, ½ cup | 89 |

**Plum:**

| | |
|---|---|
| fresh, whole, 1 lb. | 235 |
| fresh, pitted, sliced, ½ cup | 46 |
| fresh, Japanese or hybrid, 1 medium, 2⅛" diam. | 36 |
| canned: | |
| halves or whole, unpeeled (*S&W/Nutradiet*), ½ cup | 52 |
| purple, in water, ½ cup | 51 |
| purple, in water, 3 plums and 2 tbsp. liquid | 39 |
| purple, in juice, ½ cup | 73 |
| purple, in juice, 3 plums and 2 tbsp. liquid | 55 |
| purple, in juice, whole (*Featherweight*), ½ cup | 80 |
| purple, in light syrup, ½ cup | 79 |
| purple, in light syrup, 3 plums and 2¾ tbsp. liquid | 83 |
| purple, in light syrup (*Stokely*), ½ cup | 100 |
| purple, in heavy syrup, ½ cup | 115 |
| purple, in heavy syrup, 3 plums and 2¾ tbsp. liquid | 119 |
| purple, in heavy syrup (*Stokely*), ½ cup | 130 |
| purple, in extra heavy syrup (*S&W* Fancy), ½ cup | 135 |

**Plum sauce:**

| | |
|---|---|
| tangy (*La Choy*), 1 oz. | 45 |

**Poi:**

| | |
|---|---|
| ½ cup | 134 |

**Pokeberry shoots:**

| | |
|---|---|
| raw, trimmed, ½ cup | 18 |
| boiled, drained, ½ cup | 16 |

| FOOD AND MEASURE | CALORIES |
|---|---|
| **Polenta mix,** prepared: | |
| (*Fantastic Polenta*), ½ cup | 106 |
| **Polish sausage** (*see also* "Kielbasa"): | |
| (*Hillshire Farm* Links), 2 oz. | 190 |
| (*Hormel),* 2 links | 170 |
| (*Pilgrim's Pride*), 3 oz. | 131 |
| smoked (*Eckrich Lite* Sausage Links), 1 link | 180 |
| **Pollock,** meat only: | |
| Atlantic, raw, 4 oz. | 104 |
| Walleye, raw, 4 oz. | 91 |
| Walleye, baked, broiled, or microwaved, 4 oz. | 128 |
| **Pomegranate:** | |
| 1 medium, 3⅜" × 3¾", 9.7 oz. | 104 |
| **Pompano,** Florida, meat only: | |
| raw, 4 oz. | 185 |
| baked, broiled, or microwaved, 4 oz. | 239 |
| ***Ponderosa:*** | |
| entrees: | |
| chicken breast, 5.5 oz. | 98 |
| chicken wings, 2 pieces | 213 |
| fish, bake 'r broil, 5.2 oz. | 230 |
| fish, fried, 3.2 oz. | 190 |
| fish nuggets, 1 piece | 31 |
| halibut, broiled, 6 oz. | 170 |
| hot dog, 1.6 oz. | 144 |
| Kansas City Strip steak, 5 oz. precooked | 138 |
| New York Strip steak, choice, 8 oz. precooked | 314 |
| New York Strip steak, choice, 10 oz. precooked | 384 |
| porterhouse steak, choice, 16 oz. precooked | 640 |
| rib-eye steak, choice, 6 oz. precooked | 282 |
| rib-eye steak, nongraded, 5 oz. precooked | 219 |
| roughy, broiled, 5 oz. | 138 |
| salmon, broiled, 6 oz. | 192 |
| scrod, baked, 7 oz. | 120 |
| swordfish, broiled, 5.9 oz. | 271 |
| trout, broiled, 5 oz. | 228 |

| FOOD AND MEASURE | CALORIES |
| --- | --- |
| shrimp, fried, 7 pieces | 231 |
| shrimp, mini, 6 pieces | 47 |
| sirloin steak, choice, 7 oz. precooked | 241 |
| sirloin tips, choice, 5 oz. precooked | 473 |
| steak, chopped, 4 oz. precooked | 225 |
| steak, chopped, 5.3 oz. precooked | 296 |
| steak kabobs, meat only, 3 oz. precooked | 153 |
| steak sandwich, 4 oz. | 408 |
| steak teriyaki, 5 oz. precooked | 174 |
| T-bone steak, choice, 10 oz. precooked | 444 |
| T-bone steak, nongraded, 8 oz. precooked | 178 |
| side dishes, sauces, and condiments: | |
| BBQ sauce, 1 tbsp. | 25 |
| beans, baked, 4 oz. | 170 |
| cauliflower, breaded, 4 oz. | 115 |
| cheese, herb, garlic spread, 1 tbsp. | 100 |
| cheese sauce, 2 oz. | 52 |
| gravy, brown or turkey, 2 oz. | 25 |
| macaroni and cheese, 1 oz. | 17 |
| okra, breaded, 4 oz. | 124 |
| onion rings, breaded, 4 oz. | 213 |
| potatoes, baked, 7.2 oz. | 145 |
| potatoes, french fried, 3 oz. | 120 |
| potatoes, mashed, 4 oz. | 62 |
| potato wedges, 3.5 oz. | 130 |
| rice pilaf, 4 oz. | 160 |
| rolls, dinner, 1 piece | 184 |
| rolls, sourdough, 1 piece | 110 |
| shells, pasta, 2 oz. | 78 |
| spaghetti, 2 oz. | 78 |
| spaghetti sauce, 4 oz. | 110 |
| stuffing, 4 oz. | 230 |
| sweet/sour sauce, 1 oz. | 37 |
| zucchini, breaded, 4 oz. | 102 |
| desserts: | |
| banana pudding, 1 oz. | 52 |
| ice milk, chocolate, 3.5 oz. | 152 |
| ice milk, vanilla, 3.5 oz. | 150 |
| mousse, chocolate, 1 oz. | 78 |
| mousse, strawberry, 1 oz. | 74 |
| sprinkles, chocolate, .18 oz. | 24 |

| FOOD AND MEASURE | CALORIES |
|---|---|
| *Ponderosa, desserts, continued* | |
| sprinkles, rainbow, .18 oz. | 24 |
| strawberry glaze, 1 oz. | 37 |
| topping, caramel, 1 oz. | 100 |
| topping, chocolate, 1 oz. | 89 |
| topping, strawberry, 1 oz. | 71 |
| topping, whipped, 1 oz. | 80 |
| wafer, vanilla, 2 cookies | 35 |

**Popcorn,** popped, except as noted:

| | |
|---|---|
| (*Bachman*), ½ oz. | 80 |
| (*Bachman* Lite), ½ oz. | 50 |
| (*Bearitos* Organic Lite), 1 oz. | 132 |
| (*Bearitos* Organic No Salt), 1 oz. | 108 |
| (*Bearitos* Organic Traditional), 1 oz. | 140 |
| (*Frito-Lay's*), ½ oz. | 70 |
| (*Jiffy Pop* Pan Popcorn), 4 cups | 130 |
| (*Laura Scudder's* Tender Baby White Corn), ½ oz. | 80 |
| (*Orville Redenbacher* Natural), 3 cups | 80 |
| (*Orville Redenbacher* Natural Salt Free), 3 cups | 90 |
| (*Weight Watchers* Lightly Salted), .66-oz. pkg. | 80 |
| (*Wise* Tender Baby White Corn), ½ oz. | 80 |
| (*Wise* Tender Eating Baby Popcorn), ½ oz. | 70 |
| butter flavor (*Jiffy Pop* Pan Popcorn), 4 cups | 130 |
| butter flavor (*Orville Redenbacher*), 3 cups | 80 |
| butter flavor (*Wise*), ½ oz. | 80 |
| caramel-coated, see "Candy" | |
| cheese and cheese flavor: | |
| (*Bachman*), ½ oz. | 90 |
| (*Bearitos* Organic), 1 oz. | 137 |
| (*Frito-Lay's*), ½ oz. | 80 |
| cheddar (*Orville Redenbacher*), 3 cups | 160 |
| cheddar, white (*Bachman*), ½ oz. | 70 |
| cheddar, white (*Cape Cod*), ½ oz. | 80 |
| cheddar, white (*Clover Club*), ½ oz. | 70 |
| cheddar, white (*Keebler* Deluxe) | 140 |
| cheddar, white (*Laura Scudder's*), ½ oz. | 70 |
| cheddar, white (*Smartfood*), ½ oz. | 80 |
| cheddar, white (*Weight Watchers*), .66-oz. bag | 100 |
| cheddar, white (*Wise*), ½ oz. | 70 |

| FOOD AND MEASURE | CALORIES |
|---|---|
| microwave, 3 cups, except as noted: | |
| (*Featherweight* Natural Low Salt) | 80 |
| (*Weight Watchers*), 1 oz. or 1 pkg. | 100 |
| butter flavor (*Featherweight* Low Salt) | 100 |
| natural or butter flavor (*Jiffy Pop*), 4 cups | 140 |
| natural or butter flavor (*Jolly Time*) | 150 |
| natural or butter flavor (*Orville Redenbacher* Lite) | 50 |
| natural or butter flavor (*Pillsbury*) | 210 |
| natural or butter flavor (*Planters*) | 140 |
| natural or butter flavor (*Pop•Secret*) | 100 |
| natural or butter flavor (*Pop•Secret* Light) | 70 |
| natural or butter flavor (*Pop Weaver's*), 4 cups | 140 |
| natural or butter flavor (*Pops-Rite*) | 90 |
| cheddar cheese flavor (*Jolly Time*) | 180 |
| cheese flavor (*Pop•Secret*), ⅓ pkg. unpopped | 170 |
| frozen (*Pillsbury* Salt-Free) | 170 |
| white (*Jolly Time*), 4 cups | 75 |
| white or yellow, air-popped (*Pops-Rite*), 1 oz. kernels | 100 |
| white or yellow, oil-popped (*Pops-Rite*), 1 oz. kernels | 220 |
| yellow (*Jolly Time*), 4 cups | 88 |

**Popcorn seasoning:**

| | |
|---|---|
| (*McCormick/Schilling Parsley Patch*), 1 tsp. | 10 |

**Poppyseed:**

| | |
|---|---|
| 1 tsp. | 15 |

**Porgy,** see "Scup"

**Pork,** canned:

| | |
|---|---|
| (*Hormel*), 3 oz. | 240 |
| chopped (*Hormel*), 3 oz. | 200 |

**Pork, cured** (see also "Ham"):

| | |
|---|---|
| arm (picnic), roasted: | |
| lean and fat, 4 oz. | 318 |
| lean and fat, chopped or diced, 1 cup not packed | 392 |
| lean only, 4 oz. | 193 |
| lean only, chopped or diced, 1 cup not packed | 238 |
| blade roll, lean and fat, unheated, 1 oz. | 76 |
| blade roll, lean and fat, roasted, 4 oz. | 325 |

| FOOD AND MEASURE | CALORIES |
|---|---|
| **Pork,** fresh, boneless, 4 oz., except as noted: | |
| leg, see "Ham" | |
| loin (see also "top loin," below): | |
| blade, braised, separable lean and fat | 465 |
| blade, braised, lean only | 355 |
| blade, roasted, separable lean and fat | 413 |
| blade, roasted, lean only | 316 |
| center, braised, separable lean and fat | 401 |
| center, braised, lean only | 308 |
| center, roasted, separable lean and fat | 346 |
| center, roasted, lean only | 272 |
| center rib, braised, separable lean and fat | 416 |
| center rib, braised, lean only | 314 |
| center rib, roasted, separable lean and fat | 361 |
| center rib, roasted, lean only | 278 |
| sirloin, broiled, separable lean and fat | 375 |
| sirloin, broiled, lean only | 276 |
| sirloin, roasted, separable lean and fat | 330 |
| sirloin, roasted, lean only | 268 |
| shoulder: | |
| arm (picnic), braised, separable lean and fat | 391 |
| arm (picnic), braised, lean only | 281 |
| arm (picnic), roasted, separable lean and fat | 375 |
| arm (picnic), roasted, lean only | 259 |
| Boston blade, braised, separable lean and fat | 421 |
| Boston blade, braised, lean only | 333 |
| Boston blade, broiled, separable lean and fat | 397 |
| Boston blade, broiled, lean only | 311 |
| Boston blade, roasted, lean only | 290 |
| spareribs, braised, 6.3 oz. (1 lb. raw w/bone) | 703 |
| tenderloin, lean only, roasted | 188 |
| top loin, broiled, separable lean and fat | 408 |
| top loin, broiled, lean only | 293 |
| top loin, roasted, separable lean and fat | 374 |
| top loin, roasted, lean only | 278 |
| **Pork, variety meats,** see specific listings | |
| **Pork dinner,** frozen: | |
| loin of (*Swanson*), 10¾ oz. | 280 |

| FOOD AND MEASURE | CALORIES |
|---|---|
| **Pork entree,** canned: | |
| chow mein (*La Choy* Bi-Pack), ¾ cup | 80 |
| **Pork entree,** frozen or refrigerated: | |
| barbecued: | |
| back ribs (*John Morrell Pork Classics*), 4.75 oz. | 240 |
| chops, center cut (*John Morrell Pork Classics*), 4.5 oz. | 230 |
| loin, thin sliced (*John Morrell Pork Classics*), 5 slices or 3 oz. | 150 |
| spare ribs (*John Morrell Pork Classics*), 4.5 oz. | 250 |
| tenderloin (*John Morrell Pork Classics*), 3 oz. | 130 |
| steak, breaded (*Hormel*), 3 oz. | 220 |
| sweet and sour (*Chun King*), 13 oz. | 400 |
| **Pork gravy:** | |
| canned (*Franco-American*), 2 oz. | 40 |
| canned (*Heinz*), 2 oz. or ¼ cup | 25 |
| canned w/chunky pork (*Hormel Great Beginnings*), 5 oz. | 140 |
| mix, prepared (*French's*), ¼ cup | 20 |
| mix, prepared (*McCormick/Schilling*), ¼ cup | 20 |
| **Pork luncheon meat** (see also "Pork, canned"): | |
| (*Eckrich* Slender Sliced), 1 oz. | 45 |
| **Pork rind snack:** | |
| (*Baken-ets*), 1 oz. | 160 |
| **Pork seasoning and coating mix:** | |
| (*Shake'n Bake* Original Recipe/Barbecue), ⅛ pouch | 40 |
| extra crispy (*Shake'n Bake Oven Fry*), ¼ pouch | 120 |
| chop (*McCormick/Schilling* Bag'n Season), 1 pkg. | 103 |
| **Pork and beans,** see "Beans, baked" | |
| **Pot roast,** see "Beef dinner" and "Beef entree" | |
| **Pot roast seasoning mix:** | |
| (*Lawry's* Seasoning Blends), 1 pkg. | 122 |
| (*McCormick/Schilling* Bag'n Season), 1 pkg. | 55 |
| **Potato:** | |
| raw, unpeeled, 1 lb. | 269 |
| raw, peeled, diced, ½ cup | 59 |

| FOOD AND MEASURE | CALORIES |
|---|---|
| *Potato, continued* | |
| baked in skin, 1 medium, 4¾" × 2⅓" diam. | 220 |
| baked in skin, pulp only, ½ cup | 57 |
| baked in skin, skin only, 2 oz. | 112 |
| boiled in skin, pulp only, ½ cup | 68 |
| boiled w/out skin, 1 medium, 2½" diam. | 116 |
| boiled w/out skin, ½ cup | 67 |
| microwaved in skin, 1 medium, 4¾" × 2⅓" diam. | 212 |
| microwaved in skin, pulp only, ½ cup | 78 |
| microwaved in skin, skin only, 2 oz. | 75 |

**Potato,** canned (see also "Potato dishes, canned"):

| | |
|---|---|
| (*Stokely*), ½ cup | 50 |
| whole, new, extra small (*S&W*), ½ cup | 45 |
| whole or sliced, w/liquid (*Del Monte*), ½ cup | 45 |
| sliced, diced or double diced (*Allens*), ½ cup | 45 |
| sliced or diced (*Taylor's Brand*), ½ cup | 45 |

**Potato,** frozen (see also "Potato dishes, frozen"):

| | |
|---|---|
| whole, small (*Ore-Ida*), 3 oz. | 70 |
| whole, white (*Southern*), 3.5 oz. | 69 |
| whole, white, boiled (*Seabrook*), 3.2 oz. | 60 |
| diced and hash shred (*Seabrook*), 4 oz. | 80 |
| fried and french-fried: | |
| (*Heinz* Deep Fries), 3 oz. | 160 |
| (*MicroMagic*), 3 oz. | 290 |
| (*Ore-Ida Country Style Dinner Fries*), 3 oz. | 110 |
| (*Ore-Ida Crispers!*), 3 oz. | 230 |
| (*Ore-Ida Crispy Crowns*), 3 oz. | 160 |
| (*Ore-Ida Golden Fries*), 3 oz. | 120 |
| (*Ore-Ida* Lites), 3 oz. | 90 |
| (*Seabrook*), 3 oz. | 120 |
| cottage-cut (*Ore-Ida*), 3 oz. | 120 |
| cottage-cut (*Seabrook*), 2.8 oz. | 110 |
| crinkle-cut (*Heinz* Deep Fries), 3 oz. | 150 |
| crinkle-cut (*Ore-Ida Golden Crinkles*), 3 oz. | 120 |
| crinkle-cut (*Ore-Ida* Lites), 3 oz. | 90 |
| crinkle-cut (*Ore-Ida* Microwave), 3.5 oz. | 180 |
| crinkle-cut (*Ore-Ida Pixie Crinkles*), 3 oz. | 140 |
| crinkle-cut (*Quick'n Crispy*), 4 oz. | 370 |
| crinkle-cut (*Seabrook*), 3 oz. | 120 |

| FOOD AND MEASURE | CALORIES |
|---|---|
| w/onions (*Ore-Ida Crispy Crowns*), 3 oz. | 170 |
| shoestring (*Heinz* Deep Fries), 3 oz. | 200 |
| shoestring (*Ore-Ida*), 3 oz. | 140 |
| shoestring (*Ore-Ida* Lites), 3 oz. | 90 |
| shoestring (*Quick'n Crispy*), 4 oz. | 390 |
| shoestring (*Seabrook*), 3 oz. | 140 |
| skinny (*MicroMagic*), 3 oz. | 350 |
| thin cuts (*Quick'n Crispy*), 4 oz. | 370 |
| wedges (*Ore-Ida Home Style Potato Wedges*), 3 oz. | 100 |
| hash brown: | |
| (*Ore-Ida Golden Patties*), 2.5 oz. | 140 |
| (*Ore-Ida* Microwave), 2 oz. | 130 |
| (*Ore-Ida* Southern Style), 3 oz. | 70 |
| w/butter and onions (*Heinz* Deep Fries), 3 oz. | 110 |
| w/cheddar (*Ore-Ida Cheddar Browns*), 3 oz. | 90 |
| shredded (*Ore-Ida*), 3 oz. | 70 |
| O'Brien (*Ore-Ida*), 3 oz. | 60 |
| puffs (*Ore-Ida Tater Tots* Microwave), 4 oz. | 200 |
| puffs, plain or flavored (*Ore-Ida Tater Tots*), 3 oz. | 140 |
| sticks (*MicroMagic* Tater Sticks), 4 oz. | 390 |
| wedges (*Quick'n Crispy*), 4 oz. | 280 |

**Potato, mix**[1], ½ cup, except as noted:

| | |
|---|---|
| (*Betty Crocker Potato Buds*) | 130 |
| all varieties (*Betty Crocker* Potato Medleys) | 140 |
| au gratin: | |
| (*Betty Crocker*)[2] | 150 |
| (*Idahoan*) | 130 |
| (*Kraft* Potatoes & Cheese) | 130 |
| broccoli (*Kraft* Potatoes & Cheese) | 150 |
| tangy (*French's*) | 130 |
| bacon and cheddar (*Betty Crocker* Twice Baked) | 210 |
| butter, herbed (*Betty Crocker* Twice Baked) | 220 |
| cheddar, mild, w/onion (*Betty Crocker* Twice Baked) | 190 |
| cheddar, smoky (*Betty Crocker*) | 140 |
| cheddar, spicy (*Idahoan*) | 140 |
| cheddar and bacon (*Betty Crocker*) | 140 |
| cheddar and bacon casserole (*French's*) | 130 |

[1]Prepared according to package directions, except as noted.
[2]Prepared with margarine and skim milk.

| FOOD AND MEASURE | CALORIES |
|---|---|
| *Potato, mix, continued* | |
| cheese, two (*Kraft* Potatoes & Cheese 2-Cheese) | 130 |
| hash brown (*Idahoan* Quick One-Pan) | 140 |
| hash brown, w/onions (*Betty Crocker*) | 160 |
| herb and butter (*Idahoan*) | 150 |
| julienne (*Betty Crocker*)[1] | 130 |
| mashed: | |
| (*Country Store* Flakes), ⅓ cup flakes | 70 |
| (*French's Idaho*) | 130 |
| (*French's Idaho* Spuds) | 140 |
| (*Hungry Jack* Flakes) | 140 |
| (*Idahoan*) | 140 |
| microwave (*Idahoan Instamash*), ¼ pkg. or ½ cup | 80 |
| pancake, see "Potato pancake" | |
| scalloped: | |
| (*Betty Crocker*) | 140 |
| (*Idahoan*) | 140 |
| (*Kraft* Potatoes & Cheese) | 140 |
| cheese, real (*French's*) | 140 |
| cheesy (*Betty Crocker*) | 140 |
| creamy Italian (*French's*) | 120 |
| crispy top, w/savory onion mix (*French's*) | 140 |
| and ham (*Betty Crocker*) | 160 |
| w/ham (*Kraft* Potatoes & Cheese) | 150 |
| sour cream and chives (*Betty Crocker*) | 140 |
| sour cream w/chives (*Kraft* Potatoes & Cheese) | 150 |
| sour cream and onion (*Betty Crocker* Twice Baked) | 200 |
| sour cream and onion (*French's*) | 150 |
| sour cream and onion (*Idahoan*) | 130 |
| Stroganoff, creamy (*French's*) | 130 |
| western (*Idahoan*) | 120 |

**Potato chips and crisps,** 1 oz.:

| | |
|---|---|
| (*Bachman/Bachman* Unsalted/Ridge/Ruffled) | 160 |
| (*Bachman* Kettle Cooked/Saratoga Style) | 140 |
| (*Cottage Fries* No Salt Added) | 160 |
| (*Munchos*) | 150 |
| (*Ruffles* Light) | 130 |
| all varieties (*Cape Cod*) | 150 |
| all varieties (*Eagle*) | 150 |

[1]Prepared with margarine and skim milk.

| FOOD AND MEASURE | CALORIES |
|---|---|
| all varieties (*Health Valley*) | 160 |
| all varieties, except sour cream and onion (*Lay's*) | 150 |
| all varieties (*O'Boisies*) | 150 |
| all varieties (*Pringles*) | 170 |
| all varieties (*Pringles* Light) | 150 |
| all varieties, except mesquite and ranch (*Ruffles*) | 150 |
| all varieties (*Snacktime Krunchers!*) | 150 |
| all varieties, except hot and sour cream and onion (*Wise*) | 150 |
| all varieties (*Zapp's*) | 150 |
| barbecue, hot, sour cream and onion, or vinegar (*Bachman*) | 150 |
| hot or sour cream and onion (*Wise*) | 160 |
| mesquite barbecue (*Ruffles* Mesquite Grille) | 160 |
| ranch (*Ruffles*) | 160 |
| skins, all varieties (*Tato Skins*) | 150 |
| sour cream and onion (*Lay's*) | 160 |
| sour cream and onion (*Wise Ridgies*) | 160 |

**Potato dishes,** canned:

| | |
|---|---|
| au gratin (*Green Giant Pantry Express*), ½ cup | 120 |
| scalloped, and ham (*Hormel Micro-Cup*), 7.5 oz. | 260 |

**Potato dishes,** frozen:

| | |
|---|---|
| au gratin (*Birds Eye For One*), 5.5 oz. | 240 |
| au gratin (*Freezer Queen Family Side Dish*), 4 oz. | 100 |
| au gratin (*Green Giant* One Serving), 5.5 oz. | 200 |
| au gratin (*Stouffer's*), ⅓ of 11.5-oz. pkg. | 110 |
| and broccoli, w/cheese sauce (*Freezer Queen Family Side Dishes*), 5.5 oz. | 140 |
| and broccoli, in cheese-flavored sauce (*Green Giant* One Serving), 5.5 oz. | 130 |
| cheddared (*The Budget Gourmet* Side Dish), 5 oz. | 230 |
| cheddared, and broccoli (*The Budget Gourmet*), 5 oz. | 130 |
| nacho (*The Budget Gourmet* Side Dish), 5 oz. | 180 |
| new, in sour cream sauce (*The Budget Gourmet*), 5 oz. | 120 |
| scalloped (*Stouffer's*), ⅓ of 11.5-oz. pkg. | 90 |
| shredded, 'n vegetables, in cheese sauce (*Stokely Singles*), 4.5 oz. | 130 |
| sliced, 'n bacon, in cheddar cheese sauce (*Stokely Singles*), 4.5 oz. | 150 |
| stuffed, w/cheddar cheese (*Oh Boy!*), 6 oz. | 142 |
| stuffed, w/real bacon (*Oh Boy!*), 6 oz. | 116 |

| FOOD AND MEASURE | CALORIES |
|---|---|
| *Potato dishes, frozen, continued* | |
| stuffed, w/sour cream & chives (*Oh Boy!*), 6 oz. | 129 |
| stuffed, baked: | |
| broccoli and cheese (*Weight Watchers*), 10.5 oz. | 290 |
| cheese-flavored topping (*Green Giant*), 5 oz. | 200 |
| chicken divan (*Weight Watchers*), 11 oz. | 280 |
| ham Lorraine (*Weight Watchers*), 11 oz. | 250 |
| sour cream and chives (*Green Giant*), 5 oz. | 230 |
| turkey, homestyle (*Weight Watchers*), 12 oz. | 300 |
| three cheese (*The Budget Gourmet*), 5.75 oz. | 230 |

**Potato pancake,** mix, prepared:

| | |
|---|---|
| (*French's Idaho*), 3 cakes, 3" each | 90 |

**Potato salad,** canned:

| | |
|---|---|
| German (*Joan of Arc/Read*), ½ cup | 120 |
| homestyle (*Joan of Arc/Read*), ½ cup | 340 |

**Potato starch:**

| | |
|---|---|
| (*Featherweight*), 1 cup | 620 |

**Potato sticks,** canned:

| | |
|---|---|
| shoestring (*Allens* Regular/No Salt Added), 1 oz. | 140 |

**Poultry,** see specific listings

**Poultry seasoning:**

| | |
|---|---|
| 1 tsp. | 5 |

**Pout, ocean,** meat only:

| | |
|---|---|
| raw, 4 oz. | 90 |

**Praline pecan mousse,** frozen:

| | |
|---|---|
| (*Weight Watchers*), ½ pkg., 2.71 oz. | 190 |

**Preserves,** see "Jam and preserves"

**Pretzels,** 1 oz., except as noted:

| | |
|---|---|
| (*A & Eagle*) | 110 |
| all varieties: | |
| (*Bachman*) | 110 |
| (*Keebler* Butter Pretzels) | 110 |
| (*Rokeach*) | 110 |

| FOOD AND MEASURE | CALORIES |
|---|---|
| (*Rold Gold*) | 110 |
| except Dutch and twists (*Mr. Salty*) | 110 |
| beer (*Quinlan*) | 110 |
| cheddar flavor (*Combos*), 1.8 oz. | 240 |
| Dutch (*Mr. Salty*), 2 pieces | 110 |
| logs (*Quinlan*) | 103 |
| oat bran (*Quinlan*) | 115 |
| rice bran (*Quinlan* No-Salt) | 101 |
| rods, butter (*Seyfert's*) | 110 |
| sticks (*Quinlan*) | 105 |
| thins (*Quinlan*) | 104 |
| thins (*Quinlan* Ultra Thins) | 106 |
| thins, tiny (*Quinlan*) | 109 |
| thins, tiny (*Quinlan* No-Salt) | 115 |
| twists (*Mr. Salty*), 5 pieces | 110 |
| **Prickly pear:** | |
| 1 medium, 4.8 oz. | 42 |
| **Prosciutto:** | |
| boneless (*Hormel*), 1 oz. | 90 |
| **Prune:** | |
| canned, in heavy syrup, pitted, ½ cup | 123 |
| canned, in heavy syrup, 5 medium and 2 tbsp. syrup | 90 |
| dehydrated, uncooked, ½ cup | 224 |
| dried, uncooked: | |
| (*Del Monte/Del Monte* Moist Pak), 2 oz. | 120 |
| (*Sunsweet*), 2 oz. | 120 |
| w/pits, ½ cup | 193 |
| pitted, 10 medium | 201 |
| pitted (*Del Monte*), 2 oz. | 140 |
| pitted (*Sunsweet*), 2 oz. | 140 |
| dried, cooked, stewed, unsweetened, w/pits, ½ cup | 113 |
| dried, cooked, stewed, unsweetened, pitted, 4 oz. | 121 |
| **Prune juice,** 6 fl. oz.: | |
| (*Del Monte* Unsweetened) | 120 |
| (*Lucky Leaf*) | 150 |
| (*Mott's/Mott's* Country Style) | 130 |
| (*S&W* Unsweetened) | 120 |
| (*Sunsweet*) | 130 |

| FOOD AND MEASURE | CALORIES |
|---|---|

**Pudding,** frozen:

butterscotch or vanilla (*Rich's*), 3 oz. .......... 130
chocolate (*Rich's*), 3 oz. .......... 140

**Pudding, ready-to-serve:**

all flavors:
(*Estee*), ½ cup .......... 70
(*Featherweight*), ½ cup .......... 100
(*Hunt's Snack Pack* Lite), 4 oz. .......... 100
(*Jell-O* Light Pudding Snacks), 4 oz. .......... 100
(*Swiss Miss* Lite), 4 oz. .......... 100
except chocolate (*Del Monte* Pudding Cup), 5 oz. .......... 180
banana (*Lucky Leaf/Musselman's*), 4 oz. .......... 150
butterscotch (*Crowley*), 4.5 oz. .......... 150
butterscotch (*Lucky Leaf/Musselman's*), 4 oz. .......... 170
butterscotch (*White House*), 3.5 oz. .......... 113
butterscotch-chocolate-vanilla swirl (*Jell-O* Pudding Snacks), 4 oz. .......... 180
chocolate:
(*Crowley*), 4.5 oz. .......... 190
(*Hershey's* Chocolate Bar Flavor), 4 oz. .......... 180
(*Hunt's Snack Pack*), 4.25 oz. .......... 160
(*Jell-O* Pudding Snacks), 5.5 oz. .......... 230
(*Swiss Miss*), 4 oz. .......... 180
(*White House*), 3.5 oz. .......... 120
regular or fudge (*Del Monte* Pudding Cup), 5 oz. .......... 190
regular or fudge (*Jell-O* Pudding Snacks), 4 oz. .......... 170
regular or fudge (*Lucky Leaf/Musselman's*), 4 oz. .......... 180
milk (*Jell-O* Pudding Snacks), 4 oz. .......... 170
swirl, all varieties (*Jell-O* Pudding Snacks), 4 oz. .......... 170
chocolate-vanilla swirl (*Jell-O* Pudding Snacks), 5.5 oz. .......... 240
lemon (*White House*), 3.5 oz. .......... 152
rice (*Crowley*), 4.5 oz. .......... 125
rice (*Lucky Leaf/Musselman's*), 4 oz. .......... 120
rice (*White House*), 3.5 oz. .......... 111
tapioca:
(*Crowley*), 4.5 oz. .......... 135
(*Hunt's Snack Pack*), 4.25 oz. .......... 160
(*Jell-O* Pudding Snacks), 4 oz. .......... 170
(*Lucky Leaf/Musselman's*), 4 oz. .......... 140

| FOOD AND MEASURE | CALORIES |
|---|---|
| (*Swiss Miss*), 4 oz. | 150 |
| (*White House*), 3.5 oz. | 131 |
| vanilla: | |
| (*Crowley*), 4.5 oz. | 140 |
| (*Hunt's Snack Pack*), 4.25 oz. | 170 |
| (*Jell-O* Pudding Snacks), 5.5 oz. | 250 |
| (*Jell-O* Pudding Snacks), 4 oz. | 180 |
| (*Lucky Leaf/Musselman's*), 4 oz. | 170 |
| (*Swiss Miss*), 4 oz. | 160 |
| (*White House*), 3.5 oz. | 111 |
| vanilla-chocolate swirl (*Jell-O* Pudding Snacks), 4 oz. | 180 |

**Pudding bar,** frozen, 1 bar:

| | |
|---|---|
| all flavors (*Jell-O Pudding Pops*) | 80 |

**Pudding mix**[1], ½ cup:

| | |
|---|---|
| all varieties, except chocolate, custard, or flan (*Royal*) | 160 |
| banana (*Jell-O* Instant Sugar Free)[2] | 80 |
| banana creme (*Jell-O* Instant) | 160 |
| banana creme (*Jell-O* Microwave) | 150 |
| banana creme (*Royal* Instant) | 180 |
| butter almond, toasted (*Royal* Instant) | 170 |
| butter pecan (*Jell-O* Instant) | 170 |
| butterscotch: | |
| (*Jell-O*) | 170 |
| (*Jell-O* Instant) | 160 |
| (*Jell-O* Instant Sugar Free)[2] | 90 |
| (*Jell-O* Microwave) | 170 |
| (*Royal* Instant) | 180 |
| (*Royal* Instant Sugar Free)[2] | 100 |
| butterscotch or vanilla (*D-Zerta*)[3] | 70 |
| chocolate: | |
| (*D-Zerta*)[3] | 60 |
| (*Jell-O* Microwave) | 170 |
| (*Jell-O* Sugar Free/Instant Sugar Free)[2] | 90 |

[1]Prepared according to package directions, with whole milk, except as noted.

[2]Prepared with 2% lowfat milk.

[3]Prepared with skim milk.

| FOOD AND MEASURE | CALORIES |
|---|---|
| *Pudding mix, chocolate, continued* | |
| (*Royal* Instant Sugar Free)[1] | 110 |
| (*Weight Watchers* Instant)[2] | 90 |
| all varieties (*Jell-O*) | 160 |
| all varieties (*Jell-O* Instant) | 180 |
| all varieties (*Royal*) | 180 |
| all varieties (*Royal* Instant) | 190 |
| fudge (*Jell-O* Instant Sugar Free)[1] | 100 |
| milk (*Jell-O* Microwave) | 160 |
| chocolate mint (*Royal* Instant) | 190 |
| coconut, toasted (*Royal* Instant) | 170 |
| coconut cream (*Jell-O* Instant) | 180 |
| custard (*Royal*) | 150 |
| custard, egg, golden (*Jell-O Americana*) | 160 |
| flan (*Jell-O*) | 150 |
| flan, w/caramel sauce (*Royal*) | 150 |
| lemon (*French's*) | 110 |
| lemon (*Jell-O* Instant) | 170 |
| lemon (*Royal* Instant) | 180 |
| pistachio (*Jell-O* Instant) | 170 |
| pistachio (*Jell-O* Instant Sugar Free)[1] | 90 |
| pistachio nut (*Royal* Instant) | 170 |
| raspberry or strawberry (*Salada Danish Dessert*) | 130 |
| rennet custard, all flavors (*Junket*) | 120 |
| rice (*Jell-O Americana*) | 170 |
| tapioca, vanilla (*Jell-O Americana*) | 160 |
| vanilla: | |
| (*Jell-O*/*Jell-O* Microwave) | 160 |
| (*Jell-O* French/*Jell-O* Instant) | 170 |
| (*Jell-O* Instant Sugar Free)[1] | 90 |
| (*Jell-O* Sugar Free)[1] | 80 |
| (*Royal* Instant) | 180 |
| (*Royal* Instant Sugar Free)[1] | 100 |
| French (*Jell-O* Instant) | 160 |

[1]Prepared with 2% lowfat milk.
[2]Prepared with skim milk.

| FOOD AND MEASURE | CALORIES |
|---|---|
| **Puff pastry,** frozen: | |
| sheets (*Pepperidge Farm*), ¼ sheet | 260 |
| shells, mini (*Pepperidge Farm*), 1 shell | 50 |
| shells, patty (*Pepperidge Farm*), 1 shell | 210 |
| **Pummelo:** | |
| 1 medium, 5½" diam. | 228 |
| sections, ½ cup | 36 |
| **Pumpkin:** | |
| fresh, raw, 1" cubes, ½ cup | 15 |
| fresh, boiled, drained, mashed, ½ cup | 24 |
| canned (*Del Monte*), ½ cup | 35 |
| canned (*Libby's*), ½ cup | 42 |
| canned (*Stokely*) ½ cup | 40 |
| **Pumpkin flower:** | |
| raw, trimmed, ½ cup | 3 |
| boiled, drained, ½ cup | 10 |
| **Pumpkin leaf:** | |
| raw, trimmed, ½ cup | 4 |
| boiled, drained, ½ cup | 7 |
| **Pumpkin pie filling or mix,** see "Pie filling" and "Pie mix" | |
| **Pumpkin pie spice:** | |
| 1 tsp. | 6 |
| **Pumpkin seed:** | |
| roasted, whole, in shell, 1 oz. | 126 |
| roasted, shelled, 1 oz. | 148 |
| dried, in shell, 1 oz. | 114 |
| dried, shelled, 1 oz. | 154 |
| **Purslane:** | |
| raw, trimmed, ½ cup | 4 |
| boiled, drained, ½ cup | 10 |

# Q

| FOOD AND MEASURE | CALORIES |
|---|---|
| **Quail,** fresh, raw: | |
| meat w/skin, 1 quail, 3.8 oz. (4.3 oz. w/bone) | 210 |
| meat w/skin, 1 oz. | 54 |
| meat only, 1 oz. | 38 |
| **Quince:** | |
| whole, 1 medium, 5.3 oz. | 53 |
| ***Quincy's:*** | |
| catfish fillets, 2 pieces, 6.9 oz. | 309 |
| chicken breast, grilled, 5 oz. | 145 |
| chicken strips, 4 pieces, 4.5 oz. | 318 |
| hamburger, ¼ lb., 6.7 oz. | 403 |
| hamburger, ¼ lb., w/cheese, 7.2 oz. | 451 |
| shrimp, 7 pieces, 3.9 oz. | 248 |
| steak: | |
| chopped, 5.8 oz. | 466 |
| chopped, luncheon, 4 oz. | 350 |
| country style, w/mushroom sauce, 6 oz. | 288 |
| fillet, 5.6 oz. | 331 |
| rib eye, 7.3 oz. | 665 |
| sirloin, 5.9 oz. | 649 |
| sirloin, large, 7.7 oz. | 852 |
| sirloin, petite, 4 oz. | 446 |
| sirloin club, 4.8 oz. | 283 |
| sirloin tips, 4 oz. | 236 |
| T-Bone, 7.8 oz. | 1,045 |
| side dishes: | |
| coleslaw, 2.1 oz. | 60 |
| cornbread, 1.9 oz. | 178 |
| mushroom sauce, 3 oz. | 27 |
| peppers and onions, 4 oz. | 80 |
| potato, baked, w/out butter, 8.8 oz. | 181 |
| steak fries, 5.5 oz. | 426 |

| FOOD AND MEASURE | CALORIES |
|---|---|
| soups: | |
| broccoli, cream of, 9.2 oz. | 193 |
| chili, w/beans, 9.2 oz. | 346 |
| clam chowder, 9.2 oz. | 198 |
| vegetable beef, 8.6 oz. | 78 |

## Quinoa:

| | |
|---|---|
| 1 oz. | 106 |

## Quinoa seed:

| | |
|---|---|
| (*Arrowhead Mills*), 2 oz. | 200 |

# R

| FOOD AND MEASURE | CALORIES |
| --- | --- |
| **Rabbit,** domesticated, meat only: | |
| roasted, 4 oz. | 175 |
| stewed, 4 oz. | 234 |
| stewed, diced, 1 cup | 288 |
| **Radish:** | |
| 10 medium, ¾″–1″ diam. | 7 |
| sliced, ½ cup | 10 |
| **Radish, Oriental:** | |
| raw, 1 medium, 7″ × 2¼″ diam. | 62 |
| raw, sliced, ½ cup | 8 |
| dried, ½ cup | 157 |
| **Radish, white icicle:** | |
| 1 medium, .6 oz. | 2 |
| sliced, ½ cup | 7 |
| **Raisins:** | |
| natural (*Del Monte*), 3 oz. | 250 |
| seeded, ½ cup not packed | 214 |
| seedless: | |
| ½ cup not packed | 217 |
| (*Cinderella* Thompson), ½ cup | 250 |
| (*Dole*), ½ cup | 260 |
| (*Sun-Maid*), ½ cup | 290 |
| golden, ½ cup not packed | 219 |
| golden (*Del Monte*), 3 oz. | 260 |
| golden (*Dole*), ½ cup | 260 |
| **Raspberry:** | |
| fresh, trimmed, ½ cup | 31 |
| canned, red, in heavy syrup, ½ cup | 117 |
| frozen, sweetened, ½ cup | 128 |
| frozen, in light syrup (*Birds Eye* Quick Thaw Pouch), 5 oz. | 100 |

| FOOD AND MEASURE | CALORIES |
|---|---|
| **Raspberry danish,** 1 piece: | |
| (*Awrey's* Square), 3 oz. | 260 |
| fried (*Hostess Breakfast Bake Shop*) | 390 |
| frozen (*Pepperidge Farm*), 2.25 oz. | 220 |
| **Raspberry fruit roll:** | |
| (*Flavor Tree*), 1 piece | 75 |
| **Raspberry juice:** | |
| blend (*Dole Pure & Light* Country Raspberry), 6 fl. oz. | 87 |
| red (*Smucker's* Naturally 100%), 8 fl. oz. | 120 |
| **Raspberry juice cocktail:** | |
| (*Welch's Orchard*), 10-fl.-oz. bottle | 160 |
| **Raspberry mousse mix,** prepared: | |
| (*Weight Watchers*), ½ cup | 60 |
| **Raspberry turnover,** frozen: | |
| (*Pepperidge Farm*), 1 piece | 310 |
| **Raspberry-vanilla swirl,** frozen: | |
| (*Pepperidge Farm* Dessert Lights), 3¼ oz. | 160 |
| **Ravioli,** canned: | |
| beef (*Chef Boyardee Microwave*), 7.5 oz. | 190 |
| beef (*Estee*), 7.5 oz. | 230 |
| beef, in meat sauce (*Franco-American* RavioliO's), 7.5 oz. | 250 |
| beef, in tomato sauce (*Hormel Micro-Cup*), 7.5 oz. | 247 |
| cheese, in meat sauce (*Chef Boyardee* Microwave), 7.5 oz. | 200 |
| cheese, in sauce (*Buitoni*), 7.5 oz. | 190 |
| meat, in sauce (*Buitoni*), 7.5 oz. | 180 |
| **Ravioli,** frozen: | |
| (*Celentano*), 6.5 oz. | 380 |
| cheese (*Buitoni*), ¼ pkg. or 4 oz. | 360 |
| mini (*Celentano*), 4 oz. | 250 |
| **Ravioli entree,** frozen: | |
| cheese (*The Budget Gourmet* Slim Selects), 10 oz. | 260 |
| cheese, baked (*Weight Watchers*), 9 oz. | 290 |
| **Red snapper,** see "Snapper" | |

| FOOD AND MEASURE | CALORIES |
|---|---|
| **Redfish,** see "Ocean perch" | |
| **Refried beans,** see "Beans, refried" | |
| **Relish:** | |
| dill (*Vlasic*), 1 oz. | 2 |
| hamburger or piccalilli (*Heinz*), 1 oz. | 30 |
| hot dog, India, or sweet (*Heinz*), 1 oz. | 35 |
| hot dog (*Vlasic*), 1 oz. | 40 |
| jalapeño (*Old El Paso*), 2 tbsp. | 16 |
| pickle (*Claussen*), 1 oz. | 26 |
| sweet (*Vlasic*), 1 oz. | 30 |
| **Rhubarb:** | |
| fresh, raw, diced, ½ cup | 13 |
| frozen, cooked, sweetened, ½ cup | 139 |
| **Rib sauce:** | |
| (*Dip n'Joy* Saucey Rib), 1 oz. | 60 |
| **Rice, brown**[1]**:** | |
| basmati (*Fantastic Foods*), ½ cup | 102 |
| long grain, raw (*Arrowhead Mills*), 2 oz. | 200 |
| long grain: | |
| (*Carolina*), ½ cup | 110 |
| (*Mahatma/River*), ½ cup | 110 |
| (*S&W*), 3.5 oz. | 119 |
| (*Uncle Ben's* Whole Grain), ⅔ cup | 130 |
| quick (*S&W*), 3.5 oz. | 110 |
| medium grain, raw (*Arrowhead Mills*), 2 oz. | 200 |
| medium grain, ½ cup | 109 |
| precooked (*Uncle Ben's*), ½ cup | 90 |
| **Rice, white**[1]**:** | |
| basmati (*Fantastic Foods*), ½ cup | 103 |
| basmati, long grain (*Texmati*), ½ cup | 82 |
| glutinous, 1 cup | 234 |
| long grain (*Carolina/Mahatma/River*), ½ cup | 100 |
| long grain (*Uncle Ben's* Natural Whole Grain), ⅔ cup | 130 |

[1]Cooked according to package directions, without salt and butter, except as noted.

| FOOD AND MEASURE | CALORIES |
|---|---|
| long grain (*Water Maid*), ½ cup | 100 |
| long grain, parboiled, 1 cup | 199 |
| long grain, parboiled (*Uncle Ben's Converted*), ⅔ cup | 120 |
| long grain, precooked or instant: | |
| (*Carolina/Mahatma* Instant Enriched), ½ cup | 110 |
| (*Minute Rice/Minute Rice* Premium), ⅔ cup | 120 |
| (*Minute Rice* Boil-in-Bag), ½ cup | 90 |
| (*S&W*), 3.5 oz. | 106 |
| (*Success* Boil-in-Bag Enriched), ½ cup | 100 |
| (*Uncle Ben's* Boil-in-Bag), ½ cup | 90 |
| (*Uncle Ben's Rice In An Instant*), ⅔ cup | 120 |
| medium or short grain, ½ cup | 133 |

**Rice, wild,** see "Wild rice"

**Rice beverage,** flavored:

| | |
|---|---|
| chocolate (*Rice Dream*), 6 fl. oz. | 170 |

**Rice bran:**

| | |
|---|---|
| crude, 1 cup | 262 |

**Rice bran oil:**

| | |
|---|---|
| 1 tbsp. | 120 |

**Rice cake,** 1 piece, except as noted:

| | |
|---|---|
| all varieties, except mini (*Hain*) | 40 |
| all varieties (*Lundberg*) | 60 |
| plain (*Quaker* Regular/Unsalted) | 35 |
| plain, apple cinnamon, or cheese, mini (*Hain*), ½ oz. | 60 |
| barbecue, mini (*Hain*), ½ oz. | 70 |
| brown rice (*Konriko* Original Unsalted) | 30 |
| cheese, nacho, mini (*Hain*), ½ oz. | 70 |
| corn (*Quaker/Mother's*) | 35 |
| honey nut, mini (*Hain*), ½ oz. | 60 |
| multigrain (*Quaker/Mother's*) | 34 |
| ranch, mini (*Hain*), ½ oz. | 70 |
| sesame (*Quaker/Mother's* Regular/Unsalted) | 35 |
| teriyaki, mini (*Hain*), ½ oz. | 50 |

**Rice dishes,** canned:

| | |
|---|---|
| fried (*La Choy*), ¾ cup | 180 |
| Spanish (*Featherweight*), 7.5 oz. | 140 |

| FOOD AND MEASURE | CALORIES |
|---|---|
| *Rice dishes, canned, continued* | |
| Spanish (*Heinz*), 7.25 oz. | 150 |
| Spanish (*Old El Paso*), ½ cup | 70 |
| Spanish (*Van Camp's*), 1 cup | 160 |

## **Rice dishes,** frozen:

| | |
|---|---|
| and broccoli: | |
| au gratin (*Birds Eye For One*), 5.75 oz. | 180 |
| in cheese sauce (*Green Giant* One Serving), 5.5 oz. | 180 |
| in flavored cheese sauce (*Green Giant Rice Originals*), ½ cup | 120 |
| country-style (*Birds Eye* International Recipes), 3.3 oz. | 90 |
| French-style (*Birds Eye* International Recipes), 3.3 oz. | 110 |
| fried, w/chicken (*Chun King*), 8 oz. | 260 |
| fried, w/pork (*Chun King*), 8 oz. | 270 |
| Italian blend, and spinach, in cheese sauce (*Green Giant Rice Originals*), ½ cup | 140 |
| medley (*Green Giant Rice Originals*), ½ cup | 100 |
| Oriental (*The Budget Gourmet* Side Dish), 5.75 oz. | 210 |
| peas and mushrooms, sauce (*Green Giant* One Serving), 5.5 oz. | 130 |
| pilaf (*Green Giant Rice Originals*), ½ cup | 110 |
| pilaf w/green beans (*The Budget Gourmet* Side Dish), 5.5 oz. | 240 |
| Spanish-style (*Birds Eye* International Recipes), 3.3 oz. | 110 |
| white and wild rice (*Green Giant Rice Originals*), ½ cup | 130 |
| wild, sherry (*Green Giant* Microwave Garden Gourmet), 1 pkg. | 210 |

## **Rice dishes, mix**[1], ½ cup, except as noted:

| | |
|---|---|
| Alfredo (*Country Inn*)[2] | 140 |
| amandine (*Hain* 3-Grain Side Dish) | 130 |
| asparagus, w/hollandaise sauce (*Lipton* Rice and Sauce)[3] | 170 |
| asparagus au gratin (*Country Inn*)[2] | 130 |
| au gratin, herbed (*Country Inn*)[2] | 140 |
| au gratin herb (*Success*)[4] | 100 |
| beef flavor: | |
| (*Lipton* Rice and Sauce)[4] | 150 |
| (*Mahatma*) | 100 |

[1]Prepared according to package directions, except as noted.
[2]Prepared without butter or margarine.
[3]Prepared with 2 tbsp. butter.
[4]Prepared with 1 tbsp. butter.

| FOOD AND MEASURE | CALORIES |
|---|---|
| (*Minute* Microwave Family Size) | 160 |
| (*Minute* Microwave Single Size) | 150 |
| (*Rice-A-Roni*) | 150 |
| (*Success*)[1] | 100 |
| and vermicelli (*Make-it-Easy*), 1.3 oz. dry | 130 |
| beef and mushroom (*Rice-A-Roni*) | 150 |
| broccoli, stir-fry (*Suzi Wan* Dinner Recipe), 7.5 oz. | 370 |
| broccoli amandine or au gratin (*Country Inn*)[1] | 130 |
| broccoli au gratin (*Rice-A-Roni Savory Classics*) | 180 |
| brown and wild (*Success*)[1] | 120 |
| brown and wild (*Uncle Ben's*) | 150 |
| brown and wild, regular or mushroom recipe (*Uncle Ben's*)[1] | 130 |
| Cajun (*Lipton* Rice and Sauce)[2] | 150 |
| cauliflower au gratin (*Country Inn*)[1] | 130 |
| cauliflower au gratin (*Rice-A-Roni Savory Classics*) | 170 |
| cheddar, zesty (*Rice-A-Roni Savory Classics*) | 180 |
| cheddar and broccoli (*Minute* Microwave Family/Single Size) | 160 |
| chicken, and chicken flavor: | |
| (*Lipton* Rice and Sauce)[2] | 150 |
| (*Mahatma*) | 100 |
| (*Minute* Microwave Family Size) | 160 |
| (*Minute* Microwave Single Size) | 150 |
| (*Rice-A-Roni*) | 150 |
| (*Success*)[1] | 110 |
| and broccoli (*Rice-A-Roni*) | 150 |
| and broccoli (*Suzi Wan*)[1] | 120 |
| creamy, and mushroom (*Country Inn*)[1] | 140 |
| drumstick (*Minute*) | 150 |
| Florentine (*Rice-A-Roni Savory Classics*) | 130 |
| homestyle, and vegetables (*Country Inn*)[1] | 140 |
| honey-lemon (*Suzi Wan* Dinner Recipe), 7.5 oz.[3] | 200 |
| honey-lemon (*Suzi Wan* Dinner Recipe), 7.5 oz. | 370 |
| and mushroom (*Rice-A-Roni*) | 180 |
| and mushroom, creamy (*Country Inn*)[1] | 140 |
| royale (*Country Inn*)[1] | 120 |
| stock (*Country Inn*)[1] | 130 |

[1]Prepared without butter or margarine.
[2]Prepared with 1 tbsp. butter.
[3]Prepared without added ingredients.

| FOOD AND MEASURE | CALORIES |
|---|---|
| *Rice dishes, mix, chicken, and chicken flavor, continued* | |
| and vegetables (*Rice-A-Roni*) | 140 |
| and vegetables (*Suzi Wan*)[1] | 120 |
| and vermicelli (*Make-it-Easy*), 1.3 oz. dry | 130 |
| Florentine (*Country Inn*)[1] | 140 |
| fried (*Minute*) | 160 |
| fried (*Rice-A-Roni*) | 110 |
| green bean amandine (*Rice-A-Roni Savory Classics*) | 210 |
| green bean amandine casserole (*Country Inn*)[1] | 120 |
| herb, au gratin, see "au gratin," above | |
| herb and butter (*Lipton* Rice and Sauce)[2] | 150 |
| herb and butter (*Rice-A-Roni*) | 130 |
| long grain and wild: | |
| (*Mahatma*) | 100 |
| (*Minute*) | 150 |
| (*Near East*) | 130 |
| (*Rice-A-Roni* Original) | 130 |
| (*Uncle Ben's* Original) | 120 |
| (*Uncle Ben's* Original/Fast Cooking)[1] | 100 |
| (*Uncle Ben's* Fast Cooking) | 130 |
| chicken w/almonds (*Rice-A-Roni*) | 140 |
| chicken stock sauce (*Uncle Ben's*)[1] | 140 |
| chicken stock sauce (*Uncle Ben's*) | 160 |
| original or mushroom and herb (*Lipton* Rice and Sauce)[2] | 150 |
| pilaf (*Rice-A-Roni*) | 130 |
| Mexican (*Old El Paso*) | 140 |
| mushroom, creamy, and wild rice (*Country Inn*)[1] | 140 |
| Oriental (*Hain* 3-Grain Goodness) | 120 |
| Parmesan, creamy, and herbs (*Rice-A-Roni Savory Classics*) | 170 |
| pilaf: | |
| (*Casbah*), 1 oz. dry or ½ cup cooked | 90 |
| (*Lipton* Rice and Sauce)[3] | 170 |
| (*Near East*) | 140 |
| (*Rice-A-Roni*) | 150 |
| (*Success*)[1] | 120 |
| beef-flavored (*Near East*) | 140 |

[1]Prepared without butter or margarine.
[2]Prepared with 1 tbsp. butter.
[3]Prepared with 2 tbsp. butter.

| FOOD AND MEASURE | CALORIES |
|---|---|
| brown, w/miso (*Quick Pilaf*)[1] | 105 |
| brown, w/miso (*Quick Pilaf*)[2] | 145 |
| chicken-flavored (*Near East*) | 140 |
| French-style (*Minute* Microwave Family Size) | 130 |
| French-style (*Minute* Microwave Single Size) | 120 |
| garden (*Rice-A-Roni Savory Classics*) | 140 |
| lentil (*Near East*) | 170 |
| nutted (*Casbah*), 1 oz. dry or ½ cup cooked | 160 |
| Spanish, brown (*Quick Pilaf*)[2] | 136 |
| vegetable (*Country Inn*)[1] | 120 |
| wheat (*Near East*) | 150 |
| rib roast (*Minute*) | 150 |
| risotto (*Rice-A-Roni*) | 200 |
| risotto, chicken and cheese (*Country Inn*)[2] | 120 |
| Spanish: | |
| (*Lipton* Rice and Sauce)[3] | 140 |
| (*Mahatma*) | 100 |
| (*Near East*) | 170 |
| (*Rice-A-Roni*) | 150 |
| pilaf (*Casbah*), 1 oz. dry or ½ cup cooked | 90 |
| Stroganoff (*Rice-A-Roni*) | 200 |
| sweet and sour: | |
| (*Suzi Wan*)[1] | 130 |
| (*Suzi Wan* Dinner Recipe), 7.5 oz.[4] | 220 |
| (*Suzi Wan* Dinner Recipe), 7.5 oz. | 340 |
| teriyaki (Suzi Wan)[1] | 120 |
| teriyaki (*Suzi Wan* Dinner Recipe), 7.5 oz.[4] | 180 |
| teriyaki (*Suzi Wan* Dinner Recipe), 7.5 oz. | 360 |
| three-flavor (*Suzi Wan*)[1] | 120 |
| vegetable medley (*Country Inn*)[1] | 140 |
| w/vegetables, broccoli and cheddar (*Lipton* Rice and Sauce)[2] | 180 |
| vegetables, spring, and cheese (*Rice-A-Roni Savory Classics*) | 170 |
| yellow (*Mahatma/Success*)[1] | 100 |
| yellow (*Rice-A-Roni*) | 140 |

[1]Prepared without butter or margarine.
[2]Prepared with 2 tbsp. butter.
[3]Prepared with 1 tbsp. butter.
[4]Prepared without added ingredients.

| FOOD AND MEASURE | CALORIES |
|---|---|
| **Rice seasoning:** | |
| Mexican (*Lawry's* Seasoning Blends), 1 pkg. | 94 |
| **Rigatoni entree,** canned: | |
| (*Chef Boyardee* Microwave), 7.5 oz. | 210 |
| **Rigatoni entree,** frozen: | |
| bake, w/meat sauce and cheese (*Lean Cuisine*), 9.75 oz. | 260 |
| **Roast, vegetarian,** frozen: | |
| (*Worthington* Dinner Roast), 2 oz. | 120 |
| **Robert sauce:** | |
| (*Escoffier* Sauce Robert), 1 tbsp. | 20 |
| **Rockfish,** Pacific, meat only: | |
| raw, 4 oz. | 107 |
| baked, broiled, or microwaved, 4 oz. | 137 |
| **Roe,** fish (see also "Caviar"): | |
| mixed species, 1 tbsp. | 22 |
| **Roll,** 1 piece, except as noted: | |
| assorted (*Brownberry* Hearth) | 124 |
| brown and serve: | |
| (*Pepperidge Farm* Hearth) | 50 |
| club (*Pepperidge Farm* Deli Classic) | 100 |
| French (*Pepperidge Farm* Deli Classic 3/pkg.), ½ piece | 120 |
| French, petite (*du Jour*) | 230 |
| gem-style or w/buttermilk (*Wonder*) | 80 |
| Italian, crusty (*du Jour*) | 80 |
| cinnamon (*Hostess Breakfast Bake Shop*) | 140 |
| cinnamon, homestyle (*Awrey's*) | 240 |
| cinnamon swirl (*Awrey's* Grande) | 340 |
| croissant, see "Croissant" | |
| dinner: | |
| (*Arnold* 24 Dinner Party) | 51 |
| (*Pepperidge Farm* Old Fashioned/Classic Country Style) | 50 |
| (*Pepperidge Farm* Party) | 30 |

| FOOD AND MEASURE | CALORIES |
|---|---|
| (*Roman Meal*) | 69 |
| (*Wonder*) | 80 |
| Black Forest or cracked wheat (*Awrey's*) | 50 |
| crusty (*Awrey's*) | 70 |
| plain or sesame seed (*Awrey's*) | 60 |
| poppy seed (*Awrey's*) | 59 |
| potato, hearty (*Pepperidge Farm* Classic) | 90 |
| wheat (*Home Pride*) | 70 |
| white (*Home Pride*) | 80 |
| egg (*Levy's* Old Country Deli), 1 oz. | 146 |
| egg, sandwich (*Arnold* Dutch) | 123 |
| finger, w/poppy seeds (*Pepperidge Farm*) | 50 |
| frankfurter, see "hot dog," below | |
| French-style (*Francisco* International) | 108 |
| French-style (*Pepperidge Farm* Deli Classic 9/pkg.) | 100 |
| hamburger: | |
| (*Arnold*) | 115 |
| (*Pepperidge Farm*) | 130 |
| (*Roman Meal* Original) | 113 |
| (*Wonder*) | 120 |
| (*Wonder* Light) | 80 |
| hoagie (*Wonder*) | 400 |
| hoagie, soft (*Pepperidge Farm* Deli Classic) | 210 |
| honey bun, see "Bun, sweet" | |
| hot dog: | |
| (*Arnold*) | 100 |
| (*Arnold* New England Style) | 108 |
| (*Country Grain*) | 100 |
| (*Pepperidge Farm*) | 140 |
| (*Roman Meal* Original) | 104 |
| (*Wonder*) | 80 |
| Dijon (*Pepperidge Farm*) | 160 |
| oat bran (*Awrey's*) | 110 |
| kaiser (*Arnold* Francisco) | 184 |
| kaiser (*Brownberry* Hearth) | 152 |
| onion (*Levy's* Old Country Deli), 1 oz. | 153 |
| pan (*Wonder*) | 80 |
| Parkerhouse (*Pepperidge Farm*) | 60 |

| FOOD AND MEASURE | CALORIES |
|---|---|
| *Roll, continued* | |
| sandwich: | |
| oat bran (*Awrey's*) | 120 |
| onion, w/poppy seeds (*Pepperidge Farm*) | 150 |
| potato (*Pepperidge Farm*) | 160 |
| salad (*Pepperidge Farm* Deli Classic) | 110 |
| w/sesame seeds (*Pepperidge Farm*) | 140 |
| soft (*Pepperidge Farm* Family) | 100 |
| sourdough, French-style (*Pepperidge Farm* Deli Classic) | 100 |
| twist, golden (*Pepperidge Farm* Deli Classic Heat & Serve) | 110 |

**Roll,** frozen:

| | |
|---|---|
| apple, sweet (*Weight Watchers*), 2.25 oz. | 160 |
| cheese, sweet (*Weight Watchers*), 2.25 oz. | 180 |
| cinnamon (*Pepperidge Farm*), 1 piece | 280 |
| cinnamon, all butter (*Sara Lee*), 2-oz. piece | 230 |
| cinnamon, all butter, icing packet (*Sara Lee*), 1 pkt. | 50 |
| Parkerhouse (*Bridgford*), 1-oz. piece | 85 |
| strawberry, sweet (*Weight Watchers*), 2.25 oz. | 170 |

**Roll,** refrigerated:

| | |
|---|---|
| butterflake (*Pillsbury*), 1 piece | 140 |
| cinnamon, iced (*Hungry Jack*), 2 pieces | 290 |
| cinnamon, iced (*Pillsbury*), 1 piece | 110 |
| crescent (*Pillsbury*), 1 piece | 100 |

**Roll mix,** prepared, hot:

| | |
|---|---|
| (*Dromedary*), 2 pieces | 239 |
| (*Pillsbury*), 2 pieces | 270 |

**Rose apple:**

| | |
|---|---|
| trimmed, 1 oz. | 7 |

**Roselle:**

| | |
|---|---|
| trimmed, 1 oz. or ½ cup | 14 |

**Rosemary,** dried:

| | |
|---|---|
| 1 tsp. | 4 |

| FOOD AND MEASURE | CALORIES |
|---|---|
| **Rotini entree,** frozen: | |
| cheddar (*Green Giant* Microwave Garden Gourmet), 1 pkg. | 230 |
| seafood (*Mrs. Paul's* Light), 9 oz. | 240 |
| **Roughy,** orange, meat only, raw: | |
| raw, 4 oz. | 143 |
| ***Roy Rogers:*** | |
| breakfast, 1 piece or serving: | |
| apple swirls | 328 |
| cheese swirls | 383 |
| cinnamon roll | 376 |
| crescent roll | 287 |
| crescent sandwich | 408 |
| crescent sandwich, bacon | 446 |
| crescent sandwich, ham | 456 |
| crescent sandwich, sausage | 564 |
| egg and biscuit platter | 557 |
| egg and biscuit platter, bacon | 607 |
| egg and biscuit platter, ham | 605 |
| egg and biscuit platter, sausage | 713 |
| pancake platter, w/butter, syrup | 386 |
| pancake platter, bacon, w/butter, syrup | 436 |
| pancake platter, ham, w/butter, syrup | 434 |
| pancake platter, sausage, w/butter, syrup | 542 |
| chicken, fried, 1 serving: | |
| breast | 412 |
| breast and wing | 604 |
| leg (drumstick) | 140 |
| leg and thigh | 436 |
| nuggets, 6 pieces | 288 |
| thigh | 296 |
| wing | 192 |
| sandwiches and burgers, 1 serving: | |
| bacon cheeseburger | 552 |
| bar burger | 573 |
| cheeseburger | 525 |
| cheeseburger, small | 275 |
| *Express*burger | 561 |
| *Express* bacon cheeseburger | 641 |
| *Express* cheeseburger | 613 |

| FOOD AND MEASURE | CALORIES |
|---|---|
| *Roy Rogers, sandwiches and burgers, continued* | |
| fish sandwich | 514 |
| hamburger | 472 |
| hamburger, small | 222 |
| roast beef sandwich | 350 |
| roast beef sandwich, w/cheese | 403 |
| roast beef sandwich, large | 373 |
| roast beef sandwich, large, w/cheese | 427 |
| side dishes, 1 serving: | |
| biscuit | 231 |
| coleslaw | 110 |
| french fries, 4 oz. | 320 |
| french fries, small, 3 oz. | 238 |
| french fries, large, 5.5 oz. | 440 |
| salad dressings, 2 tbsp.: | |
| bacon 'n tomato | 136 |
| blue cheese | 150 |
| Italian, lo-cal | 70 |
| ranch | 155 |
| Thousand Island | 160 |
| shake, chocolate | 358 |
| shake, strawberry | 315 |
| shake, vanilla | 306 |
| sundae, caramel | 293 |
| sundae, hot fudge | 337 |
| sundae, strawberry | 216 |
| *Vitari*, 1 oz. | 30 |

**Rum,** see "Liquor"

**Rutabaga:**

| | |
|---|---|
| fresh, raw, cubed, ½ cup | 25 |
| fresh, boiled, drained, cubed, ½ cup | 29 |
| fresh, boiled, drained, mashed, ½ cup | 41 |
| canned, diced (*Allens*), ½ cup | 20 |

**Rye,** whole-grain:

| | |
|---|---|
| 1 cup | 567 |
| (*Arrowhead Mills*), 2 oz. | 190 |

| FOOD AND MEASURE | CALORIES |
| --- | --- |
| **Rye cake:** | |
| (*Quaker* Grain Cakes), .32-oz. piece | 35 |
| **Rye flakes:** | |
| (*Arrowhead Mills*), 2 oz. | 190 |
| **Rye flour,** see "Flour" | |
| **Rye whiskey,** see "Liquor" | |

# S

| FOOD AND MEASURE | CALORIES |
|---|---|

**Sablefish,** meat only:

raw, 4 oz. . . . . . . . . . . . . . . . . . . . . . . . . . . . . . . . . . . . . 221
smoked, 4 oz. . . . . . . . . . . . . . . . . . . . . . . . . . . . . . . . . . 291

**Safflower seed kernel:**

dried, 1 oz. . . . . . . . . . . . . . . . . . . . . . . . . . . . . . . . . . . 147

**Safflower seed meal:**

partially defatted, 1 oz. . . . . . . . . . . . . . . . . . . . . . . . . 97

**Saffron:**

1 tsp. . . . . . . . . . . . . . . . . . . . . . . . . . . . . . . . . . . . . . . . 2

**Sage,** ground:

1 tsp. . . . . . . . . . . . . . . . . . . . . . . . . . . . . . . . . . . . . . . . 2

**Salad dip:**

egg-free (*Nasoya Vegi-Dip*), 1 oz. . . . . . . . . . . . . . . . . . . 45

**Salad dressing,** 1 tbsp., except as noted:

bacon and tomato (*Kraft*) . . . . . . . . . . . . . . . . . . . . . . . . 70
bacon and tomato or creamy bacon (*Kraft* Reduced Calorie) . . . . . . . . 30
blue cheese:
(*Roka* Brand) . . . . . . . . . . . . . . . . . . . . . . . . . . . . . . . 60
(*Roka* Brand Reduced Calorie) . . . . . . . . . . . . . . . . . . . 16
(*S&W Nutradiet*) . . . . . . . . . . . . . . . . . . . . . . . . . . . . 25
chunky (*Kraft*) . . . . . . . . . . . . . . . . . . . . . . . . . . . . . . 60
chunky (*Kraft* Reduced Calorie) . . . . . . . . . . . . . . . . . . 30
chunky (*Wish-Bone*) . . . . . . . . . . . . . . . . . . . . . . . . . . . 75
chunky (*Wish-Bone* Lite) . . . . . . . . . . . . . . . . . . . . . . . . 40
buttermilk (*Hain* Old Fashioned) . . . . . . . . . . . . . . . . . . 70
buttermilk (*Seven Seas Buttermilk Recipe*) . . . . . . . . . . . . 80
buttermilk, creamy (*Kraft*) . . . . . . . . . . . . . . . . . . . . . . 80
buttermilk, creamy (*Kraft* Reduced Calorie) . . . . . . . . . . . 30
Caesar:
(*Lawry's* Classic), 1 oz. . . . . . . . . . . . . . . . . . . . . . . . . 130

| FOOD AND MEASURE | CALORIES |
|---|---|
| (*Weight Watchers*) | 4 |
| (*Wish-Bone*) | 77 |
| creamy (*Hain* Regular/Low Salt) | 60 |
| golden (*Kraft*) | 70 |
| canola oil citrus, French mustard, or Italian (*Hain*) | 50 |
| canola oil garden tomato vinaigrette (*Hain*) | 60 |
| Chinese vinegar w/sesame, ginger (*Lawry's* Classic), 1 oz. | 145 |
| coleslaw (*Kraft*) | 70 |
| cucumber, creamy (*Kraft*) | 70 |
| cucumber, creamy (*Kraft* Reduced Calorie) | 25 |
| cucumber dill (*Hain*) | 80 |
| Dijon mustard (*Great Impressions*) | 57 |
| Dijon vinaigrette (*Hain*) | 50 |
| Dijon vinaigrette (*Wish-Bone* Classic) | 60 |
| Dijon vinaigrette (*Wish-Bone* Lite Classic) | 30 |
| dill, creamy (*Nasoya Vegi-Dressing*) | 40 |
| French: | |
| (*Catalina*) | 60 |
| (*Catalina* Reduced Calorie) | 18 |
| (*Kraft*) | 60 |
| (*Kraft Miracle*) | 70 |
| (*Kraft* Reduced Calorie) | 20 |
| (*S&W Nutradiet*) | 18 |
| (*Wish-Bone* Deluxe) | 60 |
| (*Wish-Bone* Lite) | 31 |
| (*Wish-Bone* Lite Sweet'n Spicy) | 18 |
| (*Wish-Bone* Sweet'n Spicy) | 63 |
| creamy (*Hain*) | 60 |
| creamy (*Seven Seas*) | 60 |
| garlic (*Wish-Bone*) | 55 |
| nonfat (*Kraft Free*) | 20 |
| nonfat (*Kraft Free Catalina*) | 16 |
| red (*Wish-Bone* Lite) | 17 |
| style (*Weight Watchers*) | 10 |
| style (*Wish-Bone* Lite) | 30 |
| w/green pepper (*Great Impressions*) | 64 |
| garlic: | |
| creamy (*Kraft*) | 50 |
| creamy (*Wish-Bone*) | 74 |
| French (*Wish-Bone*) | 55 |

| FOOD AND MEASURE | CALORIES |
|---|---|
| *Salad dressing, garlic, continued* | |
| herb (*Nasoya Vegi-Dressing*) | 40 |
| and sour cream (*Hain*) | 70 |
| herb, savory (*Hain* No Salt Added) | 90 |
| herb and spice (*Seven Seas Viva*) | 60 |
| honey and sesame (*Hain*) | 60 |
| Italian: | |
| (*Hain* Traditional) | 80 |
| (*Hain* Traditional No Salt Added) | 60 |
| (*Kraft Presto*) | 70 |
| (*Nasoya Vegi-Dressing*) | 40 |
| (*Ott's*) | 80 |
| (*Seven Seas Viva*) | 50 |
| (*Wish-Bone*) | 46 |
| (*Wish-Bone* Lite) | 7 |
| (*Wish-Bone* Robusto) | 47 |
| blended (*Wish-Bone*) | 37 |
| w/bleu cheese (*Lawry's* Classic), 1 oz. | 186 |
| cheese vinaigrette (*Hain*) | 55 |
| w/cheese (*Wish-Bone*) | 89 |
| creamy (*Hain* Regular/No Salt Added) | 80 |
| creamy (*Kraft* Reduced Calorie) | 25 |
| creamy (*S&W/Nutradiet*) | 10 |
| creamy (*Seven Seas*) | 70 |
| creamy (*Weight Watchers*) | 50 |
| creamy (*Wish-Bone*) | 56 |
| creamy (*Wish-Bone* Lite) | 26 |
| creamy, w/real sour cream (*Kraft*) | 50 |
| herbal (*Wish-Bone* Classics) | 70 |
| house (*Kraft*) | 60 |
| house (*Kraft* Reduced Calorie) | 30 |
| oil-free (*Kraft* Reduced Calorie) | 4 |
| oil-free (*S&W/Nutradiet*) | 2 |
| nonfat (*Kraft Free*) | 6 |
| nonfat (*Seven Seas Free Viva*) | 4 |
| w/Parmesan cheese (*Lawry's* Classic), 1 oz. | 156 |
| style (*Weight Watchers*) | 6 |
| zesty (*Kraft*) | 50 |
| zesty (*Kraft* Reduced Calorie) | 20 |
| mayonnaise type (see also "Mayonnaise"): | |
| (*Bama*) | 50 |

| FOOD AND MEASURE | CALORIES |
|---|---|
| (*Miracle Whip*) | 70 |
| (*Miracle Whip* Light) | 45 |
| (*Spin Blend*) | 60 |
| cholesterol free (*Spin Blend*) | 40 |
| nonfat (*Kraft Free*) | 12 |
| whipped (*Weight Watchers*) | 45 |
| oil and vinegar (*Kraft*) | 70 |
| olive oil, Italian (*Wish-Bone* Classic) | 34 |
| olive oil vinaigrette (*Wish-Bone*) | 28 |
| olive oil vinaigrette (*Wish-Bone* Lite) | 16 |
| onion and chive (*Wish-Bone* Lite) | 37 |
| orange marmalade fruit salad (*Great Impressions*) | 87 |
| (*Ott's Famous*) | 40 |
| (*Ott's* Reduced Calorie *Famous*) | 26 |
| poppyseed (*Great Impressions*), 2 tbsp. | 131 |
| poppyseed (*Hain* Rancher's) | 60 |
| ranch: | |
| (*Seven Seas Viva*) | 80 |
| (*Wish-Bone*) | 78 |
| (*Wish-Bone* Lite) | 42 |
| creamy (*Rancher's Choice*) | 90 |
| creamy (*Rancher's Choice* Reduced Calorie) | 30 |
| creamy (*Weight Watchers*) | 25 |
| nonfat (*Kraft Free/Seven Seas Free*) | 16 |
| red wine vinaigrette (*Wish-Bone*) | 51 |
| red wine vinegar, w/Cabernet (*Lawry's* Classics), 1 oz. | 138 |
| red wine vinegar, nonfat (*Seven Seas Free*) | 6 |
| red wine vinegar and oil (*Seven Seas Viva*) | 70 |
| Russian: | |
| (*Kraft* Reduced Calorie) | 30 |
| (*S&W Nutradiet*) | 25 |
| (*Weight Watchers*) | 50 |
| (*Wish-Bone*) | 46 |
| (*Wish-Bone* Lite) | 22 |
| creamy or w/pure honey (*Kraft*) | 60 |
| San Francisco, w/Romano cheese (*Lawry's* Classic), 1 oz. | 136 |
| sesame garlic (*Nasoya Vegi-Dressing*) | 40 |
| Swiss cheese vinaigrette (*Hain*) | 60 |
| Thousand Island: | |
| (*Hain*) | 50 |
| (*Kraft*) | 60 |

| FOOD AND MEASURE | CALORIES |
|---|---|
| *Salad dressing, Thousand Island, continued* | |
| (*Kraft* Reduced Calorie) | 20 |
| (*S&W Nutradiet*) | 25 |
| (*Weight Watchers*) | 50 |
| (*Wish-Bone*) | 63 |
| (*Wish-Bone* Lite) | 36 |
| creamy (*Seven Seas*) | 50 |
| nonfat (*Kraft Free*) | 20 |
| Thousand Island and bacon (*Kraft*) | 60 |
| tomato vinaigrette (*Weight Watchers*) | 8 |
| vinegar and oil, balsamic vinegar (*Great Impressions*) | 67 |
| vinegar and oil, red wine vinegar (*Great Impressions*) | 64 |
| vinegar and oil, red wine vinegar (*Kraft*) | 60 |
| vinegar and oil, white wine vinegar (*Great Impressions*) | 63 |
| vintage, w/sherry wine (*Lawry's* Classic), 1 oz. | 110 |
| white wine, w/Chardonnay (*Lawry's* Classic), 1 oz. | 153 |

**Salad dressing mix:**

| | |
|---|---|
| dry, bacon (*Lawry's*), 1 pkg. | 65 |
| dry, Caesar (*Lawry's*), 1 pkg. | 75 |
| dry, Italian (*Lawry's*), 1 pkg. | 45 |
| dry, Italian, w/cheese (*Lawry's*), 1 pkg. | 74 |
| prepared, 1 tbsp.: | |
| all varieties, except buttermilk and ranch (*Good Seasons*) | 70 |
| all varieties, except ranch (*Good Seasons* Lite) | 25 |
| bleu cheese (*Hain* No Oil) | 14 |
| buttermilk (*Good Seasons* Farm Style) | 60 |
| buttermilk (*Hain* No Oil) | 11 |
| Caesar or garlic and cheese (*Hain* No Oil) | 6 |
| French or Thousand Island (*Hain* No Oil) | 12 |
| herb or Italian (*Hain* No Oil) | 2 |
| Italian (*Good Seasons* No Oil) | 6 |
| ranch (*Good Seasons*) | 60 |
| ranch (*Good Seasons* Lite) | 30 |

**Salad nuggets** (see also "Crouton"):

| | |
|---|---|
| garlic'n cheese (*Flavor Tree*), ¼ cup | 167 |
| oinion (*Flavor Tree*), ¼ cup | 163 |
| sesame (*Flavor Tree* Original Sesame), ¼ cup | 160 |

**Salad seasoning:**

| | |
|---|---|
| (*McCormick/Schilling* Salad Supreme), 1 tsp. | 11 |

| FOOD AND MEASURE | CALORIES |
|---|---|
| **Salami:** | |
| beef: | |
| (*Boar's Head*), 1 oz. | 60 |
| (*Hebrew National* Original Deli Style), 1 oz. | 80 |
| (*Hormel* Perma-Fresh), 2 slices | 50 |
| (*Kahn's*), 1 slice | 70 |
| (*Kahn's* Family Pack), 1 slice | 60 |
| (*Oscar Mayer* Machiaeh Brand), .8-oz. slice | 60 |
| beer (*Eckrich*), 1-oz. slice | 70 |
| beer (*Oscar Mayer* Salami for Beer), .8-oz. slice | 50 |
| beer, beef (*Oscar Mayer* Salami for Beer), .8-oz. slice | 63 |
| cooked (*Kahn's*), 1 slice | 60 |
| cotto: | |
| (*Eckrich*), 1 oz. slice | 70 |
| (*Hormel* Chub), 1 oz. | 100 |
| (*Hormel* Perma-Fresh), 2 slices | 105 |
| (*Kahn's* Family Pack), 1 slice | 45 |
| (*Light & Lean*), 2 slices | 80 |
| (*Oscar Mayer*), .8-oz. slice | 52 |
| (*Oscar Mayer*), .5-oz. slice | 34 |
| beef (*Eckrich*), 1.3 oz. | 100 |
| beef (*Oscar Mayer*), .8-oz. slice | 45 |
| beef (*Oscar Mayer*), .5-oz. slice | 29 |
| dry or hard (*Hormel/Hormel* Sliced), 1 oz. | 110 |
| dry or hard (*Hormel* National Brand), 1 oz. | 120 |
| dry or hard (*Hormel* Perma-Fresh), 2 slices | 80 |
| dry or hard (*Oscar Mayer* Hard), .3-oz. slice | 33 |
| Genoa (*Hormel/Hormel* Gran Valore), 1 oz. | 110 |
| Genoa (*Hormel DiLusso*), 1 oz. | 100 |
| Genoa (*Hormel* San Remo Brand), 1 oz. | 118 |
| Genoa (*Oscar Mayer*), .3-oz slice | 34 |
| (*Hormel* Party), 1 oz. | 90 |
| piccolo (*Hormel* Stick), 1 oz. | 120 |
| **"Salami," vegetarian,** frozen: | |
| roll (*Worthington*), 2 slices or 1.5 oz. | 90 |
| slices (*Worthington*), 2 slices or 1.3 oz. | 80 |
| **Salisbury steak,** see "Beef dinner" and "Beef entree" | |

| FOOD AND MEASURE | CALORIES |
|---|---|

## **Salmon,** canned:

| | |
|---|---|
| chum, keta (*Bumble Bee*), 1 cup | 306 |
| coho, Alaska (*Deming's*), ½ cup | 140 |
| pink: | |
| (*Bumble Bee*), 1 cup | 310 |
| (*Del Monte*), ½ cup | 160 |
| (*Libby's*), 7.75 oz. | 310 |
| Alaska (*Deming's*), ½ cup | 140 |
| blueback (*S&W/Nutradiet*), ½ cup | 188 |
| chunk, skinless, boneless, in water (*Deming's*), 3.25 oz. | 120 |
| red, w/liquid (*Del Monte*), ½ cup | 180 |
| red, sockeye: | |
| (*Bumble Bee*), 1 cup | 376 |
| (*Libby's*), 7.75 oz. | 380 |
| (*S&W/Nutradiet*), ½ cup | 188 |
| Alaska (*Deming's*), ½ cup | 170 |
| Alaska, medium (*Deming's*), ½ cup | 150 |
| blueback (*S&W* Fancy), ½ cup | 190 |

## **Salmon,** fresh, meat only:

| | |
|---|---|
| Atlantic, raw, 4 oz. | 160 |
| Chinook, raw, 4 oz. | 104 |
| Chinook, smoked or lox, 4 oz. | 133 |
| chum, raw, 4 oz. | 136 |
| coho, raw, 4 oz. | 165 |
| coho, boiled, poached, or steamed, 4 oz. | 210 |
| pink, raw, 4 oz. | 132 |
| sockeye, raw, 4 oz. | 191 |
| sockeye, baked, broiled, or microwaved, 4 oz. | 245 |

## **Salsa,** canned or in jars:

| | |
|---|---|
| brava (*La Victoria*), 1 tbsp. | 6 |
| burrito (*Del Monte*), ¼ cup | 20 |
| casera (*La Victoria*), 1 tbsp. | 4 |
| green chili: | |
| (*La Victoria*), 1 tbsp. | 3 |
| (*Old El Paso* Thick'n Chunky), 2 tbsp. | 3 |
| hot (*Ortega*), 1 oz. | 10 |
| mild (*Del Monte*), ¼ cup | 20 |
| mild or medium (*Ortega*), 1 oz. | 8 |
| green jalapeño (*La Victoria*), 1 tbsp. | 4 |

| FOOD AND MEASURE | CALORIES |
|---|---|
| hot (*Hain*)), ¼ cup | 22 |
| mild (*Hain*), ¼ cup | 20 |
| mild, medium, or hot (*Old El Paso* Thick'n Chunky), 2 tbsp. | 6 |
| mild or hot (*Enrico's* Chunky Style), 2 tbsp. | 8 |
| omelet (*La Victoria*), 1 tbsp. | 6 |
| picante (see also "Picante sauce"): | |
| (*La Victoria*), 1 tbsp. | 4 |
| (*Ortega*), 1 oz. | 10 |
| all styles (*Old El Paso*), 2 tbsp. | 10 |
| hot (*Del Monte*), ¼ cup | 20 |
| hot and chunky (*Del Monte*), ¼ cup | 15 |
| ranchera or red jalapeño (*La Victoria*), 1 tbsp. | 6 |
| ranchera (*Ortega*), 1 oz. | 12 |
| roja, mild (*Del Monte*), ¼ cup | 20 |
| suprema or Victoria (*La Victoria*), 1 tbsp. | 4 |
| taco, hot or mild (*Ortega*), 1 oz. | 10 |
| taco, mild (*Rosarita*), 2 oz. | 27 |
| Texas (*Hot Cha Cha*), 1 oz. | 6 |
| verde (*Old El Paso* Thick'n Chunky), 2 tbsp. | 10 |

## Salsify:

| FOOD AND MEASURE | CALORIES |
|---|---|
| raw, sliced, ½ cup | 55 |
| boiled, drained, sliced, ½ cup | 46 |

## Salt, 1 tsp.:

| FOOD AND MEASURE | CALORIES |
|---|---|
| plain | 0 |
| seasoned (see also specific listings): | |
| (*Lawry's*) | 4 |
| (*Lawry's* Hot 'n Spicy) | 3 |
| (*Lawry's* Lite) | 8 |
| (*McCormick/Schilling*) | 4 |
| (*McCormick/Schilling* Salt'n Spice) | 3 |
| (*Morton*) | 4 |
| (*Morton Nature's Seasons*) | 3 |

## Salt, substitute or imitation:

| FOOD AND MEASURE | CALORIES |
|---|---|
| (*Lawry's* Salt-Free 17), 1 tsp. | 10 |
| (*Morton*), 1 tsp. | <1 |
| regular or seasoned (*Featherweight*), ¼ tsp. | 0 |
| seasoned (*Health Valley Instead of Salt*), 1 tsp. | 11 |
| seasoned (*Lawry's Salt-Free*), 1 tsp. | 3 |
| seasoned (*Morton*), 1 tsp. | 2 |

| FOOD AND MEASURE | CALORIES |
|---|---|
| **Salt pork:** | |
| raw, 1 oz. | 212 |
| **Sandwich,** see specific listings | |
| **Sandwich sauce:** | |
| (*Hunt's Manwich*), 2.5 oz. | 40 |
| **Sandwich spread:** | |
| meat (*Oscar Mayer* Chub), 1 oz. | 67 |
| relish (*Hellman's/Best Foods*), 1 tbsp. | 50 |
| relish (*Kraft*), 1 tbsp. | 50 |
| **Sapodilla:** | |
| 1 medium, 3″ × 2½″ | 140 |
| **Sapote:** | |
| 1 medium, 11.2 oz. | 301 |
| **Sardine,** canned: | |
| Atlantic, in oil, drained, 2 oz. | 118 |
| brisling, in olive oil (*Underwood*), 3.75 oz. | 260 |
| Norway, in oil, w/liquid (*Empress*), 3.75-oz. can | 460 |
| Norway, in oil, drained (*Empress*), 3.75-oz. can | 260 |
| Norwegian brisling (*S&W*), 1.5 oz. | 130 |
| in mustard sauce (*Underwood*), 3.75 oz. | 220 |
| in oil (*Featherweight*), 1⅞ oz. | 130 |
| in sild oil (*Underwood*), 3.75 oz. | 460 |
| in soya oil, drained (*Underwood*), 3 oz. | 230 |
| w/*Tabasco*, drained (*Underwood*), 3 oz. | 220 |
| in tomato sauce (*Del Monte*), ½ cup | 360 |
| in tomato sauce (*Underwood*), 3.75 oz. | 220 |
| kippered (*Brunswick Kippered Snacks*), 3.5 oz. | 185 |
| **Sauerkraut,** canned, ½ cup: | |
| (*Claussen*) | 17 |
| (*Del Monte*) | 25 |
| (*Snow Floss*) | 28 |
| (*Stokely* Bavarian) | 30 |
| shredded (*Allens*) | 21 |
| shredded and chopped (*Stokely*) | 20 |

| FOOD AND MEASURE | CALORIES |
|---|---|
| **Sauerkraut juice:** | |
| (*S&W*), 5 fl. oz. | 14 |
| **Sausage** (see also "Sausage sticks," and specific listings): | |
| beef (*Jones Dairy Farm* Golden Brown), 1 link | 75 |
| beef and cheddar (*Hillshire Farm* Flavorseal), 2 oz. | 190 |
| brown and serve: | |
| (*Hormel*), 2 links | 140 |
| (*Jones Dairy Farm* Light), 1 link | 60 |
| (*Swift Premium* Country Recipe), 1 patty or link | 130 |
| (*Swift Premium* Microwave), 1 link | 120 |
| (*Swift Premium* Original), 1 link | 130 |
| (*Swift Premium* Original), 1 patty | 120 |
| beef or w/bacon (*Swift Premium*), 1 link | 120 |
| w/ham (*Swift Premium*), 1 link | 130 |
| maple or smoke-flavored (*Swift Premium*), 1 link | 120 |
| uncooked (*Hormel*), 2 links | 180 |
| country (*Hillshire Farm* Country Recipe), 2 oz. | 180 |
| heat 'n serve (*Eckrich* Lean Supreme), 2 links | 120 |
| hot or mild, canned (*Hormel*), 1 patty | 150 |
| minced roll (*Eckrich*), 1-oz. slice | 80 |
| pickled, firecracker (*Penrose*), 1.5-oz. link | 120 |
| pickled, firecracker, giant (*Penrose*), 2.1-oz. link | 170 |
| pickled, hot, red hot, Polish, beer, or firecracker (*Penrose*), .5-oz. link | 40 |
| pork: | |
| (*Hormel Little Sizzlers*), 2 links | 103 |
| (*Hormel* Midget Links), 2 links | 143 |
| (*Jones Dairy Farm*), 1 link | 140 |
| (*Jones Dairy Farm* Golden Brown Light), 1 link | 55 |
| (*Jones Dairy Farm* Light), 1 link | 70 |
| (*Oscar Mayer Little Friers*), 1 cooked link | 82 |
| fresh, cooked, 1 link or .5 oz. (1-oz. raw link) | 48 |
| fresh, cooked, 1 patty or 1 oz. (2-oz. raw patty) | 100 |
| mild or spicy (*Jones Dairy Farm* Golden Brown), 1 link | 100 |
| patty (*Jones Dairy Farm*), 1 patty | 155 |
| patty (*Jones Dairy Farm* Golden Brown), 1 patty | 155 |
| roll (*Jones Dairy Farm* Cello Roll), 1 slice | 105 |
| smoked: | |
| (*Eckrich* Lean Supreme), 1 oz. | 70 |
| (*Eckrich Lite*), 1 link | 150 |

| FOOD AND MEASURE | CALORIES |
|---|---|

*Sausage, smoked, continued*

| | |
|---|---|
| (*Eckrich Lite* Sausage Links), 1 link | 200 |
| (*Eckrich Lite Smok-Y-Links*), 2 links | 120 |
| (*Eckrich* Skinless), 1 link | 180 |
| (*Hillshire Farm* Bun Size), 2 oz. | 180 |
| (*Hillshire Farm* Flavorseal), 2 oz. | 190 |
| (*Hillshire Farm* Links), 2 oz. | 190 |
| (*Hillshire Farm* Lite), 2 oz. | 160 |
| (*Hormel* Smokies), 2 links | 160 |
| (*Oscar Mayer* Little Smokies), .3-oz. link | 27 |
| (*Oscar Mayer* Smokie Links), 1.5-oz. link | 126 |
| beef (*Eckrich*), 1 oz. | 100 |
| beef (*Eckrich* Lean Supreme), 1 oz. | 80 |
| beef (*Hillshire Farm* Bun Size/Flavorseal), 2 oz. | 180 |
| beef (*Oscar Mayer* Smokies), 1.5-oz. link | 124 |
| beef, cheese, or ham (*Eckrich Smok-Y-Links*), 2 links | 160 |
| cheddar (*Eckrich Lite* Sausage Links), 1 link | 190 |
| cheese (*Hormel* Smokie Cheezers), 2 links | 168 |
| cheese (*Oscar Mayer* Smokies), 1.5-oz. link | 126 |
| hot (*Eckrich Smok-Y-Links*), 2 links | 150 |
| hot (*Hillshire Farm* Flavorseal), 2 oz. | 180 |
| original or maple flavor (*Eckrich Smok-Y-Links*), 2 links | 160 |
| pork (*Hormel*), 3 oz. | 290 |
| pork and beef, 1 oz. | 95 |

## "Sausage," vegetarian:

| | |
|---|---|
| canned (*Worthington Saucettes*), 2 links | 140 |
| frozen: | |
| links (*Morningstar Farms* Breakfast Links), 3 links | 190 |
| links (*Worthington Prosage*), 3 links | 190 |
| patties (*Morningstar Farms* Breakfast Patties), 2 patties | 190 |
| patties (*Worthington Prosage*), 2 patties | 210 |
| roll (*Worthington Prosage*), 2 slices, 3/8" each | 180 |

## Sausage breakfast biscuit:

| | |
|---|---|
| frozen (*Swanson Great Starts* Breakfast On a Biscuit), 4.7 oz. | 410 |
| frozen (*Weight Watchers* Microwave), 3 oz. | 220 |
| refrigerated: | |
| (*Owens Border Breakfasts*), 2 oz. | 210 |
| egg and cheese (*Owens Border Breakfasts*), 2.5 oz. | 250 |
| smoked (*Owens Border Breakfasts*), 2 oz. | 200 |

| FOOD AND MEASURE | CALORIES |
|---|---|
| **Sausage breakfast taco,** refrigerated: | |
| (*Owens Border Breakfasts*), 2.17 oz. | 190 |
| **Sausage sticks** (see also "Beef jerky"), 1 stick, except as noted: | |
| beef, pepperoni (*Pemmican*), 1.1 oz. | 170 |
| beef, *Tabasco (Pemmican*), 1.1 oz. | 120 |
| beef teriyaki (*Pemmican*), 1.1 oz. | 150 |
| smoked: | |
| (*Slim Jim Big Slim*), .52 oz. | 80 |
| (*Slim Jim Giant Slim*), 1.1 oz. | 180 |
| (*Slim Jim Jumbo Jim*), 1 oz. | 150 |
| (*Slim Jim Super Slim/Super Slim* Tabasco), .7 oz. | 110 |
| all varieties (*Slim Jim* Handi-Paks), .31 oz. | 50 |
| nacho (*Slim Jim Super Slim*), .31 oz. | 40 |
| summer sausage, smoked (*Slim Jim*), .5 oz. | 80 |
| summer sausage, regular or teriyaki (*Pemmican*), .8 oz. | 110 |
| **Savory,** ground: | |
| 1 tsp. | 4 |
| **Scallion,** see "Onion, green" | |
| **Scallop,** mixed species, meat only: | |
| fresh, raw, 4 oz. | 100 |
| frozen, fried (*Mrs. Paul's*), 3 oz. | 160 |
| **"Scallop," vegetarian,** canned: | |
| (*Worthington Vegetable Skallops*), ½ cup | 90 |
| (*Worthington Vegetable Skallops* No Salt), ½ cup | 80 |
| **Scallop and shrimp dinner,** frozen: | |
| Mariner (*The Budget Gourmet*), 11.5 oz. | 320 |
| **Scotch whisky,** see "Liquor" | |
| **Scrapple:** | |
| (*Jones Dairy Farm*), 1 slice | 65 |
| **Scrod,** see "Cod" | |
| **Scrod entree,** frozen: | |
| baked (*Gorton's Microwave Entrees*), 1 pkg. | 320 |

| FOOD AND MEASURE | CALORIES |
|---|---|
| **Scup,** meat only, raw: | |
| raw, 4 oz. | 120 |
| **Sea bass,** meat only: | |
| raw, 4 oz. | 109 |
| baked, broiled, or microwaved, 4 oz. | 141 |
| **Sea trout,** meat only: | |
| raw, 4 oz. | 117 |
| **Seafood,** see specific listings | |
| **Seafood dinner,** frozen: | |
| w/natural herbs (*Armour Classics Lite*), 10 oz. | 190 |
| **Seafood entree,** frozen: | |
| casserole (*Pillsbury Microwave Classic*), 1 pkg. | 420 |
| combination platter, breaded (*Mrs. Paul's*), 9 oz. | 600 |
| creole, w/rice (*Swanson* Homestyle Recipe), 9 oz. | 240 |
| gumbo (*Cajun Cookin'*), 17 oz. | 330 |
| Newberg (*The Budget Gourmet*), 10 oz. | 350 |
| Newberg (*Healthy Choice*), 8 oz. | 200 |
| **Seafood sauce** (See also "Cocktail sauce"): | |
| (*Progresso* Authentic Pasta Sauces), ½ cup | 190 |
| creole (*Great Impressions*), 1 tbsp. | 21 |
| dipping (*Great Impressions*), 1 tbsp. | 17 |
| dipping, Polynesian (*Great Impressions*), 1 tbsp. | 38 |
| mixed (*Progresso*), ½ cup | 110 |
| **Seafood and crabmeat salad:** | |
| (*Longacre* Saladfest), 1 oz. | 45 |
| **Seaweed,** 1 oz.: | |
| agar, raw | 7 |
| agar, dried | 87 |
| kelp, raw | 12 |
| laver, raw | 10 |
| spirulina, raw | 8 |
| spirulina, dried | 82 |
| wakame, raw | 13 |

| FOOD AND MEASURE | CALORIES |
|---|---|
| **Semolina,** whole-grain: | |
| 1 cup | 602 |
| **Sesame butter** (see also "Tahini mix"): | |
| paste, from whole sesame seeds, 1 tbsp. | 95 |
| tahini, from raw, stone-ground kernels, 1 tbsp. | 86 |
| tahini, from unroasted kernels, 1 tbsp. | 85 |
| tahini, from roasted and toasted kernels, 1 tbsp. | 89 |
| tahini, organic (*Arrowhead Mills*), 1 oz. | 170 |
| **Sesame chips:** | |
| (*Flavor Tree*), ¼ cup | 163 |
| **Sesame meal:** | |
| partially defatted, 1 oz. | 161 |
| **Sesame nut mix:** | |
| dry roasted (*Planters*), 1 oz. | 160 |
| **Sesame seasoning:** | |
| all-purpose (*McCormick/Schilling Parsley Patch*), 1 tsp. | 15 |
| **Sesame seeds:** | |
| (*Spice Islands*), 1 tsp. | 9 |
| kernels, dried, 1 tsp. | 16 |
| kernels, dried (*Arrowhead Mills*), 1 oz. | 160 |
| roasted and toasted, 1 oz. | 161 |
| **Sesame sticks:** | |
| (*Flavor Tree*), ¼ cup | 133 |
| (*Flavor Tree* No Salt), ¼ cup | 131 |
| ***7-Eleven:*** | |
| *Big Bite*, 3.4 oz. | 287 |
| *Big Bite,* super, 5.4 oz. | 460 |
| burritos, 1 serving: | |
| bean and cheese, 10 oz. | 616 |
| beef and bean, 5 oz. | 308 |
| beef and bean, green chili, 10 oz. | 617 |
| beef and bean, red chili, 5 oz. | 308 |
| beef and bean, red hot, 5 oz. | 310 |
| beef and bean, red hot, 10 oz. | 620 |

| FOOD AND MEASURE | CALORIES |
|---|---|
| *7-Eleven, burritos, continued* | |
| beef and bean, red hot, premium, 5.2 oz. | 359 |
| beef, bean, and cheese, 5.2 oz. | 395 |
| beef and potato, 5.2 oz. | 394 |
| chicken and rice, premium, 5 oz. | 244 |
| chicken, breast of, 4.8 oz. | 405 |
| chimichanga, beef, 5 oz. | 363 |
| enchilada, beef and cheese, 6.5 oz. | 369 |
| fajitas, 5 oz. | 311 |
| sandito, ham and cheese, 5 oz. | 347 |
| sandito, pizza, 5 oz. | 345 |
| tacos, soft, twin, 5.9 oz. | 399 |
| Deli-Shoppe microwave products, 1 serving: | |
| bacon cheeseburger, 6 oz. | 558 |
| bagel and cream cheese, 4 oz. | 338 |
| char sandwich, large, 8.4 oz. | 713 |
| fish sandwich w/cheese, 5.2 oz. | 433 |
| sausage, red hot, large, 9.3 oz. | 845 |
| turkey, wedge, 3.4 oz. | 193 |

## **Shad,** American, meat only:

| | |
|---|---|
| raw, 4 oz. | 223 |

## ***Shakey's:***

| | |
|---|---|
| fried chicken (3 pieces) and potatoes | 947 |
| fried chicken (5 pieces) and potatoes | 1,700 |
| *Hot Ham and Cheese* | 550 |
| pizza, *Homestyle Pan Crust,* 1/10 of 12″ pie: | |
| cheese only | 303 |
| onion, green pepper, black olives, mushrooms | 320 |
| pepperoni | 343 |
| sausage, mushroom | 343 |
| sausage, pepperoni | 374 |
| *Shakey's Special* | 384 |
| pizza, thick crust, 1/10 of 12″ pie: | |
| cheese only | 170 |
| green pepper, black olives, mushrooms | 162 |
| pepperoni | 185 |
| sausage, mushrooms | 179 |
| sausage, pepperoni | 177 |
| *Shakey's Special* | 208 |

| FOOD AND MEASURE | CALORIES |
|---|---|
| pizza, thin crust, 1⁄10 of 12″ pie: | |
| cheese only | 133 |
| onion, green pepper, black olives, mushroom | 125 |
| pepperoni | 148 |
| sausage, mushroom | 141 |
| sausage, pepperoni | 166 |
| *Shakey's Special* | 171 |
| potatoes, 15 pieces | 950 |
| *Shakey's Super Hot Hero* | 810 |
| spaghetti, w/meat sauce and garlic bread | 940 |

**Shallots:**

| | |
|---|---|
| fresh, trimmed, 1 oz. | 20 |
| fresh, chopped, 1 tbsp. | 7 |
| freeze-dried, 1 tbsp. | 3 |

**Shark,** meat only:

| | |
|---|---|
| raw, 4 oz. | 148 |

**Sheepshead,** meat only:

| | |
|---|---|
| raw, 4 oz. | 123 |
| baked, broiled, or microwaved, 4 oz. | 143 |

**Shells, stuffed,** see "Pasta dinner" and "Pasta entree"

**Sherbert** (see also "Sorbet" and "Ice"):

| | |
|---|---|
| all flavors (*Sealtest*), ½ cup | 130 |
| orange (*Bordon*), ½ cup | 110 |
| rainbow (*Baskin-Robbins*), 1 regular scoop | 160 |

**Shortening,** vegetable:

| | |
|---|---|
| regular or butter flavor (*Crisco*), 1 tbsp. | 110 |

**Shrimp:**

| | |
|---|---|
| fresh, raw, 1 oz. or 4 large | 30 |
| fresh, boiled, poached, or steamed, 4 oz. | 112 |
| fresh, boiled, poached, or steamed, 4 large | 22 |
| canned, drained, 1 cup | 154 |
| canned, drained (*Louisiana Brand*), 2 oz. | 58 |
| frozen (*SeaPak* PDQ), 3.5 oz. | 60 |
| frozen, butterfly (*Gorton's* Specialty), 4 oz. | 160 |

| FOOD AND MEASURE | CALORIES |
|---|---|
| **Shrimp, imitation** (from surimi): | |
| 4 oz. | 115 |
| **Shrimp cocktail:** | |
| (*Sau-Sea*), 4 oz. | 113 |
| **Shrimp dinner,** frozen: | |
| baby bay (*Armour Classics Lite*), 9.75 oz. | 220 |
| Creole (*Armour Classics Lite*), 11.25 oz. | 260 |
| Creole (*Healthy Choice*), 11.25 oz. | 210 |
| marinara (*Healthy Choice*), 10.5 oz. | 220 |
| **Shrimp entree,** canned: | |
| chow mein (*La Choy* Bi-Pack), ¾ cup | 50 |
| **Shrimp entree,** frozen: | |
| 'n batter (*SeaPak*), 4 oz. | 260 |
| 'n batter, w/crabmeat stuffing (*SeaPak*), 4 oz. | 260 |
| breaded, butterfly (*SeaPak* Mikado), 4 oz. | 160 |
| breaded, butterfly/round (*SeaPak*), 4 oz. | 150 |
| and chicken Cantonese, w/noodles (*Lean Cuisine*), 10⅛ oz. | 270 |
| and clams, w/linguini (*Mrs. Paul's* Light), 10 oz. | 240 |
| Creole (*Cajun Cookin'*), 12 oz. | 390 |
| crisps (*Gorton's* Specialty), 4 oz. | 280 |
| crunchy, whole (*Gorton's* Microwave Specialty), 5 oz. | 380 |
| etouffee (*Cajun Cookin'*), 7 oz. | 360 |
| and fettuccine (*The Budget Gourmet*), 9.5 oz. | 375 |
| fettuccine Alfredo (*Booth*), 10 oz. | 260 |
| w/garlic butter sauce and vegetable rice (*Booth*), 10 oz. | 400 |
| heat and serve (*SeaPak Super Valu*), 4 oz. | 210 |
| jambalaya (*Cajun Cookin'*), 12 oz. | 450 |
| w/lobster sauce (*La Choy Fresh & Lite*), 10 oz. | 240 |
| New Orleans, w/wild rice (*Booth*), 10 oz. | 230 |
| Oriental, w/pineapple rice (*Booth*), 10 oz. | 190 |
| primavera (*Right Course*), 9⅝ oz. | 240 |
| primavera, w/fettuccine (*Booth*), 10 oz. | 200 |
| scampi (*Gorton's Microwave Entrees*), 1 pkg. | 390 |
| **Shrimp salad:** | |
| (*Longacre* Saladfest), 1 oz. | 45 |
| **Shrimp and seafood salad:** | |
| (*Longacre* Saladfest), 1 oz. | 42 |

| FOOD AND MEASURE | CALORIES |
|---|---|
| **Sisymbrium seed,** whole, dried: | |
| 1 oz. | 90 |
| **Sloppy Joe seasoning:** | |
| (*Lawry's* Seasoning Blends), 1 pkg. | 126 |
| mix (*French's*), ⅛ pkg. | 16 |
| mix (*McCormick/Schilling*), ¼ pkg. | 26 |
| **Smelt,** rainbow, meat only: | |
| raw, 4 oz. | 109 |
| baked, broiled, or microwaved, 4 oz. | 141 |
| **Snack chips** (see also specific chip listings): | |
| all flavors (*Great Snackers*), 1 pouch | 60 |
| **Snack mix** (see also specific listings): | |
| (*Eagle*), 1 oz. | 140 |
| (*Flavor Tree* Party Mix Regular/No Salt), ¼ cup | 163 |
| (*Pepperidge Farm* Classic), 1 oz. | 140 |
| (*Ralston Chex* Traditional), 1 oz. | 120 |
| (*Super Snax*), 1 oz. | 137 |
| cheddar, nacho, or sour cream-onion (*Ralston Chex*), 1 oz. | 130 |
| lightly smoked (*Pepperidge Farm*), 1 oz. | 150 |
| spicy (*Pepperidge Farm*), 1 oz. | 140 |
| **Snapper,** meat only: | |
| raw, 4 oz. | 113 |
| baked, broiled, or microwaved, 4 oz. | 145 |
| **Snow peas,** see "Peas, edible-podded" | |
| **Soft drinks and mixers,** 6 fl. oz., except as noted: | |
| all flavors (*Schweppes* Royal) | 35 |
| berry, red (*Shasta*) | 79 |
| berry, wild (*Health Valley*) | 71 |
| cherry, black (*Shasta*) | 81 |
| cherry cola (*Coca-Cola*) | 76 |
| cherry cola (*Pepsi* Wild Cherry) | 82 |
| cherry cola (*Shasta*) | 70 |
| cherry-lime (*Spree*) | 79 |
| chocolate (*Yoo-Hoo*), 9 fl. oz. | 140 |

| FOOD AND MEASURE | CALORIES |
|---|---|
| *Soft drinks and mixers, continued* | |
| citrus mist (*Shasta*) | 85 |
| club soda (all brands) | 0 |
| cola: | |
| (*Coca-Cola* Regular/Caffeine-free) | 77 |
| (*Coca-Cola* Classic) | 72 |
| (*Jolt*) | 85 |
| (*Pepsi* Regular/Caffeine-free) | 80 |
| (*Shasta*) | 74 |
| (*Shasta* Free) | 76 |
| (*Spree*) | 74 |
| collins mixer (*Canada Dry*), 8 fl. oz. | 80 |
| collins mixer (*Schweppes*) | 75 |
| collins mixer (*Shasta*) | 59 |
| cream (*A&W*) | 84 |
| cream (*Shasta* Creme) | 77 |
| diet/low-calorie, except as noted (all brands) | <3 |
| (*Dr Pepper* Regular/Caffeine-free) | 75 |
| fruit punch (*Shasta*) | 87 |
| ginger ale: | |
| (*Canada Dry*), 8 fl. oz. | 90 |
| (*Canada Dry* Golden), 8 fl. oz. | 100 |
| (*Fanta*) | 63 |
| (*Health Valley*) | 77 |
| (*Shasta*) | 60 |
| (*Spree*) | 60 |
| plain or raspberry (*Schweppes*) | 65 |
| ginger beer (*Schweppes*) | 70 |
| grape (*Canada Dry* Concord), 8 fl. oz. | 130 |
| grape (*Fanta*) | 86 |
| grape (*Schweppes*) | 95 |
| grape (*Shasta*) | 89 |
| grapefruit (*Schweppes*) | 80 |
| grapefruit (*Spree*) | 77 |
| grapefruit (*Wink*), 8 fl. oz. | 120 |
| half & half (*Canada Dry*), 8 fl. oz. | 110 |
| lemon, bitter (*Schweppes*) | 82 |
| lemon sour (*Schweppes*) | 79 |
| lemon-lime: | |
| (*Diet Slice*) | 8 |

| FOOD AND MEASURE | CALORIES |
|---|---|
| (*Schweppes*) | 72 |
| (*Shasta*) | 73 |
| (*Slice*) | 75 |
| (*Spree*) | 77 |
| lemon-tangerine (*Spree*) | 83 |
| lime, Mandarin (*Spree*) | 77 |
| (*Mello Yello*) | 87 |
| (*Mello Yello* Diet) | 3 |
| (*Mountain Dew*) | 90 |
| (*Mr. Pibb*) | 71 |
| orange: | |
| (*Diet Slice*) | 6 |
| (*Fanta*) | 88 |
| (*Minute Maid*) | 87 |
| (*Minute Maid* Diet) | 3 |
| (*Shasta*) | 89 |
| Mandarin (*Slice*) | 97 |
| sparkling (*Schweppes*) | 88 |
| pop, red (*Shasta*) | 79 |
| root beer: | |
| (*A&W*) | 90 |
| (*Fanta*) | 78 |
| (*Health Valley* Old Fashioned) | 60 |
| (*Mug*) | 84 |
| (*Ramblin'*) | 88 |
| (*Schweppes*) | 76 |
| (*Shasta*) | 77 |
| (*Spree*) | 77 |
| sarsaparilla root beer (*Health Valley*) | 77 |
| seltzer (all brands) | 0 |
| (*7-Up*) | 72 |
| (*7-Up* Cherry) | 74 |
| (*Sprite*) | 71 |
| strawberry (*Shasta*) | 74 |
| tonic (*Canada Dry*), 8 fl. oz. | 90 |
| tonic (*Schweppes*) | 64 |
| tonic (*Shasta*) | 61 |
| tropical blend (*Spree*) | 73 |
| vichy water (*Schweppes*) | 0 |
| whiskey sour mixer (*Canada Dry*), 8 fl. oz. | 90 |

| FOOD AND MEASURE | CALORIES |
|---|---|
| **Sole:** | |
| fresh, see "Flatfish" | |
| frozen (*Gorton's Fishmarket Fresh*), 5 oz. | 110 |
| frozen, Atlantic (*Booth*), 4 oz. | 90 |
| frozen, fillets (*Van de Kamp's* Natural), 4 oz. | 100 |
| **Sole dinner,** frozen: | |
| au gratin (*Healthy Choice*), 11 oz. | 270 |
| **Sole entree,** frozen: | |
| breaded (*Van de Kamp's* Light), 1 piece | 250 |
| in lemon butter (*Gorton's Microwave Entrees*), 1 pkg. | 380 |
| w/lemon butter sauce (*Healthy Choice*), 8.25 oz. | 230 |
| in wine sauce (*Gorton's Microwave Entrees*), 1 pkg. | 180 |
| **Sorbet** (see also "Sherbert" and "Ice"): | |
| orange, raspberry, or strawberry (*Dole*), 4 oz. | 110 |
| peach or pineapple (*Dole*), 4 oz. | 120 |
| raspberry (*Frusen Glädjé*), 4 fl. oz. | 140 |
| and cream, all varieties, except Key lime and raspberry sorbet (*Häagen-Dazs*), 4 fl. oz. | 190 |
| and cream, Key lime sorbet (*Häagen-Dazs*), 4 fl. oz. | 200 |
| and cream, raspberry sorbet (*Häagen-Dazs*), 4 fl. oz. | 180 |
| **Sorghum syrup:** | |
| 1 tbsp. | 53 |
| **Sorrel,** see "Dock" | |
| **Soup, canned, condensed**[1]**,** 8 oz., except as noted: | |
| asparagus, cream of (*Campbell's*) | 80 |
| barley and mushroom (*Rokeach*), 1 cup | 85 |
| bean (*Campbell's Homestyle*) | 130 |
| bean w/bacon (*Campbell's/Campbell's Special Request*) | 140 |
| beef (*Campbell's*) | 80 |
| beef broth or bouillon (*Campbell's*) | 16 |
| beef consomme w/gelatin (*Campbell's*) | 25 |
| beef noodle (*Campbell's*) | 70 |
| beef noodle (*Campbell's* Homestyle) | 80 |
| broccoli, cream of (*Campbell's*) | 80 |

[1]Prepared according to package directions, with water, except as noted.

| FOOD AND MEASURE | CALORIES |
|---|---|
| broccoli, cream of, prepared w/milk (*Campbell's*) | 140 |
| celery, cream of (*Campbell's*) | 100 |
| cheese, cheddar or nacho (*Campbell's*) | 110 |
| cheese, nacho, prepared w/milk (*Campbell's*) | 180 |
| chicken, cream of (*Campbell's/Campbell's Special Request*) | 110 |
| chicken alphabet (*Campbell's*) | 80 |
| chicken barley (*Campbell's*) | 70 |
| chicken broth (*Campbell's*) | 30 |
| chicken broth and noodles (*Campbell's*) | 45 |
| chicken and dumplings (*Campbell's* Chicken 'n Dumplings) | 80 |
| chicken gumbo (*Campbell's*) | 60 |
| chicken mushroom, creamy (*Campbell's*) | 120 |
| chicken noodle (*Campbell's*) | 60 |
| chicken noodle (*Campbell's* Homestyle/Noodle-O's) | 70 |
| chicken noodle (*Campbell's Special Request*) | 60 |
| chicken rice (*Campbell's/Campbell's Special Request*) | 60 |
| chicken and stars (*Campbell's*) | 60 |
| chicken vegetable (*Campbell's*) | 70 |
| chili beef (*Campbell's*) | 140 |
| clam chowder: | |
| Manhattan (*Campbell's*) | 70 |
| Manhattan (*Doxsee*), 7.5 oz. | 70 |
| Manhattan (*Snow's*), 7.5 oz. | 70 |
| New England (*Campbell's*) | 80 |
| New England, prepared w/milk (*Campbell's*) | 150 |
| New England, prepared w/milk (*Gorton's*), ¼ can | 140 |
| New England, prepared w/milk (*Snow's*), 7.5 oz. | 140 |
| corn chowder, prepared w/milk (*Snow's*), 7.5 oz. | 150 |
| fish chowder, prepared w/milk (*Snow's*), 7.5 oz. | 130 |
| minestrone (*Campbell's*) | 80 |
| mushroom, beefy (*Campbell's*) | 60 |
| mushroom, cream of (*Campbell's/Campbell's Special Request*) | 100 |
| mushroom, golden (*Campbell's*) | 70 |
| noodle, curly, w/chicken (*Campbell's*) | 80 |
| noodle and ground beef (*Campbell's*) | 90 |
| onion, cream of (*Campbell's*) | 100 |
| onion, cream of, prepared with water and milk (*Campbell's*) | 140 |
| onion, French (*Campbell's*) | 60 |
| oyster stew (*Campbell's*) | 70 |
| oyster stew, prepared w/milk (*Campbell's*) | 140 |
| pea, green (*Campbell's*) | 160 |

| FOOD AND MEASURE | CALORIES |
|---|---|
| *Soup, canned, condensed, continued* | |
| pea, split, w/egg barley (*Rokeach*), 1 cup | 132 |
| pea, split, w/ham and bacon (*Campbell's*) | 160 |
| pepper pot (*Campbell's*) | 90 |
| potato, cream of (*Campbell's*) | 80 |
| potato, cream of, prepared w/water and milk (*Campbell's*) | 120 |
| Scotch broth (*Campbell's*) | 80 |
| seafood chowder, prepared w/milk (*Snow's*), 7.5 oz. | 140 |
| shrimp, cream of (*Campbell's*) | 90 |
| shrimp, cream of, prepared w/milk (*Campbell's*) | 160 |
| stockpot, 1 cup | 100 |
| tomato (*Campbell's/Campbell's Special Request*) | 90 |
| tomato, prepared w/milk (*Campbell's/Campbell's Special Request*) | 150 |
| tomato, zesty (*Campbell's*) | 100 |
| tomato, cream of (*Campbell's* Homestyle) | 110 |
| tomato, cream of, prepared w/milk (*Campbell's* Homestyle) | 180 |
| tomato bisque (*Campbell's*) | 120 |
| tomato rice (*Campbell's* Old Fashioned) | 110 |
| turkey noodle or turkey vegetable (*Campbell's*) | 70 |
| vegetable (*Campbell's*) | 90 |
| vegetable (*Campbell's* Homestyle/Old Fashioned) | 60 |
| vegetable (*Campbell's Special Request*) | 90 |
| vegetable, vegetarian (*Campbell's*) | 80 |
| vegetable beef (*Campbell's/Campbell's Special Request*) | 70 |
| won ton (*Campbell's*) | 40 |

## Soup, canned, ready-to-serve:

| FOOD AND MEASURE | CALORIES |
|---|---|
| bean (*Grandma Brown's*), 1 cup | 190 |
| bean, black (*Health Valley*), 7.5 oz. | 160 |
| bean w/bacon and ham (*Campbell's* Microwave Soups), 7.5 oz. | 230 |
| bean w/ham: | |
| (*Campbell's* Chunky Old Fashioned), 11-oz. can | 290 |
| (*Campbell's* Chunky Old Fashioned), 9⅝ oz. | 250 |
| (*Campbell's* Home Cookin'), 10.75 oz. | 210 |
| (*Campbell's* Home Cookin'), 9.5 oz. | 180 |
| chowder (*Hormel Micro-Cup* Hearty Soups), 1 cont. | 191 |
| beef (*Campbell's* Chunky), 10.75 oz. | 200 |
| beef (*Campbell's* Chunky), 9.5 oz. | 170 |
| beef (*Progresso*), 10.5-oz. can | 180 |
| beef (*Progresso/Progresso* Hearty), 9.5 oz. | 160 |

| FOOD AND MEASURE | CALORIES |
|---|---|
| beef, Stroganoff style (*Campbell's* Chunky), 10.75-oz. can | 320 |
| beef, barley (*Progresso*), 10.5-oz. can | 150 |
| beef, barley (*Progresso*), 9.5 oz. | 140 |
| beef broth (*College Inn*), 1 cup | 18 |
| beef broth (*Health Valley* Regular/No Salt), 7.5 oz. | 17 |
| beef broth (*Swanson*), 7.25 oz. | 18 |
| beef broth, seasoned (*Progresso*), 4 oz. | 10 |
| beef minestrone (*Progresso*), 10.5-oz. can | 180 |
| beef minestrone or beef noodle (*Progresso*), 9.5 oz. | 170 |
| beef vegetable (*Hormel Micro-Cup* Hearty Soups), 1 cont. | 71 |
| beef vegetable (*Lipton Hearty Ones*), 11-oz. cont. | 229 |
| beef vegetable (*Progresso*), 10.5-oz. can | 170 |
| beef vegetable (*Progresso*), 9.5 oz. | 150 |
| beef w/vegetables, pasta (*Campbell's* Home Cookin'), 10.75 oz. | 140 |
| beef w/vegetables, pasta (*Campbell's* Home Cookin'), 9.5 oz. | 120 |
| berry fruit, three (*Great Impressions*), 6 oz. | 107 |
| blueberry fruit (*Great Impressions*), 6 oz. | 95 |
| borscht: | |
| (*Rokeach*), 1 cup | 96 |
| (*Rokeach Diet*), 1 cup | 29 |
| (*Rokeach* Unsalted), 1 cup | 103 |
| w/beets (*Manischewitz*), 1 cup | 80 |
| low calorie (*Manischewitz*), 1 cup | 20 |
| cherry fruit (*Great Impressions*), 6 oz. | 123 |
| chickarina (*Progresso*), 9.5 oz. | 130 |
| chicken: | |
| (*Campbell's* Chunky Old Fashioned), 10.75-oz. can | 180 |
| (*Campbell's* Chunky Old Fashioned), 9.5 oz. | 150 |
| (*Progresso* Homestyle), 9.5 oz. | 110 |
| hearty (*Progresso*), 10.5-oz. can | 130 |
| hearty (*Progresso*), 9.5 oz. | 130 |
| chicken, cream of (*Progresso*), 9.5 oz. | 190 |
| chicken barley (*Progresso*), 9.25 oz. | 100 |
| chicken broth: | |
| (*Campbell's* Low Sodium), 10.5 oz. | 30 |
| (*College Inn*), 1 cup | 35 |
| (*Hain*), 8.75 oz. | 70 |
| (*Hain* No Salt Added), 8.75 oz. | 60 |
| (*Health Valley*), 7.5 oz. | 35 |
| (*Progresso*), 4 oz. | 8 |

| FOOD AND MEASURE | CALORIES |
|---|---|
| *Soup, canned, ready-to-serve, chicken broth, continued* | |
| (*Swanson*), 7.25 oz. | 30 |
| (*Swanson* Natural Goodness), 7.25 oz. | 20 |
| chicken corn chowder (*Campbell's* Chunky), 10.75 oz. | 340 |
| chicken gumbo w/sausage (*Campbell's* Home Cookin'), 10.75 oz. | 140 |
| chicken gumbo w/sausage (*Campbell's* Home Cookin'), 9.5 oz. | 120 |
| chicken minestrone (*Campbell's* Home Cookin'), 10.75 oz. | 180 |
| chicken minestrone (*Campbell's* Home Cookin'), 9.5 oz. | 160 |
| chicken minestrone (*Progresso*), 10.5-oz. can | 140 |
| chicken minestrone (*Progresso*), 9.5 oz. | 130 |
| chicken mushroom, creamy (*Campbell's* Chunky), 10.5-oz. can | 270 |
| chicken mushroom, creamy (*Campbell's* Chunky), 9⅜ oz. | 240 |
| chicken noodle: | |
| (*Campbell's* Chunky), 10.75-oz. can | 200 |
| (*Campbell's* Chunky), 9.5 oz. | 180 |
| (*Campbell's* Microwave Soups), 7.5 oz. | 100 |
| (*Hain* Regular/No Salt Added), 9.5 oz. | 120 |
| (*Hormel Micro-Cup* Hearty Soups), 1 cont. | 108 |
| (*Lipton Hearty Ones* Homestyle), 11-oz. cont. | 227 |
| (*Progresso*), 10.5-oz. can | 120 |
| (*Progresso*), 9.5 oz. | 120 |
| (*Weight Watchers*), 10.5 oz. | 80 |
| chicken w/noodles (*Campbell's* Home Cookin'), 10.75-oz. can | 140 |
| chicken w/noodles (*Campbell's* Home Cookin'), 9.5 oz. | 110 |
| chicken w/noodles (*Campbell's* Low Sodium), 10.75 oz. | 170 |
| chicken nuggets w/vegetables and noodles (*Campbell's* Chunky), 10.75-oz. can | 190 |
| chicken nuggets w/vegetables and noodles (*Campbell's* Chunky), 9.5 oz. | 170 |
| chicken w/rice (*Campbell's* Chunky), 9.5 oz. | 140 |
| chicken w/rice (*Campbell's* Microwave Soups), 7.5 oz. | 100 |
| chicken rice (*Campbell's* Home Cookin'), 10.75 oz. | 150 |
| chicken rice (*Campbell's* Home Cookin'), 9.5 oz. | 130 |
| chicken rice (*Progresso*), 10.5-oz. can | 120 |
| chicken rice (*Progresso*), 9.5 oz. | 130 |
| chicken vegetable: | |
| (*Progresso*), 10.5 oz. | 150 |
| (*Progresso*), 9.5 oz. | 140 |
| chunky (*Campbell's* Chunky), 9.5 oz. | 170 |
| chunky (*Health Valley* Regular/No Salt Added), 7.5 oz. | 125 |
| country (*Campbell's* Home Cookin'), 10.75-oz. can | 120 |

| FOOD AND MEASURE | CALORIES |
|---|---|
| country (*Campbell's* Home Cookin'), 9.5 oz. | 110 |
| and rice (*Hormel Micro-Cup* Hearty Soups), 1 cont. | 114 |
| chili beef (*Campbell's* Chunky), 11-oz. can | 290 |
| chili beef (*Campbell's* Chunky), 9.75 oz. | 260 |
| chili beef (*Campbell's* Microwave), 7.5 oz. | 190 |
| clam chowder: | |
| Manhattan (*Campbell's* Chunky), 10.75-oz. can | 160 |
| Manhattan (*Campbell's* Chunky), 9.5 oz. | 150 |
| Manhattan (*Health Valley* Regular/No Salt), 7. 5 oz. | 110 |
| Manhattan (*Progresso*), 9.5 oz. | 120 |
| New England (*Campbell's* Chunky), 10.75-oz. can | 290 |
| New England (*Campbell's* Chunky), 9.5 oz. | 260 |
| New England (*Hain*), 9.25 oz. | 180 |
| New England (*Hormel Micro-Cup* Hearty Soups), 1 cont. | 118 |
| New England (*Progresso*), 10.5-oz. can | 220 |
| corn chowder (*Progresso*), 9.25 oz. | 200 |
| Creole style (*Campbell's* Chunky), 10.75 oz. | 240 |
| Creole style (*Campbell's* Chunky), 9.5 oz. | 220 |
| escarole, in chicken broth (*Progresso*), 9.25 oz. | 30 |
| gazpacho, 1 cup | 57 |
| ham and bean (*Progresso*), 9.5 oz. | 140 |
| ham and butter bean (*Campbell's* Chunky), 10.75-oz. can | 280 |
| lemon fruit (*Great Impressions*), 6 oz. | 90 |
| lentil: | |
| (*Health Valley* Regular/No Salt), 7.5 oz. | 170 |
| (*Progresso*), 9.5 oz. | 140 |
| hearty (*Campbell's* Home Cookin'), 10.75-oz. can | 170 |
| hearty (*Campbell's* Home Cookin'), 9.5 oz. | 140 |
| vegetarian (*Hain* Regular/No Salt Added), 9.5 oz. | 160 |
| lentil w/ham, 1 cup | 140 |
| lentil w/sausage (*Progresso*), 9.5 oz. | 170 |
| macaroni and bean (*Progresso*), 10.5-oz. can | 150 |
| macaroni and bean (*Progresso*), 9.5 oz. | 140 |
| minestrone: | |
| (*Campbell's* Chunky), 9.5 oz. | 160 |
| (*Campbell's* Home Cookin'), 10.75-oz. can | 140 |
| (*Campbell's* Home Cookin'), 9.5 oz. | 120 |
| (*Hain*), 9.5 oz. | 170 |
| (*Hain* No Salt Added), 9.5 oz. | 160 |
| (*Health Valley*), 7.5 oz. | 130 |
| (*Hormel Micro-Cup* Hearty Soups), 1 cont. | 104 |

| FOOD AND MEASURE | CALORIES |
|---|---|
| *Soup, canned, ready-to-serve, minestrone, continued* | |
| (*Lipton Hearty Ones*), 11-oz. cont. | 189 |
| (*Progresso*), 10.5-oz. can | 120 |
| hearty (*Progresso*), 9.25 oz. | 110 |
| zesty (*Progresso*), 9.5 oz. | 150 |
| mushroom, cream of (*Campbell's* Low Sodium), 10.5 oz. | 210 |
| mushroom, cream of (*Progresso*), 9.25 oz. | 160 |
| mushroom, cream of (*Weight Watchers*), 10.5 oz. | 90 |
| mushroom, creamy (*Hain*), 9.25 oz. | 110 |
| mushroom barley (*Hain*), 9.5 oz. | 100 |
| mushroom barley (*Health Valley*), 7.5 oz. | 100 |
| pea, split: | |
| (*Campbell's* Low Sodium), 10.5 oz. | 230 |
| (*Grandma Brown's*), 1 cup | 208 |
| (*Hain* Regular/No Salt Added), 9.5 oz. | 170 |
| green (*Health Valley*), 7.5 oz. | 190 |
| green (*Progresso*), 10.5-oz. can | 201 |
| green (*Progresso*), 9.5 oz. | 160 |
| pea, split, w/ham: | |
| (*Campbell's* Chunky), 10.75-oz. can | 230 |
| (*Campbell's* Chunky), 9.5 oz. | 210 |
| (*Campbell's* Home Cookin'), 10.75-oz. can | 230 |
| (*Campbell's* Home Cookin'), 9.5 oz. | 200 |
| (*Progresso*), 10.5-oz. can | 160 |
| (*Progresso*), 9.5 oz. | 150 |
| pepper steak (*Campbell's* Chunky), 10.75-oz. can | 180 |
| pepper steak (*Campbell's* Chunky), 9.5 oz. | 160 |
| potato leek (*Health Valley*), 7.5 oz. | 130 |
| shav (*Gold's*), 8 oz. | 25 |
| sirloin burger (*Campbell's* Chunky), 10.75-oz. can | 220 |
| sirloin burger (*Campbell's* Chunky), 9.5 oz. | 200 |
| steak and potato (*Campbell's* Chunky), 10.75-oz. can | 200 |
| steak and potato (*Campbell's* Chunky), 9.5 oz. | 170 |
| tomato: | |
| (*Health Valley*), 7.5 oz. | 100 |
| (*Progresso*), 9.5 oz. | 120 |
| garden (*Campbell's* Home Cookin'), 10.75-oz. can | 150 |
| garden (*Campbell's* Home Cookin'), 9.5 oz. | 130 |
| w/tomato pieces (*Campbell's* Low Sodium), 10.5 oz. | 190 |
| w/tortellini (*Progresso*), 9.25 oz. | 130 |
| tomato beef w/rotini (*Progresso*), 9.5 oz. | 170 |

| FOOD AND MEASURE | CALORIES |
|---|---|
| tortellini (*Progresso*), 9.5 oz. | 90 |
| tortellini, creamy (*Progresso*), 9.25 oz. | 240 |
| turkey rice (*Hain*), 9.5 oz. | 100 |
| turkey rice (*Hain* No Salt Added), 9.5 oz. | 120 |
| turkey vegetable (*Campbell's* Chunky), 9⅜ oz. | 150 |
| turkey vegetable (*Weight Watchers*), 10.5 oz. | 70 |
| vegetable: | |
| (*Campbell's* Chunky), 10.75-oz. can | 160 |
| (*Campbell's* Chunky), 9.5 oz. | 150 |
| (*Health Valley*), 7.5 oz. | 110 |
| (*Progresso*), 9.5 oz. | 80 |
| w/beef stock (*Weight Watchers*), 10.5 oz. | 90 |
| country (*Campbell's* Home Cookin'), 9.5 oz. | 100 |
| country (*Hormel Micro-Cup* Hearty Soups), 1 cont. | 89 |
| five-bean, chunky (*Health Valley*), 7.5 oz. | 110 |
| Mediterranean (*Campbell's* Chunky), 9.5 oz. | 170 |
| vegetarian (*Hain*), 9.5 oz. | 140 |
| vegetarian (*Hain* No Salt Added), 9.5 oz. | 150 |
| vegetarian, chunky (*Weight Watchers*), 10.5 oz. | 100 |
| vegetable beef: | |
| (*Campbell's* Chunky Old Fashioned), 10.75-oz. can | 190 |
| (*Campbell's* Chunky Old Fashioned), 9.5 oz. | 160 |
| (*Campbell's* Home Cookin'), 10.75-oz. can | 140 |
| (*Campbell's* Home Cookin'), 9.5 oz. | 120 |
| (*Campbell's* Microwave Soups), 7.5 oz. | 100 |
| chunky (*Campbell's* Low Sodium), 10.75 oz. | 180 |
| vegetable broth (*Hain*), 9.5 oz. | 45 |
| vegetable broth (*Hain* Low Sodium), 9.5 oz. | 40 |
| vegetable chicken (*Hain*), 9.5 oz. | 120 |
| vegetable chicken (*Hain* No Salt Added), 9.5 oz. | 130 |
| vegetable pasta, Italian (*Hain*), 9.5 oz. | 160 |
| vegetable pasta, Italian (*Hain* Low Sodium), 9.5 oz. | 140 |

## **Soup,** frozen:

| FOOD AND MEASURE | CALORIES |
|---|---|
| asparagus, cream of (*Kettle Ready*), 6 fl. oz. | 62 |
| asparagus, cream of (*Myers*), 9.75 oz. | 152 |
| barley and bean (*Tabatchnick*), 7.5 oz. | 130 |
| bean, black, w/ham (*Kettle Ready*), 6 fl. oz. | 154 |
| bean, northern (*Tabatchnick*), 7.5 oz. | 164 |
| bean, savory, w/ham (*Kettle Ready*), 6 fl. oz. | 113 |
| beef vegetable, hearty (*Kettle Ready*), 6 fl. oz. | 85 |

| FOOD AND MEASURE | CALORIES |
|---|---|
| *Soup, frozen, continued* | |
| broccoli, cream of (*Kettle Ready*), 6 fl. oz. | 94 |
| broccoli, cream of (*Myers*), 9.75 oz. | 174 |
| broccoli, cream of (*Tabatchnick*), 7.5 oz. | 90 |
| cabbage (*Tabatchnick*), 7.5 oz. | 110 |
| cauliflower, cream of (*Kettle Ready*), 6 fl. oz. | 93 |
| cheddar, cream of (*Kettle Ready*), 6 fl. oz. | 158 |
| cheddar and broccoli, cream of (*Kettle Ready*), 6 fl. oz. | 137 |
| cheese and broccoli (*Myers*), 9.75 oz. | 325 |
| chicken (*Tabatchnick*), 7.5 oz. | 65 |
| chicken, cream of (*Kettle Ready*), 6 fl. oz. | 98 |
| chicken gumbo or noodle (*Kettle Ready*), 6 fl. oz. | 94 |
| chicken noodle (*Myers*), 9.75 oz. | 87 |
| chili, traditional (*Kettle Ready*), 6 fl. oz. | 161 |
| chili, jalapeño (*Kettle Ready*), 6 fl. oz. | 173 |
| clam chowder: | |
| Boston (*Kettle Ready*), 6 fl. oz. | 131 |
| Manhattan (*Kettle Ready*), 6 fl. oz. | 69 |
| New England (*Kettle Ready*), 6 fl. oz. | 116 |
| New England (*Myers*), 9.75 oz. | 152 |
| New England (*Stouffer's*), 8 oz. | 180 |
| corn and broccoli chowder (*Kettle Ready*), 6 fl. oz. | 102 |
| lentil (*Tabatchnick*), 7.5 oz. | 170 |
| minestrone (*Tabatchnick*), 7.5 oz. | 137 |
| minestrone, hearty (*Kettle Ready*), 6 fl. oz. | 104 |
| mushroom, cream of (*Kettle Ready*), 6 fl. oz. | 85 |
| mushroom, cream of (*Tabatchnick*), 7.5 oz. | 75 |
| mushroom barley (*Tabatchnick*), 7.5 oz. | 92 |
| mushroom barley (*Tabatchnick* No Salt), 7.5 oz. | 97 |
| onion, French (*Kettle Ready*), 6 fl. oz. | 42 |
| pea (*Tabatchnick* Regular/No Salt), 7.5 oz. | 175 |
| pea, split, w/ham (*Kettle Ready*), 6 fl. oz. | 155 |
| pea, tortellini, in tomato (*Kettle Ready*), 6 fl. oz. | 122 |
| seafood bisque (*Myers*), 9.75 oz. | 163 |
| spinach, cream of (*Myers*), 9.75 oz. | 174 |
| spinach, cream of (*Stouffer's*), 8 oz. | 210 |
| spinach, cream of (*Tabatchnick*), 7.5 oz. | 85 |
| tomato rice (*Tabatchnick*), 7.5 oz. | 73 |
| vegetable (*Tabatchnick*), 7.5 oz. | 97 |
| vegetable (*Tabatchnick* No Salt), 7.5 oz. | 92 |
| vegetable, garden (*Kettle Ready*), 6 fl. oz. | 85 |

| FOOD AND MEASURE | CALORIES |
|---|---|
| vegetable beef (*Myers*), 9.75 oz. | 120 |
| zucchini (*Tabatchnick*), 7.5 oz. | 80 |

**Soup mix**[1], 6 fl. oz., except as noted:

| | |
|---|---|
| all varieties (*Campbell's* Cup 2 Minute Soup) | 90 |
| beef or beef flavor: | |
| (*Lipton Cup-A-Soup*) | 44 |
| broth or bouillon, 1 cup | 19 |
| hearty, and noodles (*Lipton*), 7 fl. oz. | 107 |
| noodle (*Campbell's* Cup Microwave), 1 pkg. | 130 |
| noodle (*Campbell's* Ramen Noodle), 1 cup | 190 |
| noodle, w/vegetables (*Campbell's* Cup-A-Ramen), 1 cup | 270 |
| noodle, w/vegetables, low fat (*Campbell's* Cup-A-Ramen), 1 cup | 220 |
| broccoli, creamy (*Lipton Cup-A-Soup*) | 62 |
| broccoli, creamy, and cheese (*Lipton Cup-A-Soup*) | 70 |
| broccoli, golden (*Lipton Cup-A-Soup* Lite) | 42 |
| cheddar, creamy, w/noodles (*Fantastic Noodles*), 7 oz. | 178 |
| cheese (*Hain* Savory Soup & Sauce Mix) | 250 |
| cheese and broccoli (*Hain* Soup & Recipe Mix) | 310 |
| chicken or chicken flavor: | |
| broth (*Lipton Cup-A-Soup*) | 20 |
| cream of (*Lipton Cup-A-Soup*) | 84 |
| creamy, w/vegetables (*Lipton Cup-A-Soup*) | 93 |
| w/sweet corn (*Lipton Cup-A-Soup* Country Style) | 133 |
| Florentine (*Lipton Cup-A-Soup* Lite) | 42 |
| hearty (*Lipton Cup-A-Soup* Country Style) | 69 |
| hearty, supreme (*Lipton Cup-A-Soup*) | 107 |
| lemon (*Lipton Cup-A-Soup* Lite) | 48 |
| noodle (*Campbell's* Cup Microwave), 1 pkg. | 140 |
| noodle (*Campbell's* Quality Soup & Recipe), 1 cup | 100 |
| noodle (*Campbell's* Ramen Noodle), 1 cup | 190 |
| noodle (*Lipton*), 1 cup | 81 |
| noodle (*Lipton Cup-A-Soup*) | 48 |
| noodle (*Mrs. Grass* Chickeny Rich), ¼ pkg. | 70 |
| noodle, hearty (*Lipton*), 1 cup | 83 |
| noodle, hearty (*Lipton Lots-A-Noodles Cup-A-Soup*), 7 fl. oz. | 110 |
| noodle, hearty, creamy (*Lipton Lots-A-Noodles Cup-A-Soup*), 7 fl. oz. | 179 |

[1]Prepared according to package directions, with water, except as noted.

| FOOD AND MEASURE | CALORIES |
|---|---|
| *Soup mix, chicken or chicken flavor, continued* | |
| noodle, w/meat (*Lipton Cup-A-Soup*) | 46 |
| noodle, w/white meat, diced (*Lipton*), 1 cup | 81 |
| noodle, w/vegetables (*Campbell's* Cup-A-Ramen), 1 cup | 270 |
| noodle, w/vegetables, hearty (*Lipton*), 1 cup | 75 |
| noodle, w/vegetables, low fat (*Campbell's* Cup-A-Ramen), 1 cup | 220 |
| 'n rice (*Lipton Cup-A-Soup*) | 47 |
| supreme (*Lipton Cup-A-Soup* Country Style) | 107 |
| vegetable (*Lipton Cup-A-Soup*) | 47 |
| clam chowder, Manhattan (*Golden Dipt*), ¼ pkg. dry | 80 |
| clam chowder, New England (*Golden Dipt*), ¼ pkg. dry | 70 |
| lentil (*Hain* Savory Soup Mix) | 130 |
| lobster bisque (*Golden Dipt*), ¼ pkg. dry | 30 |
| minestrone (*Hain* Savory Soup Mix) | 110 |
| minestrone (*Manischewitz*) | 50 |
| mushroom: | |
| (*Estee Instant*), 6 oz. | 40 |
| (*Hain* Savory Soup & Recipe Mix) | 210 |
| (*Hain* Savory Soup & Recipe Mix No Salt Added) | 250 |
| beef flavor (*Lipton*), 1 cup | 38 |
| cream of (*Lipton Cup-A-Soup*) | 71 |
| noodle: | |
| (*Campbell's* Quality Soup & Recipe), 1 cup | 110 |
| (*Lipton Cup-A-Soup* Ring Noodle) | 47 |
| beef (*Cup O'Noodles*) 1 cup | 290 |
| beef flavor (*Oodles of Noodles/Top Ramen*), 1 cup | 390 |
| beefy, hearty, w/vegetables (*Lipton*), 1 cup | 85 |
| chicken (*Cup O'Noodles*), 1 cup | 300 |
| chicken (*Oodles of Noodles/Top Ramen*), 1 cup | 400 |
| chicken, country (*Cup O'Noodles* Hearty), 1 cup | 300 |
| w/chicken broth (*Campbell's* Cup Microwave), 1 pkg. | 130 |
| w/chicken broth (*Lipton Giggle Noodle*), 1 cup | 77 |
| w/chicken broth (*Lipton Ring-O-Noodle*), 1 cup | 71 |
| hearty (*Campbell's* Quality Soup and Recipe), 1 cup | 90 |
| hearty, w/vegetables (*Campbell's* Cup Microwave), 1 pkg. | 180 |
| hearty, w/vegetables (*Lipton*), 1 cup | 75 |
| Oriental or pork (*Oodles of Noodles/Top Ramen*), 1 cup | 390 |
| seafood, savory (*Cup O'Noodles* Hearty), 1 cup | 300 |
| shrimp (*Cup O'Noodles*), 1 cup | 300 |

| FOOD AND MEASURE | CALORIES |
|---|---|
| vegetable, beef or old-fashioned (*Cup O'Noodles* Hearty), 1 cup | 290 |
| onion: | |
| (*Campbell's* Quality Soup & Recipe), 1 cup | 30 |
| (*Hain* Savory Soup, Dip & Recipe Mix Regular/No Salt) | 50 |
| (*Lipton*), 1 cup | 20 |
| (*Lipton Cup-A-Soup*) | 27 |
| (*Mrs. Grass* Soup & Dip Mix), ¼ pkg. | 35 |
| beefy (*Lipton*), 1 cup | 29 |
| creamy (*Lipton Cup-A-Soup*) | 70 |
| golden, w/chicken broth (*Lipton*), 1 cup | 62 |
| mushroom (*Lipton*), 1 cup | 41 |
| Oriental: | |
| (*Lipton Cup-A-Soup* Lite) | 45 |
| noodle (*Campbell's* Ramen Noodle), 1 cup | 190 |
| noodle, w/vegetables (*Campbell's* Cup-A-Ramen), 1 cup | 270 |
| noodle, w/vegetables, low fat (*Campbell's* Cup-A-Ramen), 1 cup | 220 |
| pea, green (*Lipton Cup-A-Soup*) | 113 |
| pea, split (*Hain* Savory Soup Mix) | 310 |
| pea, split (*Manischewitz*) | 45 |
| pea, Virginia (*Lipton Cup-A-Soup* Country Style) | 148 |
| pork flavor noodle (*Campbell's* Ramen Noodle), 1 cup | 200 |
| potato leek (*Hain* Savory Soup Mix) | 260 |
| seafood chowder (*Golden Dipt*), ¼ pkg. dry | 70 |
| shrimp bisque (*Golden Dipt*), ¼ pkg. dry | 30 |
| shrimp flavor, w/noodles (*Campbell's* Cup-A-Ramen), 1 cup | 280 |
| shrimp flavor, w/noodles, low fat (*Campbell's* Cup-A-Ramen), 1 cup | 230 |
| tomato (*Hain* Savory Soup & Recipe Mix) | 220 |
| tomato (*Lipton Cup-A-Soup*) | 103 |
| tomato, creamy, and herb (*Lipton Cup-A-Soup* Lite) | 66 |
| vegetable: | |
| (*Campbell's* Quality Soup and Recipe), 1 cup | 40 |
| (*Hain* Savory Soup Mix Regular/No Salt Added) | 80 |
| (*Lipton*), 1 cup | 39 |
| (*Manischewitz*) | 50 |
| country (*Lipton*), 1 cup | 80 |
| curry, w/noodles (*Fantastic Noodles*), 7 oz. | 150 |
| garden (*Lipton Lots-A-Noodles Cup-A-Soup*), 7 fl. oz. | 123 |
| harvest (*Lipton Cup-A-Soup* Country Style) | 91 |

| FOOD AND MEASURE | CALORIES |
|---|---|
| *Soup mix, vegetable, continued* | |
| miso, w/noodles (*Fantastic Noodles*), 7 oz. | 152 |
| noodle w/meatballs (*Lipton Cup-A-Soup* Country Style) | 95 |
| spring (*Lipton Cup-A-Soup*) | 33 |
| tomato, w/noodles (*Fantastic Noodles*), 7 oz. | 158 |
| **Sour cream,** see "Cream, sour" | |
| **Sour cream sauce mix:** | |
| (*McCormick/Schilling*), ¼ pkg. | 44 |
| **Sour cream and onion snack sticks:** | |
| (*Flavor Tree*), ¼ cup | 127 |
| **Soursop:** | |
| 1 medium, 2.1 lb. | 416 |
| **Souse loaf:** | |
| (*Kahn's*), 1 slice | 90 |
| **Soy beverage** (see also "Soy milk"): | |
| (*Soy Moo*), 1 cup | 125 |
| almond or vanilla malted (*Westbrae Natural*), 6 fl. oz. | 250 |
| carob, chocolate, or vanilla (*Ah Soy*), 6 fl. oz. | 160 |
| carob or java malted (*Westbrae Natural*), 6 fl. oz. | 270 |
| **Soy flour,** see "Flour" | |
| **Soy meal:** | |
| defatted, raw, 1 cup | 414 |
| **Soy milk:** | |
| fluid, 8 fl. oz. | 79 |
| powder (*Soyamel*), 8 fl. oz. | 130 |
| **Soy protein:** | |
| concentrate, 1 oz. | 94 |
| **Soy sauce:** | |
| (*Kikkoman*), 1 tbsp. | 10 |
| (*Kikkoman* Lite), 1 tbsp. | 11 |
| (*La Choy/La Choy* Lite), 1 tsp. | <1 |

| FOOD AND MEASURE | CALORIES |
|---|---|

**Soybean:**

green, raw, in pods, 1 lb. .................... 353
green, raw, shelled, ½ cup .................... 188
green, boiled, drained, ½ cup .................... 127
dried, uncooked, ½ cup .................... 387
dried, boiled, ½ cup .................... 149
dried, dry-roasted, ½ cup .................... 387
dried, roasted, ½ cup .................... 405
fermented or paste, see "Miso" and Natto"

**Soybean, sprouted,** mature seeds:

raw, ½ cup .................... 45
raw, 10 sprouts, .4 oz. .................... 12
steamed, ½ cup .................... 38

**Soybean cake or curd,** see "Tofu"

**Soybean flakes:**

(*Arrowhead Mills*), 2 oz. .................... 250

**Soybean kernels,** roasted and toasted:

whole kernels, 1 cup .................... 490

**Spaghetti dinner,** frozen:

and meatballs (*Banquet*), 10 oz. .................... 290
and meatballs (*Morton*), 10 oz. .................... 200
and meatballs (*Swanson*), 12.5 oz. .................... 390

**Spaghetti dishes,** mix, prepared:

(*Kraft* Mild American Dinner), 1 cup .................... 300
w/meat sauce (*Kraft* Dinner), 1 cup .................... 360
tangy (*Kraft* Italian Style Dinner), 1 cup .................... 310

**Spaghetti entree,** canned:

in tomato sauce, w/cheese (*Franco-American*), 7⅜ oz. .................... 180
in tomato cheese sauce (*Franco-American* SpaghettiO's), 7.5 oz. .. 170
w/franks (*Franco-American* SpaghettiO's), 7⅜ oz. .................... 220
w/franks (*Van Camp's Spaghettee Weenee*), 1 cup .................... 240
and meatballs:
(*Chef Boyardee* Microwave), 7.5 oz. .................... 230
(*Estee*), 7.5 oz. .................... 240
(*Featherweight*), 7.5 oz. .................... 160

| FOOD AND MEASURE | CALORIES |
|---|---|
| *Spaghetti entree, canned, and meatballs, continued* | |
| in sauce (*Buitoni*), 7.5 oz. | 190 |
| in tomato sauce (*Franco-American*), 7⅜ oz. | 220 |
| in tomato sauce (*Franco-American* SpaghettiO's), 7⅜ oz. | 220 |
| **Spaghetti entree,** frozen: | |
| w/beef (*Dining Lite*), 9 oz. | 220 |
| w/beef and mushroom sauce (*Lean Cuisine*), 11.5 oz. | 280 |
| w/beef sauce and mushrooms (*Le Menu* LightStyle), 9 oz. | 280 |
| w/Italian meatballs (*Swanson* Homestyle Recipe), 13 oz. | 490 |
| w/meat sauce: | |
| (*Banquet* Casserole), 8 oz. | 270 |
| (*Freezer Queen* Single Serve), 10 oz. | 350 |
| (*Healthy Choice*), 10 oz. | 310 |
| (*Stouffer's*), 12⅞ oz. | 370 |
| (*Weight Watchers*), 10.5 oz. | 280 |
| w/meatballs (*Stouffer's*), 12⅝ oz. | 380 |
| **Spaghetti sauce,** see "Pasta sauce" | |
| **Spaghetti squash,** see "Squash" | |
| **Spaghettini entree,** packaged: | |
| (*Hormel Top Shelf*), 1 serving | 240 |
| **Spice loaf:** | |
| (*Kahn's* Family Pack), 1 slice | 70 |
| beef (*Kahn's* Family Pack), 1 slice | 60 |
| **Spinach:** | |
| fresh, raw, untrimmed, 1 lb. | 73 |
| fresh, raw, trimmed, 1 oz. or ½ cup chopped | 6 |
| fresh, boiled, drained, ½ cup | 21 |
| canned, ½ cup: | |
| (*Allens/Allens* Low Sodium) | 28 |
| (*Featherweight*) | 35 |
| (*S&W* Premium Northwest) | 25 |
| (*Stokely*) | 30 |
| whole or chopped (*Del Monte* Regular/No Salt Added) | 25 |
| frozen: | |
| (*Green Giant Harvest Fresh/Green Giant* Polybag), ½ cup | 25 |
| whole (*Birds Eye* Portion Pack), 3.2 oz. | 20 |

| FOOD AND MEASURE | CALORIES |
|---|---|
| whole or chopped (*Birds Eye*), 3.3 oz. | 20 |
| whole or chopped (*Southern*), 3.5 oz. | 25 |
| creamed (*Birds Eye* Combinations), 3 oz. | 60 |
| creamed (*Green Giant*), ½ cup | 70 |
| creamed (*Stouffer's*), 4.5 oz. | 170 |
| in butter sauce, cut (*Green Giant*), ½ cup | 40 |

**Spinach, mustard,** see "Mustard spinach"

**Spinach, New Zealand,** see "New Zealand spinach"

**Spinach au gratin,** frozen:

| | |
|---|---|
| (*The Budget Gourmet*), 6 oz. | 120 |

**Spinach soufflé,** frozen:

| | |
|---|---|
| (*Stouffer's*), 4 oz. | 140 |

**Spiny lobster,** meat only

| | |
|---|---|
| raw, 4 oz. | 127 |

**Spleen:**

| | |
|---|---|
| beef, braised, 4 oz. | 164 |
| lamb, braised, 4 oz. | 177 |
| pork, braised, 4 oz. | 169 |
| veal, braised, 4 oz. | 146 |

**Split peas:**

| | |
|---|---|
| raw, green (*Arrowhead Mills*), 2 oz. | 200 |
| boiled, ½ cup | 116 |

**Spot,** meat only, raw:

| | |
|---|---|
| raw, 4 oz. | 140 |

**Sprouts,** see "Bean sprouts" and specific listings

**Squash,** canned:

| | |
|---|---|
| sliced, ½ cup | 14 |
| yellow, cut (*Allens*), ½ cup | 16 |
| zucchini, Italian-style (*Progresso*), ½ cup | 50 |
| zucchini, in tomato juice, 4 oz. or ½ cup | 33 |
| zucchini, in tomato sauce (*Del Monte*), ½ cup | 30 |

| FOOD AND MEASURE | CALORIES |
|---|---|
| **Squash,** fresh: | |
| acorn, baked, cubed, ½ cup | 57 |
| acorn, boiled, mashed, ½ cup | 41 |
| banana, baked (*Frieda* of California), 4 oz. | 72 |
| butternut, raw, cubed, ½ cup | 32 |
| butternut, baked, cubed, ½ cup | 41 |
| crookneck, raw, sliced, ½ cup | 12 |
| crookneck, boiled, drained, sliced, ½ cup | 18 |
| hubbard, baked, cubed, ½ cup | 51 |
| hubbard, boiled, drained, mashed, ½ cup | 35 |
| marrow, raw, trimmed, 1 oz. | 4 |
| scallop, boiled, drained, sliced, ½ cup | 14 |
| scallop, boiled, drained, mashed, ½ cup | 19 |
| spaghetti, raw, cubed, ½ cup | 17 |
| spaghetti, baked or boiled, drained, ½ cup | 23 |
| zucchini, raw, untrimmed, 1 lb. | 62 |
| zucchini, raw, sliced, ½ cup | 9 |
| zucchini, boiled, drained, sliced, ½ cup | 14 |
| zucchini, boiled, drained, mashed, ½ cup | 19 |
| **Squash,** frozen: | |
| butternut, boiled, drained, mashed, ½ cup | 47 |
| crookneck, yellow (*Seabrook*), 3.3 oz. | 18 |
| crookneck, yellow (*Southern*), 3.5 oz. | 21 |
| winter, cooked (*Birds Eye*), 4 oz. | 45 |
| winter, cooked (*Seabrook*), 4 oz. | 45 |
| zucchini (*Seabrook*), 3.3 oz. | 16 |
| zucchini (*Southern*), 3.5 oz. | 18 |
| zucchini, breaded (*Stilwell Quickkrisp*), 3.3 oz. | 200 |
| **Squid,** meat only: | |
| raw, 4 oz. | 104 |
| dried, 1 oz. | 86 |
| dipped in flour, fried in oil, 4 oz. | 198 |
| **Star fruit,** see "Carambola" | |
| **Steak sauce,** 1 tbsp., except as noted: | |
| (*A.1*) | 12 |
| (*Estee*) | 15 |
| (*French's*) | 25 |
| (*Heinz 57*) | 17 |

| FOOD AND MEASURE | CALORIES |
| --- | --- |
| (*Heinz* Traditional) | 12 |
| (*Lea & Perrins*), 1 oz. | 40 |
| (*Steak Supreme*) | 20 |

**Steak seasoning:**

| | |
| --- | --- |
| blackened (*Tone's*), 1 tsp. | 9 |
| broiled (*McCormick/Schilling* Spice Blends), ¼ tsp. | <1 |

**Stir-fry sauce:**

| | |
| --- | --- |
| (*Kikkoman*), 1 tsp. | 6 |
| (*Lawry's*), ¼ cup | 120 |

**Stomach:**

| | |
| --- | --- |
| pork, raw, 1 oz. | 44 |

**Strawberry:**

| | |
| --- | --- |
| fresh, trimmed, ½ cup | 23 |
| canned, in heavy syrup, ½ cup | 117 |
| frozen: | |
| unsweetened, ½ cup | 26 |
| sweetened, whole, ½ cup | 100 |
| sweetened, sliced, ½ cup | 123 |
| in lite syrup, whole (*Birds Eye*), 4 oz. | 80 |
| in lite syrup, halves (*Birds Eye* Quick Thaw Pouch), 5 oz. | 90 |
| in syrup, halves (*Birds Eye* Quick Thaw Pouch), 5 oz. | 120 |

**Strawberry cobbler,** frozen:

| | |
| --- | --- |
| (*Pet-Ritz*), ⅙ pkg. | 290 |

**Strawberry danish:**

| | |
| --- | --- |
| (*Awrey's* Round), 4.5 oz. | 400 |
| miniature (*Awrey's*), 1.7 oz. | 160 |

**Strawberry flavor milk drink,** see "Milk beverages, flavored"

**Strawberry fruit snack:**

| | |
| --- | --- |
| roll (*Flavor Tree*), 1 roll | 74 |
| yogurt coated (*Sunkist Fun Fruits* Creme Supremes), 1 pouch | 114 |

**Strawberry juice drink:**

| | |
| --- | --- |
| (*Tang* Fruit Box), 8.45 fl. oz. | 120 |

**Strawberry nectar:**

| | |
| --- | --- |
| (*Libby's*), 6 fl. oz. | 110 |

| FOOD AND MEASURE | CALORIES |
| --- | --- |
| **Strawberry syrup:** | |
| (*S&W*), 1 tsp. | 4 |
| **Strawberry yogurt dessert,** frozen: | |
| (*Sara Lee Free & Light*), 1/10 pkg. | 120 |
| **String bean,** see "Beans, green" | |
| **Stroganoff entree mix,** vegetarian: | |
| creamy, prepared w/tofu (*Tofu Classics*), ½ cup | 94 |
| creamy, prepared w/tofu and butter (*Tofu Classics*), ½ cup | 127 |
| **Stroganoff sauce mix:** | |
| (*Lawry's*), 1 pkg. | 123 |
| prepared (*Natural Touch*), 4 oz. | 90 |
| **Stuffing,** 1 oz.: | |
| all varieties, except country style, country garden herb, and wild rice and mushroom (*Pepperidge Farm* Distinctive) | 110 |
| corn (*Brownberry*) | 103 |
| country style (*Pepperidge Farm*) | 100 |
| herb (*Brownberry*) | 100 |
| herb, country garden (*Pepperidge Farm* Distinctive) | 120 |
| wild rice and mushroom (*Pepperidge Farm* Distinctive) | 130 |
| **Stuffing,** frozen, ½ cup: | |
| chicken or cornbread (*Green Giant Stuffing Originals*) | 170 |
| mushroom (*Green Giant Stuffing Originals*) | 150 |
| wild rice (*Green Giant Stuffing Originals*) | 160 |
| **Stuffing mix:** | |
| dry: | |
| (*Croutettes*), .7 oz. | 70 |
| Cajun style (*Golden Dipt*), ¼ cup | 40 |
| cheddar and French (*Golden Dipt*), ¼ cup | 80 |
| chicken (*Betty Crocker*), 1/6 pkg. | 110 |
| herb, traditional (*Betty Crocker*), 1/6 pkg. | 110 |
| prepared, ½ cup: | |
| all varieties (*Golden Grain*) | 180 |
| beef or chicken flavor (*Stove Top*) | 180 |
| broccoli and cheese (*Stove Top* Microwave) | 170 |
| chicken flavor (*Betty Crocker*) | 180 |

| FOOD AND MEASURE | CALORIES |
|---|---|
| chicken flavor (*Stove Top* Flexible Serving) | 170 |
| chicken flavor (*Stove Top* Microwave) | 160 |
| cornbread or herb, savory (*Stove Top*) | 170 |
| cornbread (*Stove Top* Flexible Serving) | 180 |
| cornbread, homestyle (*Stove Top* Microwave) | 160 |
| herb, homestyle (*Stove Top* Flexible Serving) | 170 |
| herb, traditional (*Betty Crocker*) | 190 |
| long grain and wild rice or w/rice (*Stove Top*) | 180 |
| mushroom and onion (*Stove Top*) | 180 |
| mushroom and onion (*Stove Top* Microwave) | 170 |
| pork (*Stove Top/Stove Top* Flexible Serving) | 170 |
| San Francisco style (*Stove Top Americana*) | 170 |
| turkey (*Stove Top*) | 170 |

**Sturgeon,** meat only:

| | |
|---|---|
| raw, 4 oz. | 120 |
| baked, broiled, or microwaved, 4 oz. | 153 |
| smoked, 4 oz. | 196 |

**Sturgeon roe,** see "Caviar"

**Succotash:**

| | |
|---|---|
| fresh, boiled, drained, ½ cup | 111 |
| canned, w/whole-kernel corn, w/liquid | 81 |
| canned, w/cream-style corn | 102 |
| canned (*S&W* Country Style) | 80 |
| canned (*Stokely*) | 90 |
| frozen (*Seabrook*), 3.3 oz. | 100 |

**Sucker,** white, meat only:

| | |
|---|---|
| raw, 4 oz. | 104 |

**Suet,** beef:

| | |
|---|---|
| raw, 1 oz. | 242 |

**Sugar, beet or cane:**

| | |
|---|---|
| brown, 1 cup, not packed | 541 |
| brown, 1 cup, packed | 821 |
| cane baton (*Frieda* of California), 1 oz. | 21 |
| granulated, 1 cup | 770 |
| granulated, 1 tbsp. | 46 |
| granulated, 1 tsp. | 15 |

| FOOD AND MEASURE | CALORIES |
|---|---|
| *Sugar, beet or cane, continued* | |
| powdered or confectioners, 1 cup, unsifted | 462 |
| powdered or confectioners, 1 cup, sifted | 385 |
| powdered or confectioners, 1 tbsp., unsifted | 31 |
| **Sugar, dextrous:** | |
| anhydrous, 1 oz. | 104 |
| crystallized, 1 oz. | 95 |
| **Sugar, maple:** | |
| 1 oz. | 99 |
| **Sugar, substitute:** | |
| (*Equal*), 1 pkt. | 4 |
| (*Sprinkle Sweet*), 1 tsp. | 2 |
| (*Sweet 'n Low*), 1 pkt. | 4 |
| (*Weight Watchers* Sweet'ner), 1 pkt. | 4 |
| saccharin (*Featherweight*), ¼ grain tablet | 0 |
| **Sugar, turbinado:** | |
| (*Hain*), 1 tbsp. | 50 |
| **Sugar apple:** | |
| 1 medium, 2⅞" × 3¼" | 146 |
| trimmed, ½ cup | 118 |
| **Sugar cane juice:** | |
| 1 oz. | 21 |
| **Sugar snap peas,** see "Peas, edible-podded" | |
| **Summer sausage** (see also "Thuringer cervelat"): | |
| (*Eckrich*), 1-oz. slice | 80 |
| (*Hillshire Farm*), 2 oz. | 180 |
| (*Hormel* Perma-Fresh), 2 slices | 140 |
| (*Hormel* Tangy Chub/Thuringer), 1 oz. | 90 |
| (*Lean & Lite*), 1 oz. | 43 |
| (*Light & Lean*), 2 slices | 100 |
| (*Oscar Mayer*), .8-oz. slice | 69 |
| beef (*Hillshire Farm*), 2 oz. | 190 |
| beef (*Hormel* Beefy), 1 oz. | 100 |
| beef (*Oscar Mayer*), .8-oz. slice | 70 |
| w/cheese (*Hillshire Farm*), 2 oz. | 200 |

| FOOD AND MEASURE | CALORIES |
|---|---|

**Sunfish,** pumpkinseed, meat only:

| | |
|---|---|
| raw, 4 oz. | 101 |

**Sunflower seed,** kernels:

| | |
|---|---|
| dried (*Arrowhead Mills*), 1 oz. | 160 |
| dry-roasted, 1 oz. | 165 |
| dry-roasted (*Flavor House*), 1 oz. | 180 |
| oil-roasted or toasted, 1 oz. | 175 |

**Sunflower seed butter:**

| | |
|---|---|
| 1 tbsp. | 93 |

**Surimi:**

| | |
|---|---|
| from walleye pollock, 4 oz. | 112 |

**Surinam cherry,** see "Pitanga"

**Swamp cabbage:**

| | |
|---|---|
| raw, trimmed, 1 oz. or ½ cup chopped | 6 |
| boiled, drained, chopped, ½ cup | 10 |

**Sweet potato:**

| | |
|---|---|
| fresh, raw, 1 medium, 5″ × 2″ diam. | 136 |
| fresh, baked in skin, 1 medium, 5″ × 2″ diam. | 118 |
| fresh, boiled w/out skin, mashed, ½ cup | 172 |
| candied, 4 oz. | 155 |
| canned, ½ cup: | |
| in water, cut (*Allens*) | 70 |
| in light syrup (*Joan of Arc/Princella/Royal Prince*) | 110 |
| in syrup, whole and cut (*Allens*) | 90 |
| in syrup, whole and cut (*Taylor's Brand*) | 120 |
| in heavy syrup (*Joan of Arc/Princella/Royal Prince*) | 130 |
| in extra heavy syrup (*S&W* Southern) | 139 |
| in pineapple-orange sauce (*Joan of Arc/Princella/Royal Prince*) | 210 |
| candied (*Joan of Arc/Princella/Royal Prince*) | 240 |
| candied (*S&W*) | 180 |
| mashed (*Joan of Arc/Princella/Royal Prince*) | 90 |
| vacuum pack, whole (*Taylor's Brand*) | 105 |
| frozen, candied (*Mrs. Paul's*), 4 oz. | 170 |
| frozen, w/apples (*Mrs. Paul's* Sweets 'n Apples), 4 oz. | 160 |

| FOOD AND MEASURE | CALORIES |
|---|---|
| **Sweet potato leaf:** | |
| raw, chopped, ½ cup | 6 |
| steamed, ½ cup | 11 |
| **Sweet and sour drink mix:** | |
| liquid (*Holland House*), 1 fl. oz. | 34 |
| **Sweet and sour sauce:** | |
| (*Kikkoman*), 1 tbsp. | 18 |
| (*La Choy*), 1 tbsp. | 30 |
| (*Lawry's*), ¼ cup | 549 |
| (*Sauceworks*), 1 tbsp. | 25 |
| duck sauce (*La Choy*), 1 tbsp. | 26 |
| regular, hot, or Hawaiian (*Great Impressions*), 2 tbsp. | 102 |
| **Sweetbreads,** see "Pancreas" and "Thymus" | |
| **Sweetsop,** see "Sugar apple" | |
| **Swiss chard:** | |
| raw, chopped, ½ cup | 3 |
| boiled, drained, chopped, ½ cup | 18 |
| **Swiss steak,** see "Beef dinner, frozen" | |
| **Swordfish,** meat only: | |
| fresh, raw, 4 oz. | 137 |
| fresh, baked, broiled, or microwaved, 4 oz. | 176 |
| **Syrup** (see also specific listings): | |
| (*Weight Watchers* Reduced Calorie), 1 tbsp. | 25 |
| **Szechwan sauce:** | |
| hot and spicy (*La Choy*), 1 oz. | 48 |

# T

| FOOD AND MEASURE | CALORIES |
|---|---|
| **Tabbouleh mix:** | |
| (*Fantastic Foods*), prepared w/oil and tomatoes, ½ cup | 161 |
| (*Near East*), prepared, ½ cup | 170 |
| salad (*Casbah*), 1 oz. dry | 126 |
| ***Taco Bell:*** | |
| burrito: | |
| bean, 7.3 oz. | 447 |
| beef, 7.3 oz. | 493 |
| chicken, 6 oz. | 334 |
| combination, 7 oz. | 407 |
| *Supreme,* 9 oz. | 503 |
| taco: | |
| regular, 2.75 oz. | 183 |
| regular, soft, 3.25 oz. | 225 |
| *Bellgrande,* 5.7 oz. | 335 |
| chicken, 3 oz. | 171 |
| chicken, soft, 3.8 oz. | 213 |
| steak, soft, 3.5 oz. | 218 |
| *Supreme,* 3.25 oz. | 230 |
| *Supreme,* soft, 4.4 oz. | 272 |
| tostada, w/red sauce, 5.5 oz. | 243 |
| tostada, chicken, w/red sauce, 5.8 oz. | 264 |
| specialty items: | |
| chilito, 5.5 oz. | 383 |
| cinnamon twists, 1.2 oz. | 171 |
| *Enchirito,* w/red sauce, 7.5 oz. | 382 |
| *Meximelt,* 3.7 oz. | 266 |
| *Meximelt,* chicken, 3.8 oz. | 257 |
| nachos, 3.7 oz. | 346 |
| nachos *Bellgrande,* 10.1 oz. | 649 |
| nachos *Supreme,* 5.1 oz. | 367 |
| pintos and cheese, w/red sauce, 4.5 oz. | 190 |
| pizza, Mexican, 7.9 oz. | 575 |
| taco salad, 21 oz. | 905 |
| taco salad, w/out shell, 18.3 oz. | 484 |

| FOOD AND MEASURE | CALORIES |
|---|---|
| *Taco Bell, continued* | |
| side orders and condiments: | |
| green sauce, 1 oz. | 4 |
| guacamole, .75 oz. | 34 |
| jalapeño peppers, 3.5 oz. | 20 |
| nacho cheese, 2 oz. | 103 |
| pico de gallo, .7 oz. | 6 |
| ranch dressing, 2.6 oz. | 236 |
| red sauce, 1 oz. | 10 |
| salsa, .34 oz. | 18 |
| sour cream, .75 oz. | 46 |
| taco sauce, 1 pkt. | 2 |
| taco sauce, hot, 1 pkt. | 3 |

## Taco dip:

| | |
|---|---|
| (*Hain* Dip and Sauce), 4 tbsp. | 25 |
| (*Wise*), 2 tbsp. | 12 |

## *Taco John's:*

| | |
|---|---|
| apple grande, 3 oz. | 257 |
| beans, refried, 9.5 oz. | 331 |
| burrito: | |
| bean, 5 oz. | 249 |
| beef, 5 oz. | 355 |
| combo, 5 oz. | 302 |
| smothered, w/green chili, 12.3 oz. | 405 |
| smothered, w/Texas chili, 12.3 oz. | 518 |
| super, 8.3 oz. | 434 |
| chili, Texas, 9.5 oz. | 430 |
| chimi, 12 oz. | 487 |
| churro, 1.2 oz. | 122 |
| enchilada, 7 oz. | 379 |
| nachos, 4 oz. | 407 |
| nachos, super, 11.25 oz. | 657 |
| *Potato Ole Large,* 6 oz. | 414 |
| taco, regular, 4.3 oz. | 228 |
| taco, soft shell, 5 oz. | 276 |
| taco burger, 6 oz. | 332 |
| taco *Bravo,* super, 8 oz. | 485 |
| taco salad, super, 12.3 oz. | 450 |
| tostada, 4.3 oz. | 228 |

| FOOD AND MEASURE | CALORIES |
|---|---|
| **Taco mix:** | |
| (*Old El Paso*), 1 taco | 67 |
| vegetarian (*Natural Touch*), 2 tbsp. | 90 |
| **Taco salad seasoning:** | |
| (*Lawry's* Seasoning Blends), 1 pkg. | 124 |
| **Taco salad shell:** | |
| flour (*Azteca*), 1 piece | 200 |
| **Taco sauce** (see also "Salsa"): | |
| (*Estee*), 2 tbsp. | 14 |
| (*Lawry's* Sauce'n Seasoner), ¼ cup | 40 |
| (*Old El Paso* Cans), 2 tbsp. | 15 |
| chunky (*Lawry's*), ¼ cup | 22 |
| green (*La Victoria*), 1 tbsp. | 4 |
| hot or mild (*Del Monte*), ¼ cup | 15 |
| hot or mild (*Ortega*), 1 oz. | 12 |
| hot, medium, or mild (*Old El Paso* Jars), 2 tbsp. | 10 |
| mild (*Enrico's* No Salt Added), 2 tbsp. | 14 |
| mild or medium (*Heinz*), 1 tbsp. | 6 |
| red (*La Victoria*), 1 tbsp. | 6 |
| red, mild (*El Molino*), 2 tbsp. | 10 |
| western style (*Ortega*), 1 oz. | 8 |
| **Taco seasoning mix:** | |
| (*Hain*), 1/10 pkg. | 10 |
| (*Lawry's* Seasoning Blends), 1 pkg. | 118 |
| (*McCormick/Schilling*), ¼ pkg. | 31 |
| (*Old El Paso*), 1/12 pkg. | 8 |
| (*Tio Sancho*), 1.51 oz. | 132 |
| meat (*Ortega*), 1 oz. | 90 |
| meat (*Ortega*), 1 oz. prepared | 60 |
| **Taco shell,** 1 piece, except as noted: | |
| (*Gebhardt*) | 30 |
| (*Lawry's*) | 50 |
| (*Lawry's* Super) | 86 |
| (*Old El Paso*) | 55 |
| (*Old El Paso* Super Size) | 100 |
| (*Ortega*) | 50 |

| FOOD AND MEASURE | CALORIES |
|---|---|
| *Taco shell, continued* | |
| (*Rosarita*) | 45 |
| (*Tio Sancho*) | 64 |
| (*Tio Sancho* Super) | 94 |
| corn (*Azteca*) | 60 |
| miniature (*Old El Paso*), 3 pieces | 70 |
| **Taco starter:** | |
| (*Del Monte*), 8 oz. | 140 |
| **Tahini,** see "Sesame butter" | |
| **Tahini mix:** | |
| (*Casbah*), 1 oz. dry | 25 |
| **Tamale:** | |
| canned: | |
| (*Old El Paso*), 2 pieces | 190 |
| (*Wolf* Brand), 1 scant cup | 350 |
| beef (*Gebhardt*), 4 oz. | 230 |
| beef (*Hormel/Hormel* Hot'N Spicy), 2 pieces | 140 |
| w/sauce (*Van Camp's*), 1 cup | 290 |
| frozen, beef (*Hormel*), 1 piece | 140 |
| **Tamale dinner,** frozen: | |
| (*Patio*), 13 oz. | 470 |
| **Tamalito,** canned: | |
| in chili gravy (*Dennison's*), 7.5 oz. | 310 |
| **Tamarind:** | |
| 1 tamarind, 3″ × 1″ | 5 |
| ½ cup | 144 |
| **Tangerine:** | |
| fresh, 1 medium, 2⅜″ diam. | 37 |
| fresh, sections, w/out membrane, ½ cup | 43 |
| canned: | |
| (*Del Monte* Mandarin orange), 5½ oz. | 100 |
| (*S&W* Natural Style), ½ cup | 60 |
| in water (*Featherweight* Mandarin Orange), ½ cup | 35 |
| in juice, ½ cup | 46 |

| FOOD AND MEASURE | CALORIES |
|---|---|
| in light syrup (*Dole*), ½ cup | 76 |
| in light syrup (*Empress*), 5½ oz. | 100 |
| in heavy syrup (*S&W*), ½ cup | 76 |
| unsweetened (*S&W/Nutradiet*), ½ cup | 28 |

**Tangerine juice,** 6 fl. oz.:

| | |
|---|---|
| fresh, 6 fl. oz. | 80 |
| canned, sweetened, 6 fl. oz. | 94 |
| chilled (*Dole Pure & Light* Mandarin Tangerine), 6 fl. oz. | 97 |
| chilled or frozen, diluted (*Minute Maid*), 6 fl. oz. | 91 |

**Tapioca,** pearl, dry:

| | |
|---|---|
| 1 oz. | 97 |
| ¼ cup | 130 |

**Taro:**

| | |
|---|---|
| raw, sliced, ½ cup | 56 |
| cooked, sliced, ½ cup | 94 |

**Taro, Tahitian:**

| | |
|---|---|
| raw, trimmed, sliced, ½ cup | 25 |
| cooked, sliced, ½ cup | 30 |

**Taro chips:**

| | |
|---|---|
| ½ cup | 57 |
| snack (*Ray's*), 1 oz. | 139 |

**Taro leaf:**

| | |
|---|---|
| raw, ½ cup | 6 |
| steamed, ½ cup | 18 |

**Taro shoots:**

| | |
|---|---|
| raw, 1 shoot, 15½" × 1⅛" diam. | 9 |
| raw, sliced, ½ cup | 5 |
| cooked, sliced, ½ cup | 10 |

**Tarpon,** Atlantic, meat only:

| | |
|---|---|
| raw, 4 oz. | 105 |

**Tarragon,** ground:

| | |
|---|---|
| 1 tsp. | 5 |

| FOOD AND MEASURE | CALORIES |
|---|---|
| **Tartar sauce,** 1 tbsp.: | |
| (*Golden Dipt*) | 70 |
| (*Golden Dipt* Lite) | 50 |
| (*Great Impressions*) | 86 |
| (*Heinz*) | 71 |
| (*Hellmann's/Best Foods*) | 70 |
| (*Sauceworks*) | 50 |
| (*Weight Watchers*) | 35 |
| natural lemon and herb flavor (*Sauceworks*) | 70 |
| **Tea,** brewed, 8 fl. oz., except as noted: | |
| (*Nestea*), 6 fl. oz. | 0 |
| caffeine-free (*Celestial Seasonings*) | 4 |
| instant, regular or decaffeinated (*Lipton*), 6 fl. oz. | 0 |
| instant, lemon flavor (*Lipton*), 6 fl. oz. | 3 |
| flavored or special blend: | |
| all varieties (*Bigelow*), 5.25 fl. oz. | 1 |
| all varieties, except chocolate-orange (*Celestial Seasonings*) | <4 |
| chocolate-orange (*Celestial Seasonings Bavarian Chocolate Orange*) | 7 |
| herbal: | |
| all varieties except *Roastaroma* (*Celestial Seasonings*) | <6 |
| all varieties except spice (*Lipton*) | <5 |
| all varieties except apple-spice and roasted grain (*Bigelow*), 5 fl. oz. | <2 |
| (*Celestial Seasonings Roastaroma*) | 11 |
| apple-spice (*Bigelow*), 5 fl. oz. | 5 |
| grains, roasted, w/carob (*Bigelow*), 5 fl. oz. | 3 |
| spice (*Lipton Toasty Spice*) | 6 |
| **Tea, iced,** 8 fl. oz., except as noted: | |
| canned, bottled, or chilled: | |
| (*Shasta*), 12 fl. oz. | 124 |
| w/lemon: | |
| (*Lipton* Presweetened) | 83 |
| (*Lipton* Sugar Free) | <1 |
| (*Nestea* Sugar Free) | 2 |
| (*Nestea* Sugar Sweetened) | 70 |
| (*Veryfine*) | 80 |
| natural lemon flavor (*Lipton* Aseptic), 8.45 oz. | 96 |
| flavored (*Wylers* Fruit Tea Punch), 12 oz. | 118 |

| FOOD AND MEASURE | CALORIES |
|---|---|
| instant or mix, prepared: | |
| (*Crystal Light* Sugar Free Decaffeinated) | 4 |
| (*Lipton* Sugar Free Regular/Decaffeinated) | 1 |
| (*Nestea* 100%) | 2 |
| decaffeinated (*Nestea* 100%) | 0 |
| flavored, all flavors (*Nestea Ice Teasers*) | 6 |
| lemon flavor: | |
| (*Lipton* Regular/Decaffeinated), 6 fl. oz. | 55 |
| (*Nestea*) | 6 |
| (*Nestea* Presweetened) | 70 |
| (*Nestea* Sugar Free) | 4 |
| w/*Nutrasweet* (*Lipton*) | 5 |

**Teff seed:**

| | |
|---|---|
| (*Arrowhead Mills*), 2 oz. | 200 |

**Tempeh:**

| | |
|---|---|
| ½ cup | 165 |

**Tempura batter mix:**

| | |
|---|---|
| (*Golden Dipt*), 1 oz. | 100 |

**Tequila,** see "Liquor"

**Teriyaki sauce:**

| | |
|---|---|
| (*Kikkoman*), 1 tbsp. | 15 |
| (*Kikkoman* Baste & Glaze), 1 tbsp. | 27 |
| (*La Choy* Sauce and Marinade), 1 oz. | 30 |
| (*La Choy* Thick and Rich), 1 oz. | 41 |
| barbecue marinade (*Lawry's*), ¼ cup | 164 |
| ginger marinade (*Golden Dipt*), 1 fl. oz. | 120 |
| w/pineapple juice (*Lawry's*), ¼ cup | 72 |

**Thirst quencher drink,** bottled:

| | |
|---|---|
| 8 fl. oz. | 60 |

**Thuringer cervelat** (see also "Summer sausage"):

| | |
|---|---|
| (*Hillshire Farm*), 2 oz. | 180 |
| (*Hormel Old Smokehouse*/*Hormel* Viking Chub Cervelat), 1 oz. | 90 |
| (*Hormel Old Smokehouse* Chub/Sliced), 1 oz. | 100 |

**Thyme,** ground:

| | |
|---|---|
| 1 tsp. | 4 |

| FOOD AND MEASURE | CALORIES |
|---|---|
| **Thymus:** | |
| beef, braised, 4 oz. | 362 |
| veal, braised, 4 oz. | 197 |
| **Tilefish,** meat only: | |
| raw, 4 oz. | 108 |
| baked, broiled, or microwaved, 4 oz. | 167 |
| **Toaster muffins and pastries,** 1 piece: | |
| all varieties, except frosted (*Kellogg's Pop-Tarts*) | 210 |
| apple, Dutch, frosted (*Kellogg's Pop-Tarts*) | 210 |
| apple-cinnamon (*Pepperidge Farm* Croissant Toaster Tarts) | 170 |
| banana-nut (*Thomas' Toast-r-Cakes*) | 111 |
| banana-nut (*Toaster Strudel* Breakfast Pastries) | 190 |
| blueberry (*Thomas' Toast-r-Cakes*) | 108 |
| blueberry (*Toaster Strudel* Breakfast Pastries) | 190 |
| blueberry, frosted (*Kellogg's Pop-Tarts*) | 210 |
| bran (*Thomas' Toast-r-Cakes*) | 103 |
| brown sugar cinnamon, frosted (*Kellogg's Pop-Tarts*) | 210 |
| cheese (*Pepperidge Farm* Croissant Toaster Tarts) | 190 |
| cherry (*Toaster Strudel* Breakfast Pastries) | 190 |
| cherry, frosted (*Kellogg's Pop-Tarts*) | 200 |
| chocolate fudge, frosted (*Kellogg's Pop-Tarts*) | 200 |
| chocolate-vanilla creme, frosted (*Kellogg's Pop-Tarts*) | 200 |
| cinnamon (*Toaster Strudel* Breakfast Pastries) | 190 |
| corn (*Thomas' Toast-r-Cakes*) | 120 |
| grape, frosted (*Kellogg's Pop-Tarts*) | 200 |
| oat bran, w/raisins (*Awrey's* Toastums) | 130 |
| raspberry (*Toaster Strudel* Breakfast Pastries) | 190 |
| raspberry, frosted (*Kellogg's Pop-Tarts*) | 200 |
| strawberry (*Pepperidge Farm* Croissant Toaster Tarts) | 190 |
| strawberry (*Toaster Strudel* Breakfast Pastries) | 190 |
| strawberry, frosted (*Kellogg's Pop-Tarts*) | 200 |
| **Tofu:** | |
| raw, 1 oz. | 22 |
| raw, firm, 1 oz. | 41 |
| raw, pasteurized (*Freida* of California), 4.2 oz. | 86 |
| dried-frozen (koyadofu), 1 oz. | 136 |
| flavored, Chinese 5-spice or French herb (*Nasoya*), 5 oz. | 150 |
| grilled (yakidofu), 1 oz. | 25 |

| FOOD AND MEASURE | CALORIES |
|---|---|
| okara, 1 oz. | 22 |
| salted and fermented (fuyu), 1 oz. | 33 |

**Tofu dinner or entree,** see specific listings

**Tofu patty,** frozen:

| | |
|---|---|
| garden (*Natural Touch*), 2.5-oz. patty | 90 |
| okara (*Natural Touch Okara*), 2.25-oz. patty | 160 |

**Tofu spread,** canned:

| | |
|---|---|
| green chili (*Natural Touch Tofu Topper*), 2 tbsp. | 50 |
| herb and spice (*Natural Touch Tofu Topper*), 2 tbsp. | 50 |
| Mexican (*Natural Touch Tofu Topper*), 2 tbsp. | 60 |

**Tomatillo,** fresh:

| | |
|---|---|
| (*Freida* of California), 3.5 oz. | 25 |

**Tomatillo entero:**

| | |
|---|---|
| (*La Victoria*), 1 tbsp. | 4 |

**Tomato,** red, ripe:

| | |
|---|---|
| fresh, raw, 1 tomato, 2⅗" diam. | 26 |
| fresh, raw, chopped, ½ cup | 19 |
| fresh, boiled, ½ cup | 32 |
| canned, ½ cup, except as noted: | |
| (*Featherweight*) | 20 |
| whole (*Hunt's* Regular/No Salt Added), 4 oz. | 20 |
| whole (*S&W/S&W Nutradiet/S&W* Italian Style Pear) | 25 |
| whole (*Stokely*) | 25 |
| whole, peeled (*Contadina*) | 25 |
| whole, peeled, w/liquid (*Del Monte*) | 25 |
| crushed (*Hunt's*), 4 oz. | 25 |
| crushed, in puree (*Contadina*) | 30 |
| cut, peeled (*S&W* Ready-Cut) | 25 |
| diced, in rich puree (*S&W*) | 35 |
| wedges, in tomato juice | 34 |
| wedges, w/liquid (*Del Monte*) | 30 |
| aspic, supreme (*S&W*) | 60 |
| w/green chilies (*Old El Paso*), ¼ cup | 14 |
| w/jalapeños (*Ortega*), 1 oz. | 8 |
| Cajun or Italian style (*Del Monte*) | 30 |
| Italian style, pear (*Contadina*) | 25 |

| FOOD AND MEASURE | CALORIES |
|---|---|
| *Tomato, canned, continued* | |
| Mexican style (*Del Monte*) | 35 |
| pasta style, chunky (*Del Monte*) | 45 |
| stewed (*Del Monte* Regular/No Salt Added) | 35 |
| stewed (*Hunt's* Regular/No Salt Added), 4 oz. | 35 |
| stewed (*S&W* Regular/50% Salt Reduced/Italian) | 35 |
| stewed (*Stokely*) | 35 |
| stewed, all varieties (*Contadina*) | 35 |
| stewed, Mexican style (*S&W*) | 40 |

**Tomato, green:**

| | |
|---|---|
| 1 medium, 2⅗" diam. | 30 |
| pickled, kosher, in jars (*Claussen*), 1 oz. | 5 |
| kosher (*Claussen*), 1.7-oz. piece | 9 |

**Tomato juice,** canned or bottled:

| | |
|---|---|
| (*Campbell's*), 6 fl. oz. | 40 |
| (*Featherweight*), 6 fl. oz. | 35 |
| (*Hunt's*), 6 fl. oz. | 30 |
| (*Hunt's* No Salt Added), 6 fl. oz. | 45 |
| (*S&W* California/*S&W Nutradiet*), 6 fl. oz. | 35 |
| (*Stokely*), 4 fl. oz. | 20 |
| (*Welch's*), 6 fl. oz. | 35 |

**Tomato paste,** canned:

| | |
|---|---|
| (*Contadina*), 2 oz. or ¼ cup | 50 |
| (*Del Monte* Regular/No Salt Added), 6 oz. | 150 |
| (*Hunt's* Regular/No Salt Added), 2 oz. | 45 |
| (*S&W*), 6 oz. | 150 |
| Italian (*Contadina*), 2 oz. or ¼ cup | 65 |
| Italian style (*Hunt's*), 2 oz. | 50 |

**Tomato puree,** canned:

| | |
|---|---|
| (*Contadina*), ½ cup | 40 |
| (*Hunt's*), 4 oz. | 45 |
| (*S&W*), ½ cup | 60 |

**Tomato sauce** (see also "Pasta sauce"), canned or in jars:

| | |
|---|---|
| (*Contadina/Contadina* Italian Style), ½ cup | 30 |
| (*Contadina* Thick and Zesty), ½ cup | 40 |
| (*Del Monte* Regular/No Salt Added), 1 cup | 70 |
| (*Health Valley* Regular/No Salt Added), 1 cup | 70 |

| FOOD AND MEASURE | CALORIES |
|---|---|
| (*Hunt's*), 4 oz. | 30 |
| (*Hunt's* No Salt Added/*Hunt's* Special), 4 oz. | 35 |
| (*Rokeach* Italian style), 3 oz. | 60 |
| (*Rokeach* Low Sodium), 3 oz. | 50 |
| (*S&W*), ½ cup | 40 |
| (*Stokely*), ½ cup | 30 |
| w/green chilies (*Old El Paso*), ½ cup | 14 |
| Italian (*Hunt's*), 4 oz. | 60 |
| w/jalapeños (*Old El Paso*), ¼ cup | 11 |
| w/mushrooms, ½ cup | 42 |
| w/onions (*Del Monte*), 1 cup | 100 |
| Spanish-style, ½ cup | 40 |
| **Tomato-beef cocktail:** | |
| (*Beefamato*), 6 fl. oz. | 80 |
| **Tomato-chile cocktail:** | |
| (*Snap-E-Tom*), 6 fl. oz. | 40 |
| **Tomato-clam juice cocktail:** | |
| (*Clamato*), 6 fl. oz. | 96 |
| **Tom Collins mix:** | |
| bottled (*Holland House*), 1 fl. oz. | 47 |
| instant (*Holland House*), .56 oz. | 65 |
| **Tongue:** | |
| beef, simmered, 4 oz. | 321 |
| lamb, braised, 4 oz. | 312 |
| pork, braised, 4 oz. | 307 |
| pork, cured, canned (*Hormel*, 8 lb.), 3 oz. | 190 |
| veal, braised, 4 oz. | 229 |
| **Tonic water,** see "Soft drinks and mixers" | |
| **Toppings, dessert,** 2 tbsp., except as noted: | |
| all flavors, except chocolate nut (*Smucker's Magic Shell*) | 190 |
| butterscotch (*Kraft*), 1 tbsp. | 60 |
| butterscotch (*Smucker's*) | 140 |
| butterscotch-caramel (*Smucker's* Special Recipe) | 160 |
| caramel (*Kraft*), 1 tbsp. | 60 |
| caramel (*Smucker's*) | 140 |

| FOOD AND MEASURE | CALORIES |
|---|---|
| *Toppings, dessert, continued* | |
| caramel, hot (*Smucker's*) | 150 |
| chocolate: | |
| (*Kraft*), 1 tbsp. | 50 |
| dark (*Smucker's* Special Recipe) | 130 |
| fudge (*Hershey's*) | 100 |
| fudge, hot (*Kraft*), 1 tbsp. | 70 |
| fudge, hot (*Smuckers*) | 110 |
| fudge, hot (*Smucker's* Special Recipe) | 150 |
| fudge, Swiss milk chocolate (*Smucker's*) | 140 |
| fudge or syrup (*Smucker's*) | 130 |
| milk, w/almonds (*Nestlé Candytops*), 1.25 oz. | 230 |
| milk, w/crisps (*Nestlé Crunch Candytops*), 1.25 oz. | 220 |
| nut (*Smucker's Magic Shell*) | 200 |
| white, w/almonds (*Nestlé Candytops*), 1.25 oz. | 230 |
| marshmallow (*Marshmallow Fluff*), 1 heaping tsp. | 59 |
| marshmallow creme (*Kraft*), 1 oz. | 90 |
| nut (*Planters*), 1 oz. | 180 |
| peanut butter-caramel (*Smucker's*) | 150 |
| pecans, in syrup (*Smucker's*) | 130 |
| pineapple or strawberry (*Kraft*), 1 tbsp. | 50 |
| pineapple (*Smucker's*) | 130 |
| strawberry (*Smucker's*) | 120 |
| walnuts, in syrup (*Smucker's*) | 130 |
| whipped, see "Cream" and "Cream topping, nondairy" | |

**Tortellini:**

| | |
|---|---|
| frozen, meatless (*Tofutti*), 2 oz. | 220 |
| frozen, nondairy, regular or spinach (*Tofutti*), 2 oz. | 210 |
| refrigerated, 4.5 oz.: | |
| egg, w/chicken and prosciutto (*Contadina Fresh*) | 370 |
| spinach, w/chicken and prosciutto (*Contadina Fresh*) | 340 |
| egg or spinach, w/cheese or meat (*Contadina Fresh*) | 380 |

**Tortellini dinner,** frozen:

| | |
|---|---|
| cheese (*Le Menu* LightStyle), 10 oz. | 230 |
| w/meat (*Dinner Classics Lite*), 10 oz. | 250 |

**Tortellini dishes,** frozen:

| | |
|---|---|
| beef, w/marinara sauce (*Stouffer's*), 10 oz. | 360 |
| cheese: | |
| (*The Budget Gourmet* Side Dish), 5.5 oz. | 180 |

| FOOD AND MEASURE | CALORIES |
|---|---|
| (*Weight Watchers*), 9 oz. | 310 |
| in Alfredo sauce (*Stouffer's*), 8⅞ oz. | 600 |
| marinara (*Green Giant* One Serving), 5.5 oz. | 260 |
| meat sauce and (*Le Menu* LightStyle), 8 oz. | 250 |
| in tomato sauce (*Birds Eye For One*), 5.5 oz. | 210 |
| w/tomato sauce (*Stouffer's*), 9⅝ oz. | 360 |
| w/vinaigrette dressing (*Stouffer's*), 6⅞ oz. | 400 |
| Provencale (*Green Giant* Microwave Garden Gourmet), 1 pkg. | 260 |
| veal, in Alfredo sauce (*Stouffer's*), 8⅝ oz. | 500 |

**Tortellini dishes,** packaged:

| | |
|---|---|
| cheese, w/shrimp and seafood (*Hormel Top Shelf*), 10 oz. | 278 |
| in marinara sauce (*Hormel Top Shelf*), 10 oz. | 211 |

**Tortilla,** 1 piece:

| | |
|---|---|
| corn (*Azteca*) | 45 |
| flour (*Azteca*), 9″ diam. | 130 |
| flour (*Azteca*), 7″ diam. | 80 |
| flour (*Old El Paso*) | 150 |

**Tortilla chips,** see "Corn chips, puffs, and similar snacks"

**Tortilla entree,** frozen:

| | |
|---|---|
| (*Stouffer's* Grande), 9⅝ oz. | 530 |

**Tostaco shell:**

| | |
|---|---|
| (*Old El Paso*), 1 piece | 100 |

**Tostada shell,** 1 piece:

| | |
|---|---|
| (*Lawry's*) | 73 |
| (*Old El Paso*) | 55 |
| (*Ortega*) | 50 |
| (*Tio Sancho*) | 67 |

**Tree fern,** cooked:

| | |
|---|---|
| 1 frond, 6½″ long, ⅝″ diam. | 12 |
| chopped, ½ cup | 28 |

**Tripe,** beef:

| | |
|---|---|
| raw, 1 oz. | 28 |

**Triticale,** whole-grain:

| | |
|---|---|
| 1 cup | 646 |

| FOOD AND MEASURE | CALORIES |
| --- | --- |
| **Trout,** meat only: | |
| mixed species, raw, 4 oz. | 168 |
| rainbow, raw, 4 oz. | 133 |
| rainbow, baked, broiled, or microwaved, 4 oz. | 171 |
| **Trout, sea,** see "Sea trout" | |
| **Tumeric,** ground: | |
| 1 tsp. | 8 |
| **Tuna,** canned, 2 oz., except as noted: | |
| light, in oil, drained: | |
| chunk (*Bumble Bee*) | 110 |
| chunk (*S&W* Fancy) | 140 |
| chunk (*Star-Kist*) | 150 |
| solid (*Progresso*), ⅓ cup | 150 |
| solid (*Star-Kist* Prime Catch) | 150 |
| light, in water, drained: | |
| (*Empress*) | 60 |
| chunk (*Bumble Bee*) | 50 |
| chunk (*Featherweight*) | 60 |
| chunk (*S&W* Fancy) | 60 |
| chunk, in spring water (*Star-Kist*) | 60 |
| chunk, in spring water (*Star-Kist* Select/60% Less Salt) | 65 |
| chunk, in spring water (*Weight Watchers* No Salt Added) | 60 |
| chunk, diet, in distilled water (*Star-Kist*) | 65 |
| solid, in spring water (*Star-Kist/Star-Kist* Prime Catch) | 60 |
| white, in oil, drained: | |
| chunk (*Bumble Bee*) | 110 |
| chunk or solid, Albacore (*Star-Kist*) | 140 |
| solid, Albacore (*Bumble Bee*) | 100 |
| solid, Albacore (*S&W* Fancy) | 160 |
| white, in water, drained: | |
| chunk, in spring water (*Star-Kist* Select/60% Less Salt) | 70 |
| chunk, diet, in distilled water (*Star-Kist*) | 70 |
| chunk or solid, Albacore (*Bumble Bee*) | 60 |
| solid, Albacore, in spring water (*Star-Kist*) | 70 |
| solid, Albacore, in spring water (*Weight Watchers* No Salt Added) | 70 |

| FOOD AND MEASURE | CALORIES |
|---|---|
| **Tuna,** fresh, meat only: | |
| bluefin, raw, 4 oz. | 163 |
| bluefin, baked, broiled, or microwaved, 4 oz. | 209 |
| skipjack, raw, 4 oz. | 117 |
| yellowfin, raw, 4 oz. | 123 |
| **"Tuna," vegetarian,** frozen: | |
| (*Worthington Tuna*), 2 oz. | 100 |
| **Tuna entree,** frozen: | |
| noodle casserole (*Stouffer's*), 10 oz. | 310 |
| pie (*Banquet*), 7 oz. | 540 |
| **Tuna entree mix**[1]**:** | |
| au gratin (*Tuna Helper*), 6 oz. | 280 |
| fettuccine Alfredo (*Tuna Helper*), 7 oz. | 300 |
| mushroom, creamy (*Tuna Helper*), 7 oz. | 220 |
| noodle, cheesy (*Tuna Helper*), 7.75 oz. | 250 |
| noodle, creamy (*Tuna Helper*), 8 oz. | 300 |
| pot pie (*Tuna Helper*), 5.1 oz. | 420 |
| rice, buttery (*Tuna Helper*), 6 oz. | 280 |
| salad (*Tuna Helper*), 5.5 oz. | 420 |
| tetrazzini (*Tuna Helper*), 6 oz. | 240 |
| **Tuna pie,** see "Tuna entree, frozen" | |
| **Tuna salad:** | |
| (*Longacre*), 1 oz. | 58 |
| (*Longacre* Saladfest), 1 oz. | 52 |
| **Turbot,** meat only: | |
| domestic, see "Halibut, meat only, Greenland" | |
| European, raw, 4 oz. | 108 |
| **Turkey,** fresh, roasted, 4 oz., except as noted: | |
| fryer-roaster: | |
| meat w/skin | 195 |
| meat only | 170 |
| meat only, chopped or diced, 1 cup not packed | 210 |
| skin only, 1 oz. | 85 |

[1]Prepared according to package directions, with water-packed tuna.

| FOOD AND MEASURE | CALORIES |
|---|---|
| *Turkey, fryer-roaster, continued* | |
| dark meat w/skin | 206 |
| dark meat only | 184 |
| light meat w/skin | 186 |
| light meat only | 159 |
| back, meat w/skin | 231 |
| back, meat only | 193 |
| breast, meat w/skin | 174 |
| breast, meat only | 153 |
| leg, meat w/skin | 193 |
| leg, meat only | 180 |
| wing, meat w/skin | 235 |
| wing, meat only | 185 |
| young hen: | |
| meat w/skin | 247 |
| meat only | 198 |
| meat only, chopped or diced, 1 cup not packed | 244 |
| skin only, 1 oz. | 137 |
| dark meat w/skin | 263 |
| dark meat only | 218 |
| light meat w/skin | 235 |
| light meat only | 183 |
| back, meat w/skin | 288 |
| breast, meat w/skin | 220 |
| leg, meat w/skin | 242 |
| wing, meat w/skin | 270 |
| young tom: | |
| meat w/skin | 229 |
| meat only | 191 |
| meat only, chopped or diced, 1 cup not packed | 235 |
| skin only, 1 oz. | 120 |
| dark meat w/skin | 245 |
| dark meat only | 210 |
| light meat w/skin | 217 |
| light meat only | 175 |
| back, meat w/skin | 270 |
| breast, meat w/skin | 214 |
| leg, meat w/skin | 234 |
| wing, meat w/skin | 251 |

| FOOD AND MEASURE | CALORIES |
|---|---|

**Turkey, boneless and luncheon meat:**

| | |
|---|---|
| bologna, see "Turkey bologna" | |
| breast: | |
| (*Butterball* Cold Cuts), 1 oz. | 30 |
| (*Butterball Deli* No Salt Added), 1 oz. | 45 |
| (*Butterball Slice 'n Serve*), 1 oz. | 35 |
| (*Healthy Deli* Gourmet), 1 oz. | 28 |
| (*Healthy Deli* Lessalt), 1 oz. | 25 |
| (*Hormel* Perma-Fresh), 2 slices | 60 |
| (*Light & Lean*), 2 slices | 60 |
| (*Longacre* Catering/Deli/Gourmet), 1 oz. | 35 |
| (*Longacre* Gourmet Low Salt/Premium), 1 oz. | 30 |
| (*Longacre* Salt Watchers), 1 oz. | 32 |
| (*Louis Rich*), 1 oz. | 45 |
| (*Mr. Turkey*), 1 oz. | 31 |
| barbecue-seasoned (*Butterball Slice 'n Serve* BBQ), 1 oz. | 40 |
| honey (*Healthy Deli*), 1 oz. | 28 |
| honey-roasted (*Louis Rich*), 1 oz. | 32 |
| golden (*Boar's Head*), 1 oz. | 35 |
| golden, skinless (*Boar's Head*), 1 oz. | 30 |
| oven-cooked (*Healthy Deli*), 1 oz. | 26 |
| oven-roasted (*Hillshire Farm* Deli Select), 1 oz. | 31 |
| oven-roasted (*Louis Rich*), 1 oz. | 31 |
| oven-roasted (*Louis Rich* Thin Sliced), .4-oz. slice | 12 |
| oven-roasted (*Oscar Mayer*), .75-oz. slice | 23 |
| oven-roasted or smoked (*Eckrich Lite*), 1 oz. | 30 |
| roast (*Oscar Mayer* Thin Sliced), .4-oz. slice | 12 |
| roast or sliced (*Louis Rich*), 1 oz. | 40 |
| skinless (*Longacre* Gourmet/Premium), 1 oz. | 30 |
| sliced (*Longacre*), 1 oz. | 30 |
| smoked (*Butterball* Cold Cuts), 1 oz. | 35 |
| smoked (*Healthy Deli,* 3 lb.), 1 oz. | 29 |
| smoked (*Healthy Deli* Gourmet), 1 oz. | 31 |
| smoked (*Hillshire Farm* Deli Select), 1 oz. | 31 |
| smoked (*Hormel* Perma-Fresh), 2 slices | 60 |
| smoked (*Longacre*), 1 oz. | 35 |
| smoked (*Louis Rich*), .74-oz. slice | 21 |
| smoked (*Louis Rich* Thin Sliced), .4-oz. slice | 11 |
| smoked (*Oscar Mayer*), .75-oz. slice | 20 |
| smoked, hickory (*Butterball Slice 'n Serve*), 1 oz. | 35 |
| smoked, sliced (*Longacre*), 1 oz. | 26 |

| FOOD AND MEASURE | CALORIES |
|---|---|
| *Turkey, boneless and luncheon meat, continued* | |
| breast and white (*Longacre Deli Chef*), 1 oz. | 35 |
| breast and white, roasted (*Longacre Deli Chef*), 1 oz. | 40 |
| breast and white, skinless (*Longacre Deli Chef*), 1 oz. | 40 |
| diced, white and dark meat, seasoned, 1 oz. | 39 |
| ham, see "Turkey ham" | |
| luncheon loaf (*Louis Rich*), 1 oz. | 45 |
| luncheon loaf, spiced (*Mr. Turkey*), 1 oz. | 51 |
| pastrami, see "Turkey pastrami" | |
| salami, see "Turkey salami" | |
| sausage, see "Turkey sausage" | |
| smoked (*Butterball* Cold Cuts), 1 oz. | 35 |
| smoked (*Butterball Turkey Variety Pak*), ¾ oz. | 25 |
| smoked (*Louis Rich*), 1 oz. | 32 |
| summer sausage, see "Turkey summer sausage" | |

**Turkey,** canned:

| | |
|---|---|
| chunk (*Hormel*), 6¾ oz. | 230 |
| white (*Swanson*), 2½ oz. | 80 |

**Turkey,** frozen and refrigerated:

| | |
|---|---|
| breast, raw (*Longacre* Cook-N-Bag), 1 oz. | 27 |
| breast, raw (*Longacre* Ready-to-Cook), 1 oz. | 39 |
| breast, cooked: | |
| (*Land O'Lakes*), 3 oz. | 100 |
| (*Longacre* Cook-N-Bag), 1 oz. | 38 |
| (*Louis Rich*), 1 oz. | 47 |
| barbecue, quarter (*Mr. Turkey* Chub), 1 oz. | 34 |
| barbecue, hickory smoke, or honey (*Louis Rich*), 1 oz. | 33 |
| oven-prepared, quarter (*Mr. Turkey* Chub), 1 oz. | 34 |
| oven-roasted (*Louis Rich*), 1 oz. | 31 |
| roast (*Louis Rich*), 1 oz. | 42 |
| slices (*Louis Rich*), 1 oz. | 39 |
| smoked (*Louis Rich*), 1 oz. | 33 |
| smoked, quarter (*Mr. Turkey* Chub), 1 oz. | 35 |
| steaks or tenderloins (*Louis Rich*), 1 oz. | 39 |
| dark meat, skinless, roasted (*Swift Butterball*), 3.5 oz. | 195 |
| drumsticks (*Land O'Lakes*), 3 oz. | 120 |
| drumsticks (*Louis Rich*), 1 oz. cooked | 56 |
| ground, see "Turkey, ground" | |
| hindquarter roast (*Land O'Lakes*), 3 oz. | 140 |

| FOOD AND MEASURE | CALORIES |
|---|---|
| thigh (*Land O'Lakes*), 3 oz. | 150 |
| thigh (*Louis Rich*), 1 oz. cooked | 64 |
| white meat, skinless, roasted (*Swift Butterball*), 3.5 oz. | 160 |
| white and dark meat, roasted (*Swift Butterball*), 3.5 oz. | 195 |
| whole, w/out giblets, cooked (*Louis Rich*), 1 oz. | 52 |
| wings (*Land O'Lakes*), 3 oz. | 120 |
| wings (*Louis Rich*), 1 oz. cooked | 54 |
| wings (*Louis Rich* Drumettes), 1 oz. cooked | 51 |
| young (*Land O'Lakes*), 3 oz. | 130 |
| young, butter-basted (*Land O'Lakes*), 3 oz. | 140 |
| young, self-basting, broth (*Lake O'Lakes*), 3 oz. | 120 |

**Turkey, ground:**

| | |
|---|---|
| (*Hudson's*), 1 oz. | 55 |
| (*Longacre*), 1 oz. | 60 |
| (*Louis Rich*), 1 oz. cooked | 60 |
| (*Louis Rich* 90% Lean), 1 oz. cooked | 52 |
| (*Mr. Turkey*), 1 oz. | 54 |
| w/natural flavoring (*Louis Rich* 90% lean), 1 oz. | 50 |

**"Turkey," vegetarian:**

| | |
|---|---|
| canned (*Worthington* Turkee Slices), 2 slices or 2.2 oz. | 130 |
| canned, drained (*Worthington 209*), 2 slices | 120 |
| frozen, smoked, roll or slices (*Worthington*), 4 slices | 180 |

**Turkey bacon,** see "Bacon, substitute"

**Turkey bologna,** 1 oz., except as noted:

| | |
|---|---|
| (*Butterball* Cold Cuts/*Butterball Deli/Slice 'n Serve*) | 70 |
| (*Butterball Turkey Variety Pak*), ¾ oz. | 50 |
| (*Louis Rich*) | 61 |
| mild (*Louis Rich*) | 59 |
| sliced (*Longacre*) | 61 |

**Turkey dinner,** frozen:

| | |
|---|---|
| (*Banquet*), 10.5 oz. | 390 |
| (*Banquet Extra Helping*), 19 oz. | 750 |
| (*Morton*), 10 oz. | 230 |
| (*Swanson*), 11.5 oz. | 350 |
| (*Swanson Hungry Man*), 17 oz. | 550 |
| breast: | |
| (*Healthy Choice*), 10.5 oz. | 290 |

| FOOD AND MEASURE | CALORIES |
|---|---|
| *Turkey dinner, breast, continued* | |
| Dijon (*The Budget Gourmet*), 11.2 oz. | 340 |
| roast (*Stouffer's Dinner Supreme*), 10.75 oz. | 330 |
| sliced (*The Budget Gourmet*), 11.1 oz. | 290 |
| sliced, w/mushroom gravy (*Le Menu*), 10.5 oz. | 300 |
| sliced, in mushroom sauce (*Lean Cuisine*), 8 oz. | 240 |
| divan (*Le Menu* LightStyle), 10 oz. | 260 |
| w/dressing and gravy (*Armour Classics*), 11.5 oz. | 320 |
| sliced (*Freezer Queen*), 10 oz. | 280 |

**Turkey entree,** frozen:

| | |
|---|---|
| (*Tyson Gourmet Selection*), 11.5 oz. | 380 |
| à la king, w/rice (*The Budget Gourmet*), 10 oz. | 390 |
| breast, stuffed (*Weight Watchers*), 8.5 oz. | 260 |
| casserole (*Pillsbury Microwave Classic*), 1 pkg. | 430 |
| casserole, w/gravy and dressing (*Stouffer's*), 9.75 oz. | 360 |
| croquettes, gravy and (*Freezer Queen Family Suppers*), 7 oz. | 250 |
| Dijon (*Lean Cuisine*), 9.5 oz. | 270 |
| w/dressing and potatoes (*Swanson* Homestyle Recipe), 9 oz. | 290 |
| glazed (*The Budget Gourmet* Slim Selects), 9 oz. | 270 |
| glazed (*Le Menu* LightStyle), 8.25 oz. | 260 |
| and gravy (*Freezer Queen Deluxe Family Suppers*), 7 oz. | 160 |
| pie: | |
| (*Banquet*), 7 oz. | 510 |
| (*Banquet* Supreme Microwave), 7 oz. | 430 |
| (*Morton*), 7 oz. | 420 |
| (*Stouffer's*), 10 oz. | 540 |
| (*Swanson Pot Pie*), 7 oz. | 380 |
| (*Swanson Hungry Man*), 16 oz. | 650 |
| sliced: | |
| breast, in mushroom sauce (*Lean Cuisine*), 8 oz. | 240 |
| gravy and (*Banquet Cookin' Bags*), 5 oz. | 100 |
| gravy and (*Banquet Family Entrees*), 8 oz. | 150 |
| gravy and (*Freezer Queen Cook-In-Pouch*), 5 oz. | 70 |
| gravy and (*Freezer Queen Family Suppers*), 7 oz. | 110 |
| and gravy, w/dressing (*Freezer Queen* Single Serve), 9 oz. | 230 |
| in mild curry sauce, w/rice (*Right Course*), 8.75 oz. | 320 |
| tetrazzini (*Stouffer's*), 10 oz. | 380 |

| FOOD AND MEASURE | CALORIES |
|---|---|
| traditional (*Le Menu* LightStyle), 8 oz. | 200 |
| white meat, traditional (*Le Menu* LightStyle), 8.25 oz. | 200 |
| **Turkey frankfurter:** | |
| (*Butterball*), 1 link | 140 |
| (*Health Valley* Weiners), 1 link | 96 |
| (*Longacre*), 1 oz. | 66 |
| (*Louis Rich*), 1 link | 101 |
| (*Louis Rich* Bun Length), 1 link | 128 |
| (*Mr. Turkey,* 10/lb.), 1.6 oz. | 106 |
| cheese (*Louis Rich*), 1 link | 109 |
| cheese (*Mr. Turkey*), 1.6 oz. | 109 |
| **Turkey giblets:** | |
| simmered, 4 oz. | 189 |
| simmered, chopped or diced, 1 cup | 243 |
| **Turkey gizzard:** | |
| simmered, 4 oz. | 185 |
| **Turkey gravy:** | |
| canned (*Franco-American*), 2 oz. | 30 |
| canned (*Heinz*), 2 oz. or ¼ cup | 25 |
| canned, w/chunky turkey (*Hormel Great Beginnings*), 5 oz. | 138 |
| mix, prepared (*Lawry's*), 1 cup | 102 |
| mix, prepared (*McCormick/Schilling*), ¼ cup | 22 |
| **Turkey ham:** | |
| (*Butterball* Cold Cuts/*Butterball Slice 'n Serve*), 1 oz. | 35 |
| breakfast, smoked (*Mr. Turkey*), 1 oz. | 33 |
| chopped (*Louis Rich*), 1 oz. | 46 |
| chopped (*Mr. Turkey*), 1 oz. | 37 |
| chunk (*Longacre*), 1 oz. | 37 |
| cured thigh meat (*Louis Rich*), 1 oz. | 33 |
| cured thigh meat (*Louis Rich* Round), 1 oz. | 34 |
| cured thigh meat (*Louis Rich* Square), .7-oz. slice | 24 |
| cured thigh meat (*Louis Rich* Thin Sliced), .4-oz. slice | 12 |
| honey-cured (*Butterball* Cold Cuts), 1 oz. | 35 |
| honey-cured (*Butterball Slice 'n Serve*), 1 oz. | 40 |
| honey cured (*Louis Rich*), .75-oz. slice | 25 |
| honey-cured, chopped (*Butterball* Cold Cuts), 1 oz. | 35 |
| lean lite (*Longacre* Deli), 1 oz. | 37 |

| FOOD AND MEASURE | CALORIES |
|---|---|
| *Turkey ham, continued* | |
| sliced (*Butterball* Deli Thin), 1 oz. | 35 |
| sliced (*Longacre*), 1 oz. | 33 |
| smoked (*Mr. Turkey/Mr. Turkey* Buffet Style/Chub), 1 oz. | 32 |
| **Turkey ham salad:** | |
| (*Longacre*), 1 oz. | 53 |
| (*Longacre* Saladfest), 1 oz. | 58 |
| **Turkey heart,** see "Heart" | |
| **Turkey kielbasa:** | |
| (*Louis Rich* Polska), 1 oz. | 40 |
| (*Mr. Turkey* Polska), 1 oz. | 59 |
| **Turkey liver,** see "Liver" | |
| **Turkey luncheon meat,** see "Turkey, boneless and luncheon meat" | |
| **Turkey nuggets:** | |
| breaded (*Louis Rich*), 1 heated piece | 62 |
| **Turkey pastrami:** | |
| (*Butterball* Cold Cuts), 1 oz. | 30 |
| (*Butterball Slice 'n Serve*), 1 oz. | 35 |
| (*Louis Rich* Round), 1 oz. | 32 |
| (*Louis Rich* Square), .8-oz. slice | 24 |
| (*Louis Rich* Thin Sliced), .4-oz. slice | 11 |
| (*Mr. Turkey*), 1 oz. | 28 |
| sliced (*Longacre*), 1 oz. | 32 |
| **Turkey patty:** | |
| breaded (*Louis Rich*), 1 cooked patty | 209 |
| **Turkey pie,** see "Turkey entree, frozen" | |
| **Turkey pocket sandwich,** frozen: | |
| w/ham and cheese (*Hot Pockets*), 5 oz. | 320 |
| **Turkey salad:** | |
| (*Longacre*), 1 oz. | 70 |
| (*Longacre* Saladfest) 1 oz. | 68 |

| FOOD AND MEASURE | CALORIES |
|---|---|
| **Turkey salami:** | |
| (*Butterball* Cold Cuts/*Butterball Deli/Slice 'n Serve*), 1 oz. | 50 |
| (*Butterball Turkey Variety Pak*), .75 oz. | 40 |
| (*Louis Rich*), 1 oz. | 54 |
| cotto (*Louis Rich*), 1 oz. | 53 |
| cotto (*Mr. Turkey*), 1 oz. | 45 |
| sliced (*Longacre*), 1 oz. | 52 |
| **Turkey sausage:** | |
| (*Butterball*), 1 oz. | 50 |
| breakfast (*Louis Rich*), 1 oz. cooked | 56 |
| breakfast (*Mr. Turkey*), 1 oz. | 58 |
| breakfast, ground (*Hudson's*), 1 oz. | 65 |
| breakfast, links (*Louis Rich*), 1 cooked link | 46 |
| smoked (*Louis Rich*), 1 oz. | 43 |
| smoked (*Mr. Turkey*), 1 oz. | 47 |
| smoked, w/cheese (*Louis Rich*), 1 oz. | 47 |
| **Turkey spread:** | |
| chunky (*Underwood* Light), 2⅛ oz. | 75 |
| **Turkey sticks:** | |
| breaded (*Louis Rich*), 1 cooked stick | 81 |
| **Turkey summer sausage:** | |
| (*Louis Rich*), 1-oz. slice | 55 |
| **Turkey and corned beef:** | |
| (*Healthy Deli* Doubledecker), 1 oz. | 30 |
| **Turkey and ham:** | |
| (*Healthy Deli* Doubledecker), 1 oz. | 30 |
| **Turnip** | |
| fresh, raw, cubed, ½ cup | 18 |
| fresh, boiled, drained, cubed, ½ cup | 14 |
| fresh, boiled, drained, mashed, ½ cup | 21 |
| canned (*Stokely*), ½ cup | 20 |
| canned, diced (*Allens*), ½ cup | 16 |
| frozen, diced (*Southern*), 3.5 oz. | 17 |

| FOOD AND MEASURE | CALORIES |
|---|---|
| **Turnip greens:** | |
| fresh, raw, trimmed, 1 oz. or ½ cup chopped | 7 |
| fresh, boiled, drained, chopped, ½ cup | 15 |
| canned, chopped (*Allens*) | 21 |
| canned, chopped, w/diced turnips (*Allens*) | 19 |
| canned, chopped, w/diced turnips (*Stokely*) | 20 |
| frozen, chopped (*Southern*), 3.5 oz. | 25 |
| **Turnovers,** see specific listings | |

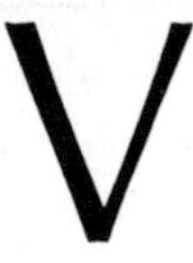

| FOOD AND MEASURE | CALORIES |
|---|---|
| **Vanilla extract:** | |
| pure (*Virginia Dare*), 1 tsp. | 10 |
| **Vanilla flavor drink,** see "Milk beverages, flavored" | |
| **Veal,** boneless, 4 oz.: | |
| cubed, leg and shoulder, braised or stewed, lean only | 213 |
| ground, broiled | 195 |
| leg (top round), roasted, separable lean and fat | 181 |
| leg (top round), roasted, lean only | 170 |
| loin, braised, separable lean and fat | 322 |
| loin, braised, lean only | 256 |
| loin, roasted, separable lean and fat | 246 |
| loin, roasted, lean only | 198 |
| rib, roasted, separable lean and fat | 259 |
| rib, roasted, lean only | 201 |
| shoulder, arm, braised, separable lean and fat | 268 |
| shoulder, arm braised, lean only | 228 |
| shoulder, blade, braised, separable lean and fat | 255 |
| shoulder, blade, braised, lean only | 224 |
| sirloin, roasted, lean and fat | 229 |
| sirloin, roasted, lean only | 191 |
| **Veal, variety meats,** see specific listings | |
| **Veal dinner,** frozen: | |
| Marsala (*Le Menu* LightStyle), 10 oz. | 230 |
| parmigiana: | |
| (*Armour Classics*), 11.25 oz. | 400 |
| (*Le Menu*), 11.5 oz. | 390 |
| (*Morton*), 10 oz. | 260 |
| (*Stouffer's Dinner Supreme*), 11.25 oz. | 350 |
| (*Swanson*), 12.25 oz. | 430 |
| (*Swanson Hungry Man*), 18.25 oz. | 590 |
| breaded (*Freezer Queen*), 5 oz. | 220 |
| platter (*Freezer Queen*), 10 oz. | 400 |

| FOOD AND MEASURE | CALORIES |
|---|---|
| **Veal entree,** frozen: | |
| parmigiana: | |
| (*Swanson* Homestyle Recipe), 10 oz. | 330 |
| breaded (*Banquet Cookin' Bags*), 4 oz. | 230 |
| breaded (*Freezer Queen Cook-In-Pouch*), 5 oz. | 220 |
| breaded (*Freezer Queen Deluxe Family Suppers*), 7 oz. | 300 |
| patty (*Banquet Family Entrees*), 8 oz. | 370 |
| patty (*Weight Watchers*), 8.44 oz. | 190 |
| primavera (*Lean Cuisine*), 9⅛ oz. | 250 |
| steak (*Hormel*), 4 oz. | 130 |
| steak, breaded (*Hormel*), 4 oz. | 240 |
| **Vegetable entree,** canned: | |
| chow mein, meatless (*La Choy*), ¾ cup | 35 |
| stew (*Dinty Moore*), 8 oz. | 170 |
| **Vegetable entree,** frozen (see also specific listings): | |
| and pasta Mornay, w/ham (*Lean Cuisine*), 9⅜ oz. | 280 |
| **Vegetable flakes,** dehydrated: | |
| (*French's*), 1 tbsp. | 12 |
| **Vegetable juice:** | |
| (*Veryfine* 100%), 6 fl. oz. | 32 |
| all varieties ("*V-8*"/"*V-8*" No Salt Added), 6 fl. oz. | 35 |
| hearty or hot and spicy (*Smucker's*), 8 fl. oz. | 58 |
| **Vegetable spread,** see "Margarine" | |
| **Vegetable stew,** see "Vegetable entree, canned" | |
| **Vegetable sticks,** breaded, frozen: | |
| (*Farm Rich*), 4 oz. | 240 |
| (*Stilwell Quickkrisp*), 3 oz. | 240 |
| **Vegetables,** see specific listings | |
| **Vegetables, mixed,** canned: | |
| (*Del Monte*), ½ cup | 40 |
| (*Green Giant* Garden Medley), ½ cup | 40 |
| (*S&W* Old Fashioned Harvest), ½ cup | 35 |
| (*Stokely* Regular/No Salt or Sugar Added), ½ cup | 40 |

| FOOD AND MEASURE | CALORIES |
|---|---|
| Chinese (*La Choy*), ½ cup | 12 |
| chop suey (*La Choy*), ½ cup | 9 |

**Vegetables, mixed,** frozen:

| | |
|---|---|
| (*Birds Eye*), 3.3 oz. | 60 |
| (*Birds Eye* Portion Pack), 3 oz. | 50 |
| (*Green Giant/Green Giant Harvest Fresh*), ½ cup | 40 |
| (*Health Valley*), ½ cup | 68 |
| (*Southern*), 3.5 oz. | 69 |
| (*Stokely Singles*), 3 oz. | 60 |
| California (*Green Giant* American Mixtures), ½ cup | 25 |
| Chinese style (*Birds Eye* Stir-Fry), 3.3 oz. | 35 |
| chow mein, in Oriental sauce (*Birds Eye Custom Cuisine*), 4.6 oz., w/out added ingredients | 80 |
| chow mein style, w/seasoned sauce (*Birds Eye* International Recipes), 3.3 oz. | 90 |
| Dutch-style (*Frosty Acres*), 3.2 oz. | 30 |
| heartland (*Green Giant* American Mixtures), ½ cup | 25 |
| Italian style, w/seasoned sauce (*Birds Eye* International Recipes), 3.3 oz. | 100 |
| Japanese style (*Birds Eye* Stir-Fry), 3.3 oz. | 30 |
| Japanese style, w/seasoned sauce (*Birds Eye* International Recipes), 3.3 oz. | 90 |
| New England (*Green Giant* American Mixtures), ½ cup | 70 |
| New England style, w/seasoned sauce (*Birds Eye* International Recipes), 3.3 oz. | 130 |
| Oriental style, w/authentic sauce for beef (*Birds Eye Custom Cuisine*), 4.6 oz., w/out added ingredients | 90 |
| Oriental style, w/seasoned sauce (*Birds Eye* International Recipes), 3.3 oz. | 70 |
| pasta primavera style, w/seasoned sauce (*Birds Eye* International Recipes), 3.3 oz. | 120 |
| San Francisco (*Green Giant* American Mixtures), ½ cup | 25 |
| San Francisco style, w/seasoned sauce (*Birds Eye* International Recipes), 3.3 oz. | 100 |
| Santa Fe (*Green Giant* American Mixtures), ½ cup | 70 |
| Seattle (*Green Giant* American Mixtures), ½ cup | 25 |
| in butter sauce (*Green Giant*), ½ cup | 60 |
| w/herb sauce for chicken or shrimp (*Birds Eye Custom Cuisine*), 4.6 oz., w/out added ingredients | 90 |

| FOOD AND MEASURE | CALORIES |
|---|---|
| *Vegetables, mixed, frozen, continued* | |
| w/mushroom sauce, creamy, for beef (*Birds Eye Custom Cuisine*), 4.6 oz., w/out added ingredients | 60 |
| w/mustard sauce, Dijon, for chicken or fish (*Birds Eye Custom Cuisine*), 4.6 oz., w/out added ingredients | 70 |
| w/tomato basil sauce for chicken (*Birds Eye Custom Cuisine*), 4.6 oz., w/out added ingredients | 110 |
| 'n rice, in teriyaki sauce (*Stokely Singles*), 4 oz. | 100 |
| 'n rotini, in cheddar cheese sauce (*Stokely Singles*), 4 oz. | 100 |
| 'n shells, in Italian style sauce (*Stokely Singles*), 4 oz. | 170 |
| stew (*Ore-Ida*), 3 oz. | 60 |
| 'n white and wild rice pilaf (*Stokely Singles*), 4 oz. | 80 |
| w/wild rice, in white wine sauce for chicken (*Birds Eye Custom Cuisine*), 4.6 oz., w/out added ingredients | 100 |
| **Vegetarian entree,** frozen (see also specific listings): | |
| (*Natural Touch* Dinner Entree), 3-oz. patty | 230 |
| **Vegetarian foods,** see specific listings | |
| **Venison,** meat only, roasted: | |
| roasted, 4 oz. | 179 |
| roasted, diced, 1 cup | 221 |
| **Vienna sausage,** canned: | |
| in barbecue sauce (*Libby's*), 2.5 oz. | 180 |
| in beef broth (*Libby's*), 3½ links | 160 |
| no broth (*Hormel*), 4 links | 200 |
| **Vine spinach:** | |
| raw, 1 lb. | 86 |
| **Vinegar:** | |
| all varieties (*Heinz*), 1 tbsp. | 2 |
| all varieties (*White House*), 2 tbsp. | 4 |
| apple cider (*Indian Summer*), 1 cup | 40 |
| apple cider or white (*Lucky Leaf/Musselman's*), 2 tbsp. | 4 |
| white (*Indian Summer*), 1 cup | 30 |
| wine, all varieties (*Regina*), 2 tbsp. | 4 |
| wine, basil, garlic, raspberry (*Great Impressions*), 1 tbsp. | 7 |
| wine, hot paprika or red (*Great Impressions*), 1 tbsp. | 6 |
| **Vodka,** see "Liquor" | |

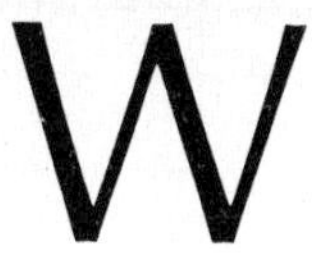

| FOOD AND MEASURE | CALORIES |
|---|---|
| **Waffle,** frozen: | |
| (*Aunt Jemima* Original), 1 piece | 173 |
| (*Downyflake*), 2 pieces | 120 |
| (*Downyflake* Hot-N-Buttery) , 2 pieces | 180 |
| (*Downyflake* Jumbo), 2 pieces | 170 |
| (*Eggo Homestyle*), 1 piece | 120 |
| (*Eggo Nutri•Grain*), 1 piece | 130 |
| (*Roman Meal*), 2 pieces | 280 |
| apple-cinnamon (*Aunt Jemima*), 1 piece | 176 |
| apple-cinnamon, blueberry, or strawberry (*Eggo*), 1 piece | 130 |
| Belgian (*Weight Watchers* Microwave), 1.5 oz. | 120 |
| blueberry (*Aunt Jemima*), 1 piece | 175 |
| blueberry (*Downyflake*), 2 pieces | 180 |
| buttermilk (*Aunt Jemima*), 1 piece | 179 |
| buttermilk (*Downyflake*), 2 pieces | 190 |
| buttermilk (*Eggo*), 1 piece | 120 |
| multigrain (*Downyflake*), 2 pieces | 250 |
| oat bran (*Eggo Common Sense*), 1 piece | 110 |
| oat bran, w/fruit and nut (*Eggo Common Sense*), 1 piece | 120 |
| raisin and bran (*Eggo Nutri•Grain*), 1 piece | 130 |
| rice bran (*Downyflake*), 2 pieces | 210 |
| whole grain wheat (*Aunt Jemima*), 1 piece | 154 |
| **Waffle breakfast,** frozen: | |
| w/bacon (*Swanson Great Starts*), 2.2 oz. | 230 |
| Belgian, and sausage (*Swanson Great Starts*), 2.85 oz. | 280 |
| Belgian, and strawberries, w/sausage (*Swanson Great Starts*), 3.5 oz. | 210 |
| **Waffle mix** (see also "Pancake and waffle mix"): | |
| prepared (*Bisquick Shake'N Pour* Complete), 2 pieces | 280 |
| **Walnut,** dried, shelled: | |
| Black, chopped, 1 cup | 759 |
| Black (*Planters*), 1 oz. | 180 |

| FOOD AND MEASURE | CALORIES |
|---|---|
| *Walnut, continued* | |
| English or Persian, halves, 1 cup | 642 |
| English or Persian (*Diamond*), 1 oz. | 192 |
| English or Persian (*Planters*), 1 oz. | 190 |
| **Wasabi:** | |
| powder, 1/4 oz. | 24 |
| **Wasabi snack chips:** | |
| (*Eden*), 1 oz. | 130 |
| **Waterchestnuts,** Chinese: | |
| 4 medium, 1.7 oz. | 38 |
| sliced, 1/2 cup | 66 |
| canned, w/liquid, sliced, 1/2 cup | 35 |
| canned (*La Choy*), 1.28 oz. | 18 |
| **Watercress:** | |
| 10 sprigs, 11/4" long, .9 oz. | 3 |
| chopped, 1/2 cup | 2 |
| **Watermelon:** | |
| 1/16 of 10"-diam. melon, 1"-thick slice | 152 |
| diced, 1/2 cup | 25 |
| **Wax beans,** see "Beans, green" | |
| **Welsh rarebit:** | |
| canned (*Snow's*), 1/2 cup | 170 |
| frozen (*Stouffer's*), 10 oz. | 350 |
| ***Wendy's,*** 1 serving: | |
| sandwiches, 1 serving: | |
| chicken, 6.9 oz. | 440 |
| chicken, grilled, 6.2 oz. | 340 |
| chicken club, 7.2 oz. | 506 |
| fish fillet, 6 oz. | 460 |
| hamburger, single, plain, 4.4 oz. | 340 |
| hamburger, single, w/everything, 7.4 oz. | 420 |
| cheeseburger, 4.4 oz. | 310 |
| Jr. bacon cheeseburger, 5.5 oz. | 430 |
| Jr. Swiss deluxe, 5.8 oz. | 360 |

| FOOD AND MEASURE | CALORIES |
|---|---|
| *Wendy's, sandwiches, continued* | |
| Kid's Meal cheeseburger, 4.1 oz. | 300 |
| Kid's Meal hamburger, 3.7 oz. | 260 |
| steak, country fried, 5.1 oz. | 440 |
| *Wendy's Big Classic,* 9.2 oz. | 570 |
| chicken nuggets, crispy, 6 pieces | 280 |
| chicken nuggets sauces: | |
| barbecue or sweet mustard, 1 oz. | 50 |
| honey, .5 oz. | 45 |
| sweet & sour, 1 oz. | 45 |
| chili and chili condiments: | |
| chili, regular, 9 oz. | 220 |
| cheddar cheese, shredded, 1 oz. | 110 |
| sour cream, 1 oz. | 60 |
| potatoes: | |
| baked, plain, 8.8 oz. | 270 |
| baked, bacon and cheese stuffed, 12.8 oz. | 520 |
| baked, broccoli and cheese stuffed, 12.3 oz. | 400 |
| baked, cheese stuffed, 11.2 oz. | 420 |
| baked, chili and cheese stuffed, 14.2 oz. | 500 |
| baked, sour cream and chives stuffed, 11.4 oz. | 500 |
| french fries, small, 3.2 oz. | 240 |
| salads, prepared: | |
| chef, 9.1 oz. | 130 |
| garden, 8.1 oz. | 70 |
| taco, 17.3 oz. | 530 |
| salad dressing, 1 tbsp.: | |
| bacon and tomato, reduced calorie | 45 |
| blue cheese | 90 |
| celery seed | 70 |
| French | 60 |
| French, sweet red | 70 |
| *Hidden Valley Ranch* | 50 |
| Italian, golden | 45 |
| Italian, reduced calorie | 25 |
| Italian Caesar | 80 |
| Thousand Island | 70 |
| SuperBar, Mexican Fiesta: | |
| cheese sauce, 2 oz. | 39 |
| picante sauce, 2 oz. | 18 |
| refried beans, 2 oz. | 70 |

| FOOD AND MEASURE | CALORIES |
|---|---|
| *Wendy's, SuperBar, Mexican Fiesta, continued* | |
| rice, Spanish, 2 oz. | 70 |
| sour topping, imitation, 1 oz. | 58 |
| taco chips, 1.4 oz. | 260 |
| taco meat, 2 oz. | 110 |
| taco sauce, 1 oz. | 16 |
| taco shells, .4 oz. shell | 45 |
| tortilla, flour, 1.3 oz. shell | 110 |
| SuperBar, pasta: | |
| Alfredo sauce, 2 oz. | 35 |
| cheese ravioli in spaghetti sauce, 2 oz. | 45 |
| cheese tortellini in spaghetti sauce, 2 oz. | 60 |
| fettuccine, 2 oz. | 190 |
| garlic toast, .6-oz. piece | 70 |
| pasta medley, 2 oz. | 60 |
| rotini, 2 oz. | 90 |
| spaghetti sauce, 2 oz. | 28 |
| spaghetti meat sauce, 2 oz. | 60 |
| dessert: | |
| chocolate chip cookie, 2.25 oz. | 275 |
| frosty, dairy, small, 8.6 oz. | 340 |

**Western dinner,** frozen:

| | |
|---|---|
| (*Banquet*), 11 oz. | 630 |
| (*Morton*), 10 oz. | 290 |
| style (*Swanson*), 11.5 oz. | 430 |

**Wheat,** whole-grain:

| | |
|---|---|
| durum, 1 cup | 650 |
| hard red spring, 1 cup | 631 |
| hard red winter, 1 cup | 628 |
| soft red, for pastry (*Arrowhead Mills*), 2 oz. | 190 |
| soft red winter, 1 cup | 556 |
| hard white, 1 cup | 656 |
| soft white, 1 cup | 571 |

**Wheat, sprouted:**

| | |
|---|---|
| 1 cup | 214 |

| FOOD AND MEASURE | CALORIES |
|---|---|
| **Wheat bran:** | |
| crude, 2 tbsp. or ¼ oz. | 15 |
| toasted (*Kretschmer*), 1 oz. or ⅓ cup | 57 |
| unprocessed (*Quaker*), 2 tbsp. or ¼ oz. | 8 |
| **Wheat cake:** | |
| (*Quaker* Grain Cakes), .32-oz. piece | 34 |
| **Wheat flakes:** | |
| (*Arrowhead Mills*), 2 oz. | 210 |
| **Wheat flour,** see "Flour" | |
| **Wheat germ:** | |
| (*Kretschmer*), 1 oz. or ¼ cup | 103 |
| crude, 1 oz. | 102 |
| honey crunch (*Kretschmer*), 1 oz. or ¼ cup | 105 |
| raw (*Arrowhead Mills*), 2 oz. | 210 |
| toasted, 1 oz. or ¼ cup | 108 |
| **Wheat gluten:** | |
| (*Arrowhead Mills* Vital), 1 oz. | 100 |
| **Wheat pilaf mix:** | |
| (*Casbah*), 1 oz. dry or ½ cup cooked | 100 |
| **Whelk,** meat only: | |
| raw, 4 oz. | 156 |
| **Whey,** fluid: | |
| acid, 1 oz. | 7 |
| sweet, 1 oz. | 8 |
| **Whipped topping,** see "Cream" and "Cream topping, nondairy" | |
| **Whiskey,** see "Liquor" | |
| **Whiskey sour mix:** | |
| bottled (*Holland House*), 1 fl. oz. | 37 |
| instant (*Holland House*), .56 oz. dry | 64 |
| instant, prepared w/whiskey (*Bar-Tender's*), 3.5 fl. oz. | 177 |

| FOOD AND MEASURE | CALORIES |
|---|---|
| ***White Castle:*** | |
| cheeseburger, 2.3 oz. | 200 |
| chicken sandwich, 2.25 oz. | 186 |
| fish sandwich, w/out tartar sauce, 2.1 oz. | 155 |
| french fries, 3.4 oz. | 301 |
| hamburger, 2.1 oz. | 161 |
| onion chips, 3.3 oz. | 329 |
| onion rings, 2.1 oz. | 245 |
| sausage sandwich, 1.7 oz. | 196 |
| sausage and egg sandwich, 3.4 oz. | 322 |
| **White sauce mix:** | |
| prepared w/whole milk, ½ cup | 121 |
| **Whitefish,** meat only: | |
| raw, 4 oz. | 152 |
| smoked, 4 oz. | 122 |
| **Whiting,** meat only: | |
| fresh, raw, 4 oz. | 102 |
| fresh, baked, broiled, or microwaved, 4 oz. | 130 |
| **Wiener,** see "Frankfurter" | |
| **Wild rice:** | |
| raw, 1 oz. | 101 |
| cooked (*Fantastic Foods*), ½ cup | 83 |
| **Wine:** | |
| dessert, 3.5 fl. oz. | 140 |
| table, dry, red, 3.5 fl. oz. | 75 |
| table, dry, white or champagne, 3.5 fl. oz. | 80 |
| **Wine, cooking:** | |
| burgundy or Sauterne (*Regina*), ¼ cup | 2 |
| Marsala (*Holland House*), 1 fl. oz. | 9 |
| red (*Holland House*), 1 fl. oz. | 6 |
| sherry (*Holland House*), 1 fl. oz. | 5 |
| sherry (*Holland House*), 1 fl. oz. | 20 |
| vermouth or white (*Holland House*), 1 fl. oz. | 2 |
| **Wine vinegar,** see "Vinegar" | |

| FOOD AND MEASURE | CALORIES |
|---|---|
| **Winged bean:** | |
| fresh, raw, sliced, ½ cup | 11 |
| fresh, boiled, drained, ½ cup | 12 |
| dried, raw, ½ cup | 372 |
| dried, boiled, ½ cup | 126 |
| **Wolf fish,** Atlantic, meat only: | |
| raw, 4 oz. | 109 |
| **Wonton skin:** | |
| (*Nasoya*), 1 piece | 23 |
| **Worcestershire sauce:** | |
| (*Heinz*), 1 tbsp. | 5 |
| (*Lea & Perrins*), 1 tsp. | 5 |
| regular or smoky (*French's*), 1 tbsp. | 10 |
| white wine (*Lea & Perrins*), 1 tsp. | 3 |

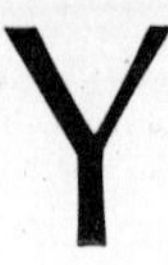

| FOOD AND MEASURE | CALORIES |
|---|---|
| **Yam:** | |
| fresh, raw, cubed, ½ cup | 89 |
| fresh, baked or boiled, drained, ½ cup | 79 |
| canned or frozen, see "Sweet potato" | |
| **Yam, mountain,** Hawaiian: | |
| raw, 1 medium, 8¼" × 2½" diam. | 282 |
| raw, cubed, ½ cup | 46 |
| steamed, cubed, ½ cup | 59 |
| **Yam bean tuber:** | |
| raw, trimmed, sliced, ½ cup | 25 |
| boiled, drained, 4 oz. | 52 |
| **Yeast,** baker's: | |
| (*Fleischmann's* Active Dry/RapidRise), ¼ oz. | 20 |
| fresh or household (*Fleischmann's*), .6 oz. | 15 |
| **Yellow squash,** see "Squash, crookneck" | |
| **Yellowtail,** meat only: | |
| raw, 4 oz. | 165 |
| **Yogurt:** | |
| plain: | |
| (*Colombo*), 8 oz. | 160 |
| (*Colombo* Nonfat Lite), 8 oz. | 110 |
| (*Crowley*), 1 cup | 160 |
| (*Crowley* Lowfat), 1 cup | 140 |
| (*Crowley* Nonfat), 1 cup | 120 |
| (*Dannon* Lowfat), 8 oz. | 140 |
| (*Dannon* Nonfat), 8 oz. | 110 |
| (*Friendship* Lowfat 1.5%), 1 cup | 150 |
| (*Lite-Line* Swiss Style 1.5%), 1 cup | 140 |
| (*Meadow Gold* Lowfat 2%), 1 cup | 160 |
| (*Mountain High*), 1 cup | 200 |

| FOOD AND MEASURE | CALORIES |
|---|---|
| (*Weight Watchers* Nonfat), 1 cup | 90 |
| (*Yoplait*), 6 oz. | 130 |
| (*Yoplait* Nonfat), 8 oz. | 120 |
| all flavors: | |
| (*Dannon* Fresh Flavors), 8 oz. | 200 |
| (*Dannon* Fruit-on-the-Bottom), 8 oz. | 240 |
| (*Dannon* Fruit-on-the-Bottom), 4.4 oz. | 130 |
| (*Friendship* Lowfat), 1 cup | 210 |
| (*New Country* Regular/Lowfat/Supreme), 6 oz. | 150 |
| (*Ripple 70*), 6 oz. | 70 |
| (*Weight Watchers Ultimate 90*), 1 cup | 90 |
| (*Yoplait Custard Style*), 4 oz. | 130 |
| (*Yoplait* Fat Free), 6 oz. | 150 |
| except vanilla (*Dannon* Hearty Nuts & Raisins), 8 oz. | 260 |
| all fruit flavors: | |
| (*Colombo* Fruit on the Bottom), 8 oz. | 230 |
| (*Colombo* Nonfat Fruit on the Bottom), 8 oz. | 190 |
| (*Colombo* Nonfat Lite Minipack), 4.4 oz. | 100 |
| (*Crowley* Nonfat, Aspartame-sweetened), 1 cup | 100 |
| (*Crowley* Sundae Style), 1 cup | 250 |
| (*Crowley* Swiss Style), 1 cup | 240 |
| (*Yoplait*), 6 oz. | 190 |
| (*Yoplait*), 4 oz. | 120 |
| (*Yoplait* Light), 6 oz. | 90 |
| (*Yoplait* Light), 4 oz. | 60 |
| except cherry and berries (*Yoplait Custard Style*), 6 oz. | 190 |
| berries, mixed (*Dannon* Extra Smooth), 4.4 oz. | 130 |
| berries, mixed (*Yoplait Breakfast Yogurt*), 6 oz. | 210 |
| berries or cherry (*Yoplait Custard Style*), 6 oz. | 180 |
| blueberry, natural flavors (*Mountain High*), 1 cup | 220 |
| cherry w/almonds (*Yoplait Breakfast Yogurt*), 6 oz. | 200 |
| cherry-vanilla (*Lite-Line* Swiss Style 1%), 1 cup | 240 |
| fruit, tropical (*Yoplait Breakfast Yogurt*), 6 oz. | 210 |
| peach (*Lite-Line* Swiss Style 1%), 1 cup | 230 |
| raspberry (*Meadow Gold* Lowfat 1.5%), 1 cup | 250 |
| strawberry (*Colombo*), 8 oz. | 210 |
| strawberry (*Crowley* Nonfat), 1 cup | 190 |
| strawberry (*Dannon* Extra Smooth), 4.4 oz. | 130 |
| strawberry (*Lite-Line* Lowfat 1%), 1 cup | 240 |
| strawberry-almond (*Yoplait Breakfast Yogurt*), 6 oz. | 200 |
| strawberry-banana (*Yoplait Breakfast Yogurt*), 6 oz. | 220 |

| FOOD AND MEASURE | CALORIES |
|---|---|
| *Yogurt, continued* | |
| vanilla: | |
| (*Colombo* Nonfat Lite), 8 oz. | 160 |
| (*Crowley* Lowfat), 1 cup | 200 |
| (*Dannon* Fresh Flavors), 4.4 oz. | 110 |
| (*Yoplait/Yoplait Custard Style*), 6 oz. | 180 |
| (*Yoplait* Nonfat), 8 oz. | 180 |
| French (*Colombo*), 8 oz. | 215 |
| w/wheat, nuts, and raisins (*Dannon* Hearty Nuts & Raisins), 8 oz. | 270 |
| yogurt drink, all flavors (*Dan'up*), 8 oz. | 190 |

## **Yogurt,** frozen:

| FOOD AND MEASURE | CALORIES |
|---|---|
| plain, soft-serve (*Crowley* Peaks of Perfection), 3.5 fl. oz. | 90 |
| all flavors: | |
| (*Crowley*), 3 fl. oz. | 80 |
| (*Dreyer's Inspirations*), 3 oz. | 80 |
| except cherry and chocolate (*Sealtest Free*), ½ cup | 100 |
| except chocolate, soft-serve (*Dannon*), ½ cup | 100 |
| soft-serve (*Bresler's* Gourmet), 1 oz. | 29 |
| soft-serve (*Bresler's* Lite), 1 oz. | 27 |
| soft-serve (*Crowley* Peaks of Perfection), 3.5 fl. oz. | 100 |
| soft-serve (*Dannon* Nonfat), ½ cup | 90 |
| caramel pecan chunk (*Colombo* Gourmet), 3 fl. oz. | 120 |
| cheesecake, wild raspberry (*Colombo* Gourmet), 3 fl. oz. | 100 |
| cherry, black (*Breyers*), ½ cup | 120 |
| cherry, black, or chocolate (*Sealtest Free*), ½ cup | 110 |
| chocolate: | |
| (*Bison*), 3½ fl. oz. | 94 |
| (*Breyers*), ½ cup | 120 |
| (*Häagen-Dazs*), 3 fl. oz. | 130 |
| chunk, Bavarian (*Colombo* Gourmet), 3 fl. oz. | 120 |
| soft-serve (*Dannon*), ½ cup | 120 |
| *Heath* bar crunch (*Colombo* Gourmet), 3 fl. oz. | 130 |
| mocha Swiss almond (*Colombo* Gourmet), 3 fl. oz. | 120 |
| peach (*Breyers*), ½ cup | 110 |
| peach (*Häagen-Dazs*), 3 fl. oz. | 120 |
| peanut butter cup (*Colombo* Gourmet), 3 fl. oz. | 140 |
| raspberry, red (*Breyers*), ½ cup | 120 |
| strawberry (*Häagen-Dazs*), 3 fl. oz. | 120 |
| strawberry or strawberry-banana (*Breyers*), ½ cup | 110 |

| FOOD AND MEASURE | CALORIES |
|---|---|
| strawberry passion (*Colombo* Gourmet), 3 fl. oz. | 100 |
| vanilla (*Breyers*), ½ cup | 120 |
| vanilla (*Häagen-Dazs*), 3 fl. oz. | 130 |
| vanilla dream (*Colombo* Gourmet), 3 fl. oz. | 90 |
| vanilla-almond crunch (*Häagen-Dazs*), 3 fl. oz. | 150 |

**Yogurt and fruit bar,** see "Fruit bar"

**Yokan:**

| | |
|---|---|
| 1 oz. | 74 |
| 1 slice, ¼" thick, .5 oz. | 36 |

# Z

| FOOD AND MEASURE | CALORIES |
|---|---|
| **Ziti,** frozen: | |
| in marinara sauce (*The Budget Gourmet* Side Dish), 6.25 oz. | 220 |
| **Zucchini,** see "Squash" | |
| **Zucchini, combinations,** frozen: | |
| carrots, pearl onions, and mushrooms (*Birds Eye* Farm Fresh), 4 oz. | 30 |
| **Zucchini lasagna,** see "Lasagna entree, frozen" | |